AF559581

ENVIRONMENTAL STUDIES

About the Authors

R.P. Singh is the Principal, Bareilly College, Bareilly. He is an aminent academician and dynamic administrator. Among the positions he has are as follows :

1. Reader, Department of Geography, Hindu College, Moradabad.
2. Principal, S.M. College, Dhampur.
3. Principal, K.G.K. College, Moradabad.
4. Member, U.P. Higher Education Service Commission, Allahabad.
5. Vice Chancellor, C.C.S. University, Meerut.

He has written and edited half a dozen books on Practical Geography. Tourism Geography, Geography of India, Economy of Geography, Resource Geography, Environmental Geography and has been a frequent contributor to the professional journals. His role in the strengthening of geography research is widely acknowledged.

Zubairul Islam is Head, Department of Geography, Bareilly College, Bareilly. He has edited books on Geog. of India, Eco. Geog. and Practical Geography. He is also working as co-Investigator in the U.G.C. sponsored major project entitled "Municipal GIS resource mapping and planning : A case Study of Bareilly Municipal Corporation."

ENVIRONMENTAL STUDIES

By

R.P. Singh

D. Litt. (Geography)

Principal, Bareilly College, Bareilly,

Former Member of U.P. Higher Education Service Commission Allahabad, and

Former Vice Chancellor, C.C.S. University, Meerut, Uttar Pradesh

&

Zubairul Islam

UGC.NET, UPSLET, Ph.d. (Geography)

Head, Department of Geography

Bareilly College, Bareilly, Uttar Pradesh

CONCEPT PUBLISHING COMPANY PVT. LTD.

NEW DELHI-110059

ISBN-13 : 978-81-8069-774-6 (HB)

First Published 2012

Published and Printed by

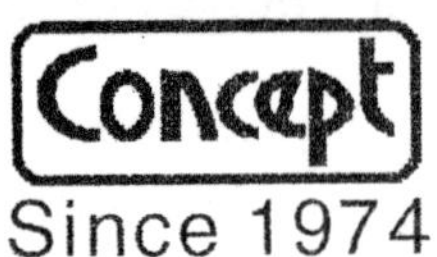

Concept Publishing Company Pvt. Ltd.
Regd. Office:
A/15-16, Commercial Block, Mohan Garden
New Delhi-110059 (India)
Phones : 25351460, 25351794, *Fax* : 091-11-25357109
Email : publishing@conceptpub.com
Website: www.conceptpub.com

Editorial Office:
H-13, Bali Nagar, New Delhi-110 015, India

Cataloging in Publication Data--*Courtesy:* D.K. Agencies (P) Ltd. <docinfo@dkagencies.com>

Singh, R. P., *Principal.*
Environmental studies / by R.P. Singh & Zubairul Islam.
p. cm.
Includes index.
ISBN 9788180697746

1. Human ecology--Study and teaching--India. 2. Environmental sciences--India. 3. Natural resources--India. I. Islam, Zubairul, joint author. II. Title.

DDC 304.2071054 22

PREFACE

After schools, it is now the turn of universities across the country to go green. With the University Grants Commission (UGC) finally coming out for implementation of a "compulsory" course on Environmental Studies as per Supreme Court ruling in colleges across the country, conservation may finally manage to get its due space in higher education.

In line with the Supreme Court ruling that directed the UGC to formulate a basic course on environment meant for every college student, the Commission had decided on the formulation of a six-month core module course in environmental studies that could be taught by Universities across the country.

Following the setting up of an Expert Committee headed by Erach Bharucha, the Director of Bharati Vidyapeeth Institute of Environmental Studies, a Core Module Syllabus for Environmental Studies for undergraduate courses of all branches of higher education was framed.

Although the UGC maintains that the success of the course would eventually depend on the "initiative and drive of teachers and students", The Expert Committee includes Prof. C. Manoharachary of Osmania University, S. Thayumanavan of Anna University's Centre for Environmental Studies; D.C. Goswami of Guwahati University's Department of Environmental Science; R. Mehta from the Ministry of Environment and Forests; and N.K. Jain from the UGC.

Divided into eight units covering 50 lectures, the core module syllabus for Environmental Studies includes classroom teaching and fieldwork. While the first seven units will cover 45 lectures through classroom teaching to enhance knowledge, skills and attitude towards the environment, the eighth one will be based on field activities and would be covered over five lecture hours to provide students with first-hand knowledge on various local environmental aspects.

Although the UGC has mentioned that Universities can make use of outside expertise for teaching purposes, they would have to utilize the course material provided by the UGC.

The course covers a range of topic from water resources, mineral resources and food resources to energy resources and land resources. Clearly an attempt to give students a crash course in the very basics of environment and its concerns, the course will also look at biodiversity at the global, national and local levels as well present pollution case studies and disaster management, it will also take a look at AIDS, women and child welfare and other interlinked subjects.

ACKNOWLEDGEMENTS

We are thankful to Professor M.H. Qureshi (CRDS, JNU, New Delhi), Professor Sant Bahadur Singh (BHU), Professor Aabha Laxmi Singh (Dean, Science Faculty, AMU), Professor Ali Mohammad (AMU), Professor S.K. Shukla (Satna University, M.P.), for their guidance and suggestions at every stage of this work.

We are also grateful to a number of learned people who have been of assistance during the preparation of this book. They include : Professor Manhas (Jammu University), Professor Ishtyaq Ahamad (JMI University, New Delhi), Professor Mazhar (JMI University, New Delhi), Professor G.L. Shah (Kumaon University, Uttarakhand), Dr. Sarfaraz Asghar (Jammu University), and Dr. Bahar Uddin Shah (Manipur).

Dr. Uma Vyas has been helpful at various stages in final planning of the book and making available some recent literature on the subject.

We are also thankful to all members of our families Dr. Usha Singh, Deep Shikha Singh, Dr. Ritu Singh, Mrs. Zaheena Begum, Haji Rafiq Ahamad, Mr. Ajaz Ahamad, Mrs. Salma Begum, Mr. Shamshul Islam, Mr. Bazrul Qumar, Femi, Zainab, Hira, Sayyada, Musheer, Sameer, Ruby and Arisha.

R.P. Singh
Zubairul Islam

CORE MODULE SYLLABUS FOR ENVIRONMENTAL STUDIES FOR UNDER GRADUATE COURSES OF ALL BRANCHES OF HIGHER EDUCATION

Unit 1 : The multidisciplinary nature of environmental studies (2 lectures)

- Definition, scope and importance; and
- Need for public awareness.

Unit 2 : Natural Resources : (8 Lectures)

Renewable and Non-renewable resources :

- Natural resources and associated problems :
  (a) **Forest resources** : Use and over-exploitation, deforestation, case studies. Timber extraction, mining, dams and their effects on forests and tribal people.
  (b) **Water resources** : Use and over-utilization of surface and ground water, floods, drought, conflicts over water, dams-benefits and problems.
  (c) **Mineral resources** : Use and exploitation, environmental effects of extracting and using mineral resources, case studies.
  (d) **Food resources** : World food problems, changes caused by agriculture and overgrazing, effects of modern agriculture, fertilizer-pesticide problems, waterlogging, salinity, case studies.
  (e) **Energy resources** : Growing energy needs, renewable and non-renewable energy sources, use of alternate energy sources, case studies.
  (f) **Land resources** : Land as a resource, land degradation, man induced landslides, soil erosion and desertification.
- Role of an individual in conservation of natural resources.
- Equitable use of resources for sustainable lifestyles.

Unit 3 : Ecosystems (6 Lectures)

- Concept of an ecosystem.
- Structure and function of an ecosystem.
- Producers, consumers and decomposers.

- Energy flow in the ecosystem.
- Ecological succession.
- Food chains, food webs and ecological pyramids.
- Introduction, types, characteristic features, structure and function of the following ecosystem :
  - (a) Forest ecosystem
  - (b) Grassland ecosystem
  - (c) Desert ecosystem
  - (d) Aquatic ecosystems (ponds, streams, lakes, rivers, ocean estuaries)

Unit 4 : Biodiversity and its Conservation (8 Lectures)

- Introduction – Definition : genetic, species and ecosystem diversity.
- Biogeographical classification of India.
- Value of biodiversity : consumptive use, productive use, social, ethical aesthetic and option values.
- Biodiversity at global, national and local levels.
- India as a mega-diversity nation.
- Hot-spots of biodiversity.
- Threats to biodiversity: habitat loss, poaching of wildlife, man wildlife conflicts.
- Endangered and endemic species of India.
- Conservation of biodiversity : *In-situ* and *Ex-situ* conservation of biodiversity.

Unit 5 : Environmental Pollution (8 Lectures)

Definition

- Causes, effects and control measures of :
  - (a) Air pollution,
  - (b) Water pollution,
  - (c) Soil pollution,
  - (d) Marine pollution,
  - (e) Noise pollution,
  - (f) Thermal pollution, and
  - (g) Nuclear pollution
- Solid waste management : Causes, effects and control measures of urban and industrial wastes.
- Role of an individual in prevention of pollution.
- Pollution case studies.
- Disaster management : floods, earthquake, cyclone and landslides.

Unit 6 : Social Issues and the Environment (7 Lectures)

- From unsustainable to sustainable development.
- Urban problems and related to energy.
- Water conservation, rain water harvesting, watershed management.
- Resettlement and rehabilitation of people; its problems and concerns. Case studies.
- Environmental ethics : Issues and possible solutions
- Climate change, global warming, acid rain, ozone layer depletion, nuclear accidents and holocaust. Case studies.
- Wasteland reclamation.
- Consumerism and waste products.
- Environmental Protection Act.
- Air (Prevention and Control of Pollution) Act.
- Water (Prevention and Control of Pollution) Act.
- Wildlife Protection Act.
- Forest Conservation Act.
- Issues involved in enforcement of environmental legislation.
- Public awareness.

Unit 7 : Human Population and the Environment (6 Lectures)

- Population growth, variation among nations.
- Population explosion – Family Welfare Programmes.
- Environment and human health.
- Human Rights.
- Value Education.
- HIV/AIDS.
- Women and Child Welfare.
- Role of Information Technology in Environment and Human Health.
- Case Studies.

Unit 8 : Field Work

- Visit to a local area to document environmental assets river/forest/grassland/hill/mountain.
- Visit to a local polluted site – Urban/Rural/Industrial/Agricultural.
- Study of common plants, insects, birds.
- Study of simple ecosystems—pond, river, hill slopes, etc. (Field work equal to 5 lecture hours).

CONTENTS

Preface *v*
Acknowledgements *vi*

UNIT - 1 : ENVIRONMENT 1-13

I. Introduction *1*
II. Multidisciplinary Nature of Environmental Studies *1*
III. Environmental Education *2*
IV. Biosphere *5*
V. Need for Public Awareness *8*
VI. The Earth *9*

UNIT - 2 : NATURAL RESOURCES 14-106

I. Definition *14*
II. Classification of Resources *14*
III. Forest Resources *16*
(a) Definitions *16*
(b) Importance of forest resources *17*
(c) Global Situation of Forest Resources *19*
(d) Forest in India *23*
(e) Forest Conservation. *27*

IV. Water Resources *28*

(a) Forms of Water *29*
(b) Importance of Water *29*
(c) Distribution of Water on the Earth *32*
(d) Water Resources in India *33*
(e) Floods *38*
(f) Drought *38*
(g) Conflicts over Water *39*
(h) Interlinking of Rivers *40*
(i) Dams *41*

(j) Conservation of Water Resources 42

V. Mineral Resources 45

(a) Classification of Minerals 45
(b) Uses and Exploitation of Major Minerals in the World 45
(c) Environmental Damages caused by Mining Activities 49
(d) Mineral Resources in India 50
(e) Conservation of Mineral Resources 51

VI. Food Resources 52

(a) World Food Problems/Food Crises 52
(b) Sources of Food 54
(c) Agriculture 55
(d) Effects of Modern Agriculture 59
(e) Food Demand in India 61

VII. Energy Resources 64

(a) Energy Consumption 64
(b) Types of Energy Resources 67
- Non-Renewable Sources of Energy 67
  - (1) Coal 68
  - (2) Petroleum 69
  - (3) Nuclear Energy 70
- Renewable Energy Resources 71
  - (1) Solar Energy 71
  - (2) Wind Energy 76
  - (3) Water Power 76
  - (4) Geothermal Energy 79
  - (5) Biogas 80
  - (6) Biofuel 82
  - (7) Liquid Biofuel 82
  - (8) Solid Biomass 83
  - (9) Hydrogen as a Biofuel 83

VIII. Land Resources 85

(a) Land as a Resource 85
(b) Land Degradation 86
(c) Soils 89
- Formation of Soil 90
- The Soil Profile 90
- Soils in India 91

1. Soil Erosion 91
2. Desertification 97
3. Landslides 99
(d) Management of Soil 99
IX. Role of an Individual in Conservation of Natural Resources 100
X. Equitable use of Resources for Sustainable Lifestyles. 101

UNIT - 3 : ECOSYSTEM 107-149

I. Concept of Ecosystems 107
II. Structure of Ecosystems 108
III. Functions of Ecosystems 111
(a) Trophic Level 111
(b) Food Chain 112
(c) Food Web 114
(d) Ecological Pyramid 115
(e) Energy Flow 117
IV. Nutrient/Biogeochemical Cycles 119
(a) Nitrogen Cycle 119
(b) Carbon Cycle 120
V. Balance in Ecosystem 121
VI. Ecological Succession/Adoption 122
VII. Benefits of Ecosystem 123
VIII. Major Types of Ecosystem 124
(a) Forest Ecosystem 126
(b) Grassland Ecosystem 130
(c) Desert Ecosystem 131
(d) Tundra Ecosystem 134
(e) Aquatic Ecosystem 135
IX. Polar Regions 141
(a) Arctic 143
(b) Antarctica 143
X. Conversion of Natural Ecosystem 144

UNIT - 4 : BIODIVERSITY AND ITS CONSERVATIONS 150-189

I. Introduction 150
(a) Levels of Biodiversity 151
(b) Value of Biodiversity 152
(c) Evolution of Biodiversity 153

II. Global Biodiversity 157
(a) Distribution on the Earth 157
(b) Global Biodiversity Losses 159

III. Biodiversity in India *166*
- (a) India as a Mega Diversity Nation *166*
- (b) Biodiversity Hotspots of India *166*
- (c) Eco-regions in India *168*
- (d) Wildlife in India *180*
- (e) Conservation of Biodiversity in India *183*

UNIT - 5 : ENVIRONMENTAL POLLUTION **190-240**

I. Definition *190*
II. Pollutants *190*
III. Types of Pollution *191*
- (a) Air Pollution *192*
- (b) Noise Pollution *199*
- (c) Water Pollution *204*
- (d) Soil Pollution *211*
- (e) Marine Pollution *212*
- (f) Thermal Pollution *214*

IV. Critical Pollution Problem Areas in India *218*
V. Role of Man in Prevention of Pollution *219*
VI. Solid Waste *220*
- (a) Major Types of Solid Waste *220*
- (b) Health Impacts of Solid Waste *221*
- (c) Solid Waste in India *221*
- (d) Preventive Measures of Solid Waste at Household Level 225

VII. Disasters *225*
- (a) Earthquake *226*
- (b) Landslides *229*
- (c) Cyclones *231*
- (d) Disasters Planning and Management in India *236*

UNIT - 6 : SOCIAL ISSUES AND ENVIRONMENT **241-272**

I. Sustainable Development *241*
- (a) Concept of Sustainable Development *241*
- (b) Sustainable Development in India *242*

II. Global Warming *248*
- (a) History of Global Warming *248*
- (b) Causes Global Warming *249*

(c) Effects of Global Warming *250*
(d) Measures to Control Global Warming *251*

III. Acid Rain *251*
(a) Causes of Acid Rains *252*
(b) Effects and Problems of Acid Rains *252*
(c) Possible Solutions of Acid Rain *253*

IV. Ozone Depletion *255*
(a) Ozone Layer *255*
(b) Industrial Production of Ozone *255*
(c) Applications of Ozone *256*
(d) Ozone as a Pollutant *257*

V. Environment and Consumerism *258*

VI. Environmental Laws in India *259*
(a) Forest Laws *260*
(b) Laws to Protect the Wild Life *260*
(c) Water Pollution Preventionlaws *260*
(d) Air Prevention and Control of Pollution *261*
(e) The Environmental Protection Act (EPA) of (1986) *261*
(f) Noise Pollution (Regulation and Control) Rules, 2000 *262*
(g) Coastal Zone *262*
(h) Hazardous Subsistences Act *262*

VII. Major Environmental Treaties *263*

VIII. Public Environmental Awareness *267*

UNIT - 7 : HUMAN POPULATION AND ENVIRONMENT 273-309

I. Population Growth *273*

II. Population Characteristics and Variations among Nations *275*
(a) Exponential Growth *275*
(b) Doubling Time *275*
(c) Total Fertility Rate *275*
(d) Infant Mortality Rate *276*
(e) Age Structure *276*
(f) Zero Population Growth *277*
(g) Life Expectancy *277*
(h) Urbanization *277*
(i) Demographic Transition *278*

III. Overpopulation/Population Explosion *280*

IV. Family Welfare Programmes *284*
V. Planning to Reduce Fertility, Mortality and Population Growth in India *290*
VI. Environment and Human Health *291*
VII. HIV/AIDS *294*
VIII. Human Rights *297*
IX. Information Technology and Environment *305*

UNIT - 8 : FIELD WORK (Practical) 310-317

I. Study of River/Forest/Grassland/Hill/Mountain. *310*
II. Visit to Some Local Polluted Site. *314*
III. Study of Common Plants, Insects and Birds. *316*

GLOSSARY **318-333**
INDEX **334-**

Unit-1

Environment

"Everything that is not me, is environment"

— *Einstein*

I. Introduction

The word 'environment' is derived from the French word *"environ"* which means to encircle or surround. In general an environment is a complex of surrounding circumstances, conditions, or influences in which a thing is situated or is developed, or in which a person or organism lives, modifying and determining the life or character.

In other words environment means all of the external factors affecting an organism. These factors may be living organisms (biotic factors) or non-living variables (abiotic factors), such as temperature, rainfall, day length, wind, and ocean currents. The interactions of organisms with biotic and abiotic factors form an ecosystem.

Organisms and their environment constantly interact, and both are changed by this interaction. Like all other living creatures, humans have clearly changed their environment, but they have done so generally on a larger scale than have all other species. Some of these human-induced changes such as the destruction of the world's tropical rain forests to create farms or grazing land for cattle have led to altered climate patterns. In turn, altered climate patterns have changed the way animals and plants are distributed in different ecosystems.

II. The Multidisciplinary Nature of Environmental Studies

Environmental Science is the study of the interactions among the physical, chemical and biological components of the environment; with a focus on pollution and degradation of the environment related due to human activities; and the impact on biodiversity and sustainability from local and global development.

It is inherently an interdisciplinary field that draws upon not only its core scientific areas, but also applies knowledge from other non-scientific studies such as economics, law and social sciences. Physics is used to understand the flux of material and energy interaction and to construct mathematical models of environmental phenomena. Chemistry is applied to understand the molecular interactions in natural systems. Biology is fundamental to describing the effects within the plant and animal kingdoms.

The concept of environmental science has existed for centuries, it came alive as a substantive, active field of scientific investigation in the 1960's and 1970's driven by the following factors :

(a) The need for a large multi-disciplined team to analyze complex environmental problems;
(b) The arrival of substantive environmental laws requiring specific environmental protocols of investigation; and
(c) The growing public awareness of a need for action in addressing environmental problems.

Environmental science encompasses issues such as climate change, conservation, biodiversity, groundwater and soil contamination, use of natural resources, waste management, sustainable development, air pollution and noise pollution. Due to the inherent interdisciplinary nature of environmental science, teams of professionals commonly work together to conduct environmental research or to produce Environmental Impact Statements. There are professional organizations that engender work in environmental science and aid in communication among the diverse sciences; the earliest known such organization, the Association of Environmental Professionals was founded in the United States; thereafter, a variety of other countries and states have formed such associations.

III. Environmental Education

Environmental education is a process of learning about the existing situation through which sufficient knowledge can be gained to understand environmental problems and contribute towards solving them.

Environmental education constitute two major categories :

1. *The Formal Education* : Including pre-school, primary, secondary and higher education as well as teachers and environmental professionals in training and retraining.
2. *The Non-Formal Education* : It deals with masses including youth and adults, individually or collectively from all segments of the population, such as the family, workers, managers, and decision-makers, in environmental as well as non-environmental fields.

Environmental education provides :

- A comprehensive knowledge with working of nature and environment.
- An experience in evaluating environmental quality and quantity.
- An understanding of the impact on environmental quality and quantity.
- A source of guidance to the people to act as more responsible citizens with an increased civic sense.

➢ Scope of Environmental Education

Sope of the environmental studies is broad based, which encompasses a large number of areas and aspects as follows :

- *Natural Resources*
  - Natural resources and associated problems;
  - Role of an individual in conservation of natural resources; and
  - Equitable use of resources for sustainable lifestyles.
- *Ecology and Biodiversity*
  - Concept, structure, functional attributes and types of ecosystems; and
  - Definition, value, distribution, threat and conservation of biodiversity.
- *Environmental Pollutions*
  - Definition;
  - Causes, effects and control measures of environmental pollutions;
  - Causes, effects and control measures of Solid waste management; and
  - Disaster management such as floods, earthquake, cyclone and landslides.
- *Social Issues and Environment*
- *Human Population and its Effects on Environment*

➢ Objectives of Environmental Education

The objectives formulated by UNESCO in 1977 to help social groups and individuals are as following :

- *Awareness* : To acquire an awareness of and sensitivity to the total environment and its allied problems.

- *Attitude* : To acquire a set of values and feeling of concern for the environment and the motivation for active participation in environmental improvement and protection.
- *Knowledge* : To gain a variety of experiences and acquire a basic understanding of the environment and the associated problems.
- *Skill* : To acquire skills for identifying and solving environmental problems.
- *Evaluation* : To evaluate environmental measures and education programmes in terms of ecological, economic, social, aesthetic and educational factors.
- *Participation* : To provide an opportunity to be actively involved at all levels in working towards the resolution of environmental problems.

➤ Importance of Environmental Education

There is a Chinese proverb *"If you plan for one year, plant rice, if you plan for 10 years, plant trees and if you plan for 100 years educate people."*

In general, environmental education focuses on making people aware of environmental issues and promotes an understanding of the relationship between humans and their surrounding environment. As people gain a greater understanding of environmental issues, it is hoped that concern for these issues will follow. One clear example of success can be seen from Rachel Carson's book, *Silent Spring,* which helped to make people aware of the negative effects of pesticides on the environment. This work played a large part in gaining public support to push for an end to DDT use in the United States.

Take the case of CFC emissions and ozone layer depletion. Scientists were able to identify the problem of a hole in the ozone layer and then conduct studies to understand the cause. It was then necessary for other individuals to develop an effective policy solution to address this problem. The Montreal Protocol serves as an example of an international policy agreement to address the problem of ozone depletion. Under this agreement, countries banned the use of CFCs, which had been shown by scientists to have negative effects on stratospheric ozone. This example shows that there is a need for individuals who understand different components of the environment in order to promote the effective development of programmes to address existing and future environmental problems.

Furthermore, there is a need to develop a more extensive and effective environmental education strategy to better prepare the public to understand and take action regarding current and future environmental issues. NGOs have offered the majority of support and resources for environmental education, but it is becoming increasingly important for this area to be a focus of standard educational institutions.

IV. Biosphere

The biosphere is that portion of the earth, which is occupied by life. Biosphere extends from 11,000 metres below sea level to 15,000 metres above. It reaches well into the following three spheres.

(a) The hydrosphere (sphere of water);
(b) The lithosphere (sphere of soils and rocks); and
(c) The atmosphere (sphere of the air).

It is thought that life first developed in the hydrosphere, at shallow depths, in the photic zone. Terrestrial life developed later, after the ozone layer protecting living beings from UV (ultraviolet) rays formed in the atmosphere. Diversification of terrestrial species is thought to be increased by the continents drifting apart.

(a) Hydrosphere

Hydrosphere is the collective mass of water found on, under, and over the surface of a planet. The abundance of water on Earth is a unique feature that distinguishes our "Blue Planet" from others in the solar system. Approximately 70.8 per cent of the Earth is covered by water and only 29.2 per cent is terra firma.

Water on the Earth	
Oceans	*97.60 %*
Ice / Glaciers	*1.87 %*
Groundwater	*0.50 %*
Rivers/ Lakes	*0.02 %*
Soil Moisture	*0.01%*

The hydrosphere consists chiefly of the oceans, but technically includes all water surfaces in the world, including inland seas, lakes, rivers, and underground waters. The average depth of the oceans is 3,794 m (12,447 ft), more than five times the average height of the continents. The mass of the oceans is approximately 1.35×10^{18} tonnes, or about 1/4400 of the total mass of the Earth.

This global, interconnected body of salt water, called the World Ocean, is generally divided by the continents and archipelagos into the following bodies, from the largest to the smallest : the Pacific Ocean, the Atlantic Ocean, the Indian Ocean, and the Arctic Ocean. Smaller regions of the oceans are called seas, gulfs, straits and other names. The deepest point in the ocean is the Marianas Trench located in the Pacific Ocean near the Northern Mariana Islands. It has a maximum depth of 10,923 metres.

Oceans are divided into numerous regions depending on the physical and biological conditions of these areas. The pelagic zone includes all open ocean regions, and can be sub-divided into further regions categorised by depth and light abundance.The Photic Zone covers the oceans from surface level to 200 metres down. This is the region where photosynthesis most commonly occurs and, therefore, contains the largest biodiversity in the ocean. Since plants can only survive with photosynthesis any life found lower than this must either rely on material floating down from above or find another primary source, this often comes in the form of hydrothermal vents, this is known as the Aphotic Zone and is defined as being deeper than 200 metres down.

All currently recognized forms of life rely on an active hydrosphere. All organic chemistry indicative of life occurs with water as its solvent. The water cycle in the Earth's hydrosphere allows for the purification of salt water into fresh water. The action of both evaporation and wetland swamps serves to remove a large portion of atmospheric pollutants from the atmosphere (i.e. acid rain). Through this process the water cycle purifies the gaseous atmosphere. Although most life on the planet exists in the salt water oceans, humans are particularly interested in the hydrosphere because it provides the fresh water we depend upon.

(b) Lithosphere

The lithosphere (from the Greek for "rocky" sphere) is the solid outermost shell of a rocky planet. On the Earth, the lithosphere includes the crust and the uppermost layer of the mantle (the upper mantle or lower lithosphere) which is joined to the crust.

Table : The Composition of Crust

Oxygen	49.8%	Sodium	2.30%
Silicon	26.03%	Potassium	2.30%
Aluminium	7.28%	Magnesium	2.11%
Iron	4.12%	Hydrogen	0.97%
Calcium	3.18%	Others	1 – 2%

As the cooling surface layer of the Earth's convection system, the lithosphere thickens over time. It is fragmented into relatively strong pieces, called tectonic plates, which move independently relative to one another. This movement of lithospheric plates is described as plate tectonics.

There are two types of lithosphere.

- Continental lithosphere; and
- Oceanic lithosphere.

The continental area is all land rising above sea level which amounts to about

29 per cent of the earth's total area. More than two-thirds of the continental land area lies north of the equator. The continents, in order of size, are Eurasia (conventionally regarded as the two continents of Asia and Europe), Africa, North America, South America, Antarctica, and Australia.

Oceanic lithosphere is about 70 km thick (but can be as thin as 1.6 km at the mid-ocean ridges); while continental lithosphere is about 150 km thick (and can be considerably thicker at continental collision zones).

Oceanic lithosphere is denser than continental lithosphere, which consists predominantly of felsic rocks. New oceanic lithosphere is constantly being produced at mid-ocean ridges from mantle material and is recycled back to the mantle at subduction zones. As a result, oceanic lithosphere is much younger than continental lithosphere : the oldest oceanic lithosphere is about 200 million years old, while parts of the continental lithosphere are billions of years old. As oceanic lithosphere grows older, it gets cooler and denser, with the result that if two oceanic plates converge, the older one will subduct below the younger one.

(c) Atmosphere

Earth's atmosphere is a layer of gases surrounding the planet Earth and retained by the Earth's gravity. It contains roughly 78 per cent nitrogen and 21 per cent oxygen, trace amounts of other gases, and water vapour. This mixture of gases is commonly known as **air**. The atmosphere protects life on earth by absorbing ultraviolet solar radiation and reducing temperature extremes between day and night.

The average temperature of the atmosphere at the surface of earth is 14 °C but it varies with location and time. Atmospheric **pressure** is a direct result of the weight of the air (it decreases with increasing temperature and *vice versa*). This means that air pressure varies with location and time, because the amount and weight of air above the earth varies with location and time.

The atmosphere has no abrupt cut-off. It slowly becomes thinner and fades away into space. There is no definite boundary between the atmosphere and outer space. Three-quarters of the atmosphere's mass is within 11 km of the planetary surface. The atmospheric density decreases as the altitude increases. The average mass of the atmosphere is about 5,000 trillion metric tonnes.

➢ Layers of the Atmosphere

The temperature of the Earth's atmosphere varies with altitude; the mathematical relationship between temperature and altitude varies between the different atmospheric layers as given below :

- *Troposphere :* From the Greek word "tropos" meaning to turn or mix. The troposphere is the lowest layer of the atmosphere starting at the surface going up to between 7 km at the poles and 17 km at the equator with some

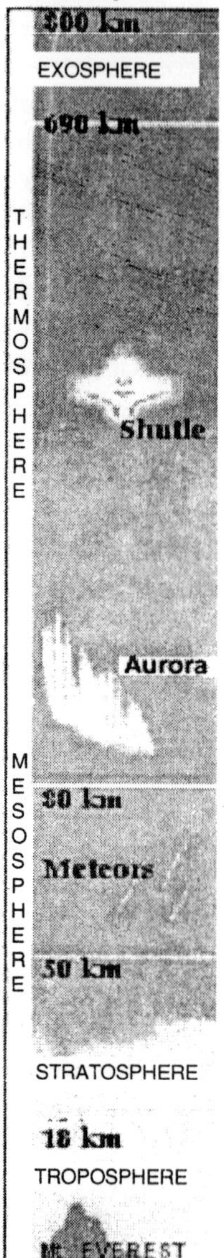

variation due to weather factors. The troposphere has a great deal of vertical mixing due to solar heating at the surface. This heating warms air masses, which then rise to release latent heat as sensible heat that further buoys the air mass. This process continues until all water vapour is removed. In the troposphere, on an average, temperature decreases with height due to expansive cooling.

- *Stratosphere :* It extends from that 7–17 km range to about 50 km, temperature increases with height.
- *Mesosphere :* From about 50 km to the range of 80 km to 85 km, temperature decreases with height.
- *Thermosphere :* From 80–85 km to more than 640 km, temperature increases with height.

The boundaries between these regions are named as the *tropopause, stratopause,* and *mesopause.*

➢ Thickness of the Atmosphere

Although the atmosphere exists at heights of 1,000 km and more, it is so thin as to be considered non-existent.

- 57.8 per cent of the atmosphere by mass is below the summit of Mount Everest.
- 72 per cent of the atmosphere by mass is below the common cruising altitude of commercial airliners (about 10,000 m).
- 99.99999 per cent of the atmosphere by mass is below an altitude of 108 km.

Therefore, most of the atmosphere (99.9999%) by mass is below 100 km, although in the rarefied region above this, there are auroras and other atmospheric effects.

V. Need for Public Awareness

Enhancing environmental awareness is essential to harmonize patterns of individual behaviour with the requirements of environmental conservation. This would minimize the demands placed on the monitoring and enforcement regimes; in fact, large scale non-compliance would simply overwhelm any feasible regulatory machinery.

Awareness relates to the general public, as well as specific sections, e.g. the youth, adolescents, urban dwellers, industrial and construction workers, municipal and other public employees, etc. Awareness involves not only internalization of environmentally responsible behaviour, but also enhanced understanding of the impacts of irresponsible actions, including to public health, living conditions, sanitation, and livelihood prospects.

Environmental education is the principal means of enhancing such awareness, both among the public at large, and among focused groups. Such education may be formal, or informal, or a combination of both. It may rely on educational institutions at different levels; the print, electronic, or live media; and various other formal and informal settings. Several steps to expand and enrich the content of the environment awareness and education programmes have been taken.

The Supreme Court has also mandated that environmental education must be imparted at all levels, including higher education in the formal system. However, there is need for further strengthening the existing programmes and making them more inclusive and participatory.

Access to environmental information is the principal means by which environmentally conscious stakeholders may evaluate compliance by the concerned parties with environmental standards, legal requirements, and covenants. They would thereby be enabled to stimulate necessary enforcement actions, and through censure, motivate compliance. Access to information is also necessary to ensure effective, informed participation by potentially impacted publics in various consultation processes, such as for preparation of environmental impact assessments, and environment management plans of development projects.

The National Natural Resources Management System (NNRMS) was set up in 1983 for optimally managing the natural resources and environment of the country using an optimal mix of remote sensing and conventional techniques. Remote Sensing and data, both satellite and aerial, is being used extensively in the country for mapping and managing the natural resources and environment, over the past three decades.

The "Reduce, Reuse, Recycle" (3R) campaigns will have a lot of success across the country.

VI. The Earth

Five billion years ago the Earth was formed by a massive conglomeration of space materials. The heat energy released by this event melted the entire planet, and it is still cooling off today. Denser materials like iron sank into the core of the Earth, while lighter silicates, other oxygen compounds, and water rose near the surface.

The earth is divided into four main layers as the inner core, outer core, mantle, and crust. The core is composed mostly of iron and is so hot that

EARTH: INTERIOR STRUCTURE

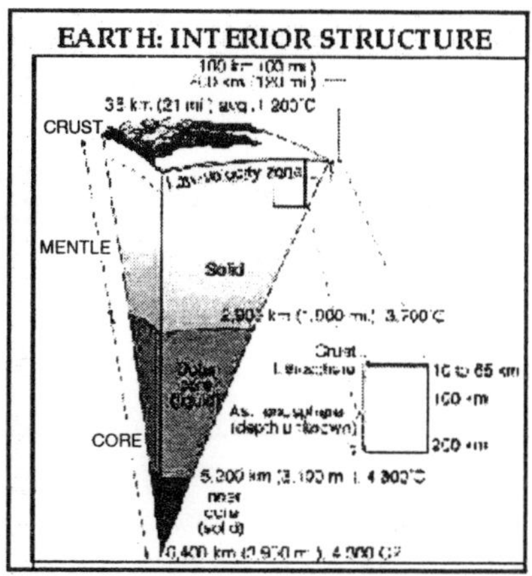

the outer core is molten, with about 10 per cent sulphur. The inner core is under such extreme pressure that it remains solid.

Most of the Earth's mass is in the mantle, which is composed of iron, magnesium, aluminum, silicon, and oxygen silicate compounds. At over 1,000 degrees C, the mantle is solid but can deform slowly in a plastic manner.

The crust is much thinner than any of the other layers, and is composed of the least dense calcium and sodium aluminium-silicate minerals. Being relatively cold, the crust is rocky and brittle, so it can fracture in earthquakes.

Table : Geological History of the Earth

Eras	*Approximate age (in years)*	*Subdivision*	*Notes*
CENOZOIC	10,000 2 M -Million 5 M 24 M 37 M 57 M 66 M	HOLOCENE PLEISTOCENE PLIOCENE MIOCENE OLIGOCENE EOCENE PALEOCENE	The beginning of the Eocene was a period when the Earth was very hot, with palm trees and alligators at the north pole. Earth was cooled by the start of the Quaternary. This period relates to today's concern about global warming. *Homo sapiens* evolved and Ice Ages occur towards the end of this time. The Little Ice Age (which is not a true ice age) occurred a few hundred years ago.
MESOZOIC	144 M 208 M 245 M	CRETACEOUS JURASSIC TRIASSIC	This is the period of the dinosaurs, which came to an end, at the end of the Cretaceous, with an asteroid impact in the Yucatan Peninsula of today's Mexico. During this time, the giant continent PANGAEA broke apart into the continents we have today.
PALEOZOIC	286 M 360 M 408 M 438 M 505 M 570 M	PERMIAN CARBONIFEROUS DEVONIAN SILURIAN ORDOVICIAN CAMBRIAN	The Cambrian period, at the beginning of the Paleozoic, was the first time that multicellular life forms flourished on Earth. By the end of the Paleozoic, and beginning of the Mesozoic, all the continents of the Earth came together to form the giant continent called PANGAEA and dinosaurs began to roam on land.
PRE-CAMBRIAN	2800 M 4800 M	PROTEROZOIC ARCHEAN	This period is about 5 times as long as the Paleozoic and Mesozoic combined, a very long time. Less is known about it than the younger time periods. The oldest fossils are of bacteria/ archaea dating from 3000 M. The oldest rock is dated at 3800 M. The Earth is thought to be 4600 M years old.

Questions

Long answer type of questions

1. Discuss the multidisciplinary nature of environmental studies.
2. What do you understand by environment? Discuss its components.
3. What is the need to study environmental issues?
4. What are the objectives of environmental studies?
5. What is the scope of environmental education?
6. Environmental awareness helps to protect our environment, discuss.

Write short notes on the following :

1. Lithosphere
2. Atmosphere
3. Hydrosphere
4. Biosphere

Fill in the blanks :

1. The word 'Environment' is derived from the French word..........................
2. Environmental science is the study of the interactions among the physical, chemical and .... components of the environment
3. This global, interconnected body of salt water, called the.....................
4. The continental area amounts to about ....% of the earth's total area.
5. Earth's atmosphere is retained by the Earth's....................
6. The mixture of gases is commonly known as....................
7. The atmosphere protects life on Earth by absorbing ....solar radiation.

Keys : 1. "Environ". 2. biological. 3. World Ocean. 4. 29. 5. Gravity. 6. Air. 7. ultraviolet.

Tick the right answer :

1. The word 'Environment' is derived from the :

   (a) Greek word.
   (b) Latin word.
   (c) German word.
   (d) French word.

2. The objectives of Environmental education was formulated by UNESCO in :

   (a) 1977
   (b) 1965
   (c) 1980
   (d) 1995

3. The average depth of the oceans is :

   (a) 5,400 m
   (b) 4,794 m
   (c) 3,794 m
   (d) 3,000 m

4. The movement of lithospheric plates is described in :

   (a) Geocyncline
   (b) Isostacy
   (c) Earth movement
   (d) Plate tectonics

5. Average thickness of oceanic lithosphere is about :

   (a) 40 km thick
   (b) 112 km thick
   (c) 70 km thick
   (d) 111 km thick

6. The National Natural Resources Management System (NNRMS) was set up in :

   (a) 1983
   (b) 1977
   (c) 1956
   (d) 1990

7. The oldest oceanic lithosphere is about :

   (a) 100 million years old
   (b) 200 million years old

(c) 300 million years old
(d) 400 million years old

Keys : - 1. d, 2. a, 3. c, 4. d, 5. c, 6. a 7.b.

True / False types of questions :

1. Approximately 70.8 per cent of the Earth is covered by water.
2. Earth's atmosphere contains roughly 78 per cent nitrogen.
3. Earth's atmosphere contains roughly 31 per cent oxygen.
4. The average temperature of the atmosphere at the surface of earth is 14 °C.
5. The biosphere sometimes described as "the fourth envelope".
6. The biosphere is only the very thin surface layer, which extends from 11,000 metres below sea level to 15,000 metres above.
7. It is thought that life first developed in the hydrosphere.

Keys : - 1. true, 2. true, 3. false, 4. true, 5. true, 6. true, 7. true

Unit - 2

NATURAL RESOURCES

"The Earth provides enough to satisfy every man's needs, but not for anybody's greed"

— *Mahatama Gandhi*

I. Definition

Natural resources are naturally occurring substances that are considered valuable in their relatively unmodified (natural) form. A commodity is generally considered a natural resource when the primary activities associated with it are extraction and purification, as opposed to creation. Thus, mining, petroleum extraction, fishing, and forestry are generally considered natural resource industries.The term "resources" was introduced to a broad audience by E.F. Schumacher in his 1970's book *Small Is Beautiful.*

Because human needs are varied and extend from basic physical requirements, such as food and shelter, to spiritual and emotional needs that are hard to define, so resources cover a vast range of items.

The intellectual resources of a society, its ideas and technologies determine which aspects of the environment meet that society's needs and, therefore, become resources. For example, in the nineteenth century uranium was used only in the manufacture of coloured glass. Today, with the development of nuclear technology, it is a military and energy resource.

II. Classification of Resources

Natural resources are often classified into Renewable and Non-renewable resources.

➢ Renewable Resources

A renewable resource is a natural resource that can be used more than once. The most common definition is that *renewable energy is from an energy resource that is replaced by a natural process at a rate that is equal to or faster than the rate at which that resource is being consumed.*

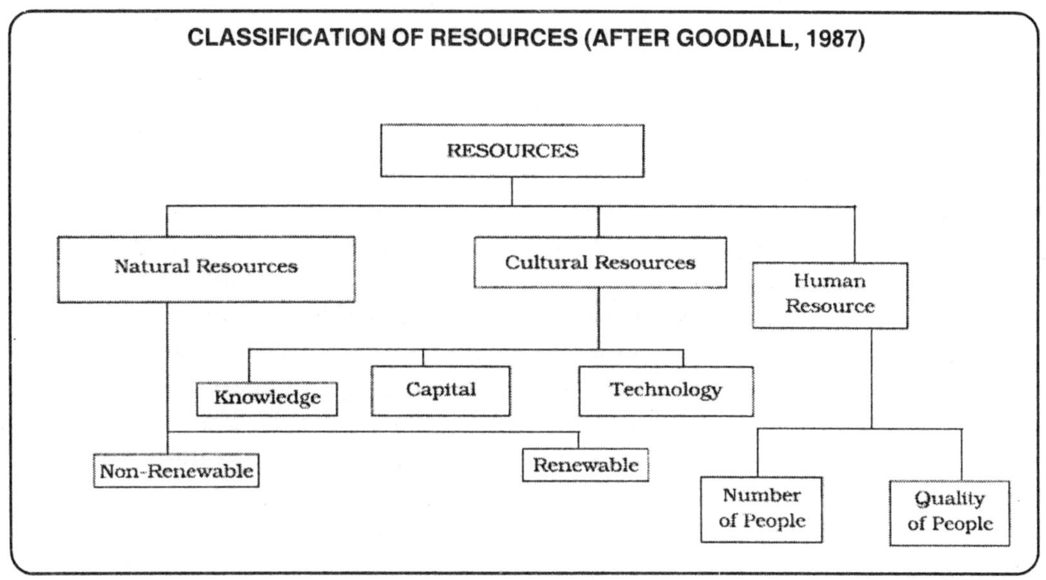

Renewable resources capture their energy from existing flows of energy, from on-going natural processes, such as sunshine, wind, wave power , flowing water (hydropower), biological processes such as anaerobic digestion, and geothermal heat flow.

Most renewable forms of energy, other than geothermal and tidal power, ultimately derive from solar energy. Energy from biomass derives from plant material produced by photosynthesis using the power of the sun. Wind energy derives from winds, which are generated by the sun's uneven heating of the atmosphere. Hydropower depends on rain which again depends on sunlight's power to evaporate water.

Renewable energy resources may be used directly, or used to create other more convenient forms of energy. Examples of direct use are solar ovens, geothermal heating, and water- and wind-mills. Examples of indirect use which require energy harvesting are electricity generation through wind turbines or photovoltaic cells (PV cells), or production of fuels such as biogas from anaerobic digestion or ethanol from biomass.

➢ Non-renewable Resources

A non-renewable resource is a natural resource that cannot be re-made or re-grown. Often fossil fuels, such as coal, petroleum and natural gas are considered non-renewable resources, as they do not naturally re-form at a rate that makes the way we use them sustainable. This is as opposed to natural resources such as timber, which re-grows naturally and can, in theory, be harvested sustainably at a constant rate without depleting the existing resource pool. In this sense, all mined resources, stone, metals, uranium, and various other materials and minerals should be considered non-renewable.

Carbon based non-renewables—Natural resources such as coal, oil, or natural gas, take millions of years to form naturally and cannot be replaced as fast as they are consumed. Eventually they will be used up. At present, the main energy sources used by humans are non-renewable; renewable resources, such as solar, tidal, wind, and geothermal power, have so far been less exploited. Fossil fuels like coal, oil, and gas generate a considerable amount of energy when they are burnt (the process of combustion). Non-renewable resources have a high carbon content because their origin lies in the photosynthetic activity of plants millions of years ago. The fuels release this carbon back into the atmosphere as carbon dioxide. The rate at which such fuels are being burnt is thus resulting in a rise in the concentration of carbon dioxide in the atmosphere, a cause of the green house effect.

Major resources are as follows :

- Forest resources,
- Water resources,
- Mineral resources,
- Food resources
- Energy resources,
- Land resources.

The detailed description of these major resources is as following :

III. Forest Resources

(a) Definitions

Forests are self sustained wooden tracks with biotic community dominated by trees. It is used to refer to land with a tree canopy cover of more than 10 per cent and area of more than 0.5 ha. Forests are determined both by the presence of trees and the absence of other predominant land uses. The trees should be able to reach a minimum height of 5 m.

Dense Forests are defined as those with a canopy cover of more than 70 per cent, open forests as those with canopy cover between 40 and 70 per cent and scrub as those with canopy cover of 10 to 40 per cent.

Evergreen Forest is described, as a forest comprising thick and dense canopy of all trees, which predominantly remain green throughout the year. It includes both coniferous and tropical broad-leafed evergreen trees.

Deciduous Forest is described as a forest predominantly comprising deciduous species and where the trees shed their leaves once in a year.

Mangrove is described as a dense thicket or woody aquatic vegetation or forest cover occurring in tidal waters, near estuaries and along the confluence of delta in coastal areas.

Degraded Forest is described as a forest where the vegetative (crown) density is less than 40 per cent of the canopy cover. It is the result of both biotic and abiotic influences. Forest blank is described as openings amidst forests without any tree cover.

(b) Importance of Forest Resources

Global forest cover is a key indicator of the health of the planet. An intact forest cycles nutrients, regulates climate, stabilizes soil, treats waste, provides habitat, and offers opportunities for recreation. By a conservative tally, these services are worth more than $ 4.7 trillion, a total equal to one-tenth of the gross world product.

Some of the life support systems of major economic and environmental importance are as following:

- Supply of timber, fuel wood, fodder, and a wide range of non-wood products.
- Natural habitat for bio-diversity and repository of genetic wealth.
- Provision of recreation and opportunity for ecotourism.
- Playing an integral part of the watershed to regulate the water regime, conserve soil, and control floods.
- Forests ensure environmental functions such as biodiversity, water and soil conservation, water supply and climate regulation.
- Mismanagement of woodlands in humid and subhumid tropical countries significantly contributes to soil losses equivalent to a 10 per cent loss of agricultural Gross Domestic Product (GDP) per year.
- Deforestation accounts for up to 20 per cent of the global greenhouse gas emissions that contribute to global warming.
- In arid environments, forests are crucial to food security in dry seasons and years.
- Forests provide habitats to about two-thirds of all species on earth.
- Deforestation of closed tropical rainforests could account for the loss of as many as 100 species a day.
- Global employment in the formal forestry sector—13 million people (2000).
- Gross value-added in the forestry sector is US$ 354 billion (2000).
- Global trade in primary wood products is US$ 186 billion (2005).
- Global roundwood production is 3,503 million cubic metres (2005).

- Countries with the highest contribution of the forestry sector to Gross Domestic Product (GDP) are Bhutan, Finland, Malaysia, Baltic States and some African countries.
- Small-scale forest product enterprises are among the top three non-farm rural commercial activities in most countries.
- Forests are home to 300 million people around the world.
- More than 1.6 billion people depend to varying degrees on forests for their livelihoods, e.g. fuel wood, medicinal plants and forest foods.
- About 60 million indigenous people are almost wholly dependent on forests.
- Some 350 million people who live within or adjacent to dense forests depend on them to a high degree for subsistence and income.
- In developing countries, about 1.2 billion people rely on agroforestry farming systems that help to sustain agricultural productivity and generate income.
- Mangrove forests, which cover about 15 million hectares worldwide, are essential to the life cycles of the majority of the world's commercial fish species.

Despite significant resource flows and national concern, the potential of forests to reduce poverty, realise economic growth, and their contribution to the local and global environment has not been fully realized. A combination of market and institutional failures has led to forests failing to contribute as significantly to rural incomes and poverty alleviation and economic growth as would be possible under good economic and technical management.

Box — Major forest products and their producers

Percentage of global production (2005)

- *Wood fuel :* India (17 per cent); China (11 per cent); Brazil (8 per cent); Ethiopia (5 per cent); Indonesia (4 per cent).
- *Industrial roundwood :* USA (26 per cent); Canada (11 per cent); Russian Federation (8 per cent); Brazil (7 per cent); China (6 per cent).
- *Sawnwood :* USA (22 per cent); Canada (14 per cent); Brazil (5 per cent); Russian Federation (5 per cent); Germany (5 per cent); Sweden (4 per cent).
- *Wood-based panels :* China (19 per cent); USA (19 per cent); Canada (8 per cent); Germany (7 per cent); Canada (7 per cent); Brazil (4 per cent).
- *Pulp for paper :* USA (29 per cent); Canada (13 per cent); China (9 per cent); Sweden (7 per cent); Finland (6 per cent); Japan (6 per cent).
- *Paper and paperboard :* USA (23 per cent); China (15 per cent); Japan (8 per cent); Canada (6 per cent); Germany (6 per cent).

Box – Leading consumers of major forest products
Percentage of global consumption (2005)

- *Industrial roundwood :* USA (25 per cent); Canada (12 per cent); China (7 per cent); Brazil (7 per cent); Sweden (6 per cent); Russian Federation (5 per cent).
- *Sawnwood :* USA (32 per cent); Japan (5 per cent); Canada (5 per cent); Brazil (5 per cent); Germany (5 per cent).
- *Wood-based panel :* USA (27 per cent); China (18 per cent); Germany (6 per cent); Japan (5 per cent); Russian Federation (3 per cent).
- *Pulp for paper :* USA (29 per cent); China (13 per cent); Canada (8 per cent); Japan (7 per cent); Sweden (5 per cent); Finland (5 per cent).
- *Paper and paperboard* : USA (25 per cent); China (17 per cent); Japan (8 per cent); Germany (5 per cent); UK (3 per cent); Italy (3 per cent); France (3 per cent).

(c) Global Situation of Forest Resources

Forests cover about 25 per cent of the world's land surface, excluding Greenland and Antarctica. Global forest cover has been reduced by at least 20 per cent since preagricultural times, and possibly by as much as 50 per cent.

Forest area has increased slightly since 1980 in industrial countries, but has declined by almost 10 per cent in developing countries. Tropical deforestation probably exceeds 130,000 km^2 per year.

Less than 40 per cent of forests globally are relatively undisturbed by human action. The great majority of forests in the industrial countries, except Canada and Russia, are reported to be in "semi-natural" condition or converted to plantations.

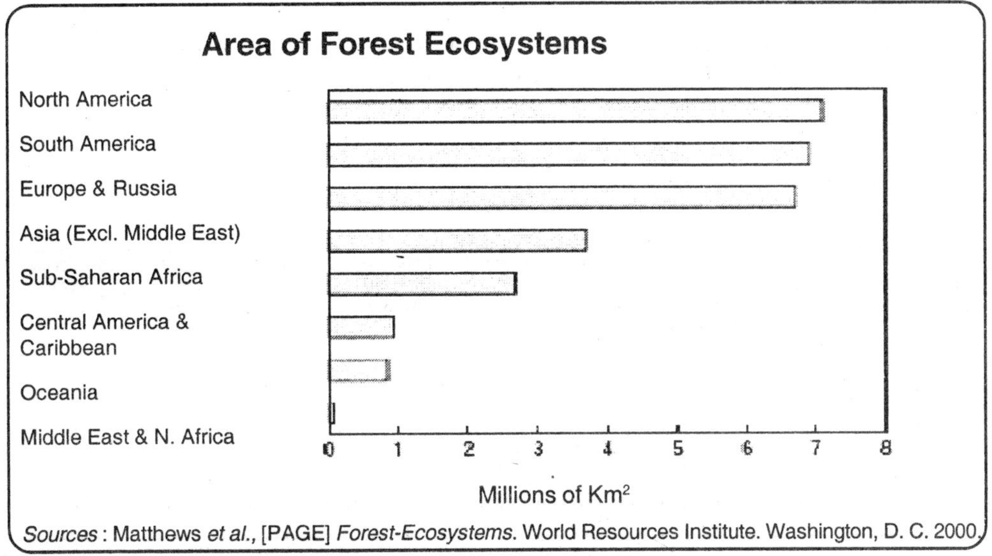

Sources : Matthews *et al.*, [PAGE] *Forest-Ecosystems.* World Resources Institute. Washington, D. C. 2000.

Many developing countries today rely on timber for export earnings. At the same time, millions of people in tropical countries still depend on forests to meet their every need.

The greatest threats to forest extent and condition today are conversion to other forms of land use and fragmentation by agriculture, logging, and road construction. Logging and mining roads open up intact forest to pioneer settlement and to increases in hunting, poaching, fires, and exposure of flora and fauna to pest outbreaks and invasive species.

➢ Deforestation in the World

Deforestation is the permanent destruction of indigenous forests and woodlands. Deforestation has resulted in the reduction of indigenous forests to four-fifths of their pre-agricultural area. Indigenous forests now cover 21 per cent of the earth's land surface.

Deforestation is brought about by the following causes :

- Conversion of forests and woodlands to agricultural land to feed growing numbers of people;
- Development of cash crops and cattle ranching, both of which earn money for tropical countries;
- Commercial logging (which supplies the world market with woods such as meranti, teak, mahogany and ebony) destroys trees as well as opening up forests for agriculture; and
- Felling of trees for firewood and building material; the heavy lopping of foliage for fodder; and heavy browsing of saplings by domestic animals like goats.

Fig. 2.1 : Change in Forest Area from 1980 to 1995

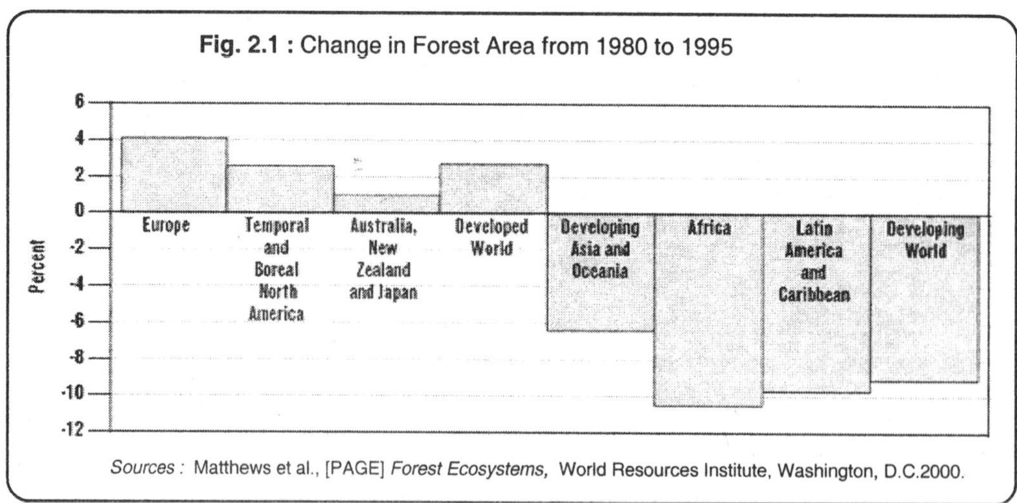

Sources : Matthews et al., [PAGE] *Forest Ecosystems,* World Resources Institute, Washington, D.C.2000.

Forests worldwide cover some 3.9 billion hectares—almost a third of the earth's land surface excluding Antarctica and Greenland. Though vast, this wooded area is only half the size of forested land at the dawn of agriculture some 11,000 years ago. Most forests are no longer in their original condition, having changed in composition and quality.

The U.N. Food and Agriculture Organization conservatively estimates that the world lost 94 million hectares of forest in the last decade of the twentieth century. This number assumes that developing countries lost 130 million hectares while the industrial world gained 36 million hectares as abandoned agricultural areas returned to forest. The yearly loss of natural forests during this period, which includes deforestation plus the conversion of natural forests to tree plantations, was 16 million hectares, 94 per cent of which occurred in the tropics.

During the 1990s, Brazil suffered the heaviest loss of forest (23 million hectares). South America as a whole saw net losses of 37 million hectares. In Africa, 52 million hectares were destroyed. Sudan, Zambia, and the Democratic Republic of the Congo account for half of Africa's forest loss. While the United States gained 4 million hectares of forests, Mexico lost over 6 million, although government reports reveal the loss may be even higher. The total net losses for North and Central America were 6 million hectares.

Table 2.1: Change in Forest Cover, 1990-2000

Continents	*Total Forest, 1990*	*Total Forest, 2000*	*Change, 1990-2000*
	Million Hectares		*Percent*
Africa	702	650	- 7.8
Asia	551	548	- 0.7
Oceania	201	198	- 1.8
Europe	1,030	1,039	+ 0.8
North and Central America	555	549	- 1.0
South America	923	886	- 4.1
Total World	3,963	3,869	- 2.2

Source: U.N. Food and Agriculture Organization, State of the World's Forests, Rome, 2001.

A massive reforestation campaign in China meant the country added an average of 1.8 million hectares each year during this period, largely because bans on deforestation near the end of the decade heightened the country's reliance on plantations and imports of forest products from other nations. In Indonesia, where tree felling destroyed 13 million hectares over the decade, forest loss has accelerated and now averages 2 million hectares each year. Over the decade, forest cover in all of Asia declined by 4 million hectares.

Although FAO data suggest that world forest loss is slowing, deforestation in tropical areas is accelerating, likely exceeding 13 million hectares each year. As tree cutting in many parts of the world accelerates, nearly half of the remaining forests are at risk. The World Resources Institute estimates that about 40 per cent of the world's intact forests will be gone within 10-20 years, if not sooner, considering current deforestation rates.

Wood consumption drives deforestation. Since 1960, global industrial wood production has risen by 50 per cent, to 1.5 billion cubic metres, four-fifths of which is from primary and secondary-growth forests. About the same quantity, 1.8 billion cubic metres, is burned directly as wood fuel each year in developing countries.

A satellite-based survey of the world's forests by the U.N. Environment Programme, along with NASA and the U.S. Geological Survey, found that 80 per cent of largely intact forests (those with a canopy closure of over 40 per cent) are located in just 15 countries. A full 88 per cent of the key closed forest areas are sparsely populated, making them hopeful targets for conservation. Short of calling for a moratorium of all logging, conservation in these 15 countries offers a reasonable starting point for forest preservation.

Consequences of Deforestation

➢ *Alteration of Local and Global Climates through Disruption of :*

(i) *The carbon cycle.* Forests act as a major carbon store because carbon dioxide (CO_2) is taken up from the atmosphere and used to produce the carbohydrates, fats, and proteins that make up the tree. When forests are cleared, and the trees are either burnt or rot, this carbon is released as CO_2. This leads to an increase in the atmospheric CO_2 concentration. CO_2 is the major contributor to the greenhouse effect. It is estimated that deforestation contributes one-third of all CO_2 releases caused by people.

(ii) *The water cycle.* Trees draw groundwater up through their roots and release it into the atmosphere (transpiration). In Amazonia over half of all the water circulating through the region's ecosystem remains within the plants. With removal of part of the forest, the region cannot hold as much water. The effect of this could be a drier climate.

- *Soil erosion :* With the loss of a protective cover of vegetation more soil is lost.
- *Silting of water courses,* lakes and dams: This occurs as a result of soil erosion.
- *Extinction of species* which depend on the forest for survival. Forests contain more than half of all species on our planet — as the habitat of these species is destroyed, so the number of species declines.
- *Desertification :* The causes of desertification are complex, but deforestation is one of the contributing factors.

(d) *Forest in India*

India has 76.50 million hectares of recorded forest area. This accounts for 23.28 per cent of geographical area. In India per capita forest availability is 0.08 ha which is much lower than the world average of 0.8 ha.

State Area as percentage of Country's Area

States/UTs	*Geog*	*Forest*	*Dense Forest*
Andhra Pradesh	8.368	6.608	6.196
Arunachal Pradesh	2.547	10.073	12.939
Assam	2.386	4.103	3.798
Bihar	2.86	0.85	0.81
Chhatisgarh	4.112	8.36	9.09
Goa	0.113	0.31	0.428
Gujarat	5.963	2.243	2.081
Haryana	1.345	0.26	0.273
Himachal Pradesh	1.694	2.126	2.502
Jammu & Kashmir	6.76	3.144	2.843
Jharkhand	2.421	3.35	2.83
Karnataka	5.834	5.476	6.275
Kerala	1.182	2.303	2.824
Madhya Pradesh	9.38	11.44	10.648
Maharashtra	9.36	7.029	7.412
Manipur	0.679	2.506	1.37
Meghalaya	0.682	2.307	1.363
Mizoram	0.641	2.59	2.144
Nagaland	0.504	1.975	1.294
Orissa	4.737	7.229	6.711
Punjab	1.532	0.36	0.372
Rajasthan	10.41	2.423	1.517
Sikkim	0.216	0.473	0.574
Tamil Nadu	3.956	3.18	2.999
Tripura	0.319	1.046	0.831
Uttar Pradesh	7.332	2.03	2.15
Uttarakhand	1.63	3.54	4.56
West Bengal	2.7	1.583	1.523
Andaman & Nicobar Islands	0.251	1.026	1.582
Chandigarh	0.003	0.001	0.001
Dadar & Nagar Haveli	0.015	0.032	0.036
Daman & Diu	0.003	0.001	0
Delhi	0.045	0.016	0.009
Lakshadweep	0.001	0.004	0.006
Pondicherry	0.015	0.005	0.008
All India	100	100	100

Source : Forest Survey of India.

The Forest Survey of India (FSI), using remote sensing technology, assesses the forest cover of the country biennially. The results of past assessments since 1987 show that the extent of forest cover in the country has stabilized though a large area still remains degraded.

The latest assessment on forest cover (FSI 1999) is as follows :

- Dense forest 37.73 m ha 11.48 per cent
- Open forest 25.51 m ha 7.76 per cent
- Mangroves 0.49 m ha 0.15 per cent

The net increase in forest cover is 3,896 sq km over the previous assessment of 1997. The dense forest has increased by 10,098 sq km and mangrove by 44 sq km, whereas open forest has decreased by 6,246 sq km during this period.

India is a large country consequently there is varying climatic conditions. Forest grows where good weathering and leaching of soil have taken place due to rain. These vary from extremely arid xerophytes to evergreen mesophytic biological forms, rich in biogenetic diversities of species and density. Over 45,000 plants including 15,000 flowering plants have been identified in India. Of these, about 5,000 are endemic to India.

The *conifer* forests of *fir, spruce, kail, deodar and chir pine* are in Himalaya. The holloc are tall broad leaf trees exceeding 50 m in height, in the rain forests.

The *deciduous sal* and *teak* grow gregariously in monsoon forests. The former in northern India and the latter in southern India, the Narmada being the divide line of the two species. Each one of the two species displays its own pattern of distribution.

Tendu, mahuwa, aonla, harra, bahera, bel, ber, pipal bar, gular adds food for the wild animals. *Tendu* leaf is the indigenous cigarette paper wrapping local tobacco for biri making and *mahuwa* flower, rich in sugar is the base for brewing local liquor. Both species have much economic value at the provincial or local levels. *Rose wood* and *Chandan* with the aromatic *hard wood* tree, grow in deciduous forests. *Semal* is the Indian silk cotton tree, *dhak* the flame of the forests, *kachnar, amaltas*, the *Indian laburnum* and *jarul* are some of the colourful flowering trees, which grow over a wide track of the country. The *khair* in the hot desert and rhododendrons in the temperate high Himalayas are flowering shrubs of bright red flowers.

➢Forest Degradation in India

The country's forest resource is under tremendous pressure. Intensified shifting cultivation, indiscriminate removal of timber, fuel wood, fodders and other forest produce, forest fire and encroachment has led to forest degradation and deforestation. Forests meet nearly 40 per cent of the country's energy needs and 30 per cent of the fodder needs. It is estimated that about 270 mt of fuelwood, 280 mt of fodder, over 12 million m^3 (cubic metre) of timber and countless non-wood forest products (NWFPs) are removed from forests annually.

At the all-India level, the area under recorded forest is about 76 million hectares accounting for 23 per cent of the total geographical area. The impact of the declining quality will be more revealing if we look at the actual degradation data in absolute terms. The estimates put the extent of degradation at 38 million hectares accounting for about 50 per cent of the recorded forest area in the country. The extent of degradation varies across States, viz., 10.8 per cent in Sikkim to 86 per cent in Rajasthan. There appears to be some problem in the case of Arunachal Pradesh where the extent of area under degraded forests is negative. The incidence of degradation is on the higher side in the north-eastern States, which may be due to the practice of *jhum* (shifting) cultivation. However, these States are not exceptions. Degradation is equally bad in States like Rajasthan, Haryana, Bihar, Tamil Nadu, Andhra Pradesh, Gujarat, etc. In a majority of the cases the incidence of degradation seems to be higher in the States where the proportion of deciduous forests is more and forest plantations are low.

In terms of changes in the area under degraded forests, there is a marginal increase at the all-India level between 1989 and 1999. However, 15 States have recorded negative growth rates while 10 States recorded an increase in the area under degraded forests. Based on the changes in the area under forests, dense forests and degraded forests during the last decade, the States can be categorized as best performers and worst performers. The States that have shown an increase in the area under dense forest along with a decline in the area under degraded forests are termed as best performers and those States recording negative growth in the area under dense forests along with an increase in the area under degraded forests are termed as worst performers. Accordingly, 13 States (Arunachal Pradesh, Gujarat, Haryana, Jammu & Kashmir, Karnataka, Kerala, Maharashtra, Manipur, Meghalaya, Nagaland, Rajasthan, Punjab and West Bengal) turned out to be best performers while 7 States (Andhra Pradesh, Assam, Bihar, Madhya Pradesh, Mizoram, Sikkim and Tamil Nadu) turned out to be worst performers. And the remaining 5 States fall in between (average performers).

Forests are consistently and seriously undervalued in economic and social terms. For example, the contribution of the forestry sector to gross domestic product (GDP) was only 1 per cent in 1996-97 (measured at constant prices of 1980- 81). A latest estimate of gross value of goods and services provided by forestry sector puts its contribution to GDP at 2.37 per cent. Though it is extremely difficult to quantify, the economic value of the eco-system services of the forests is vast. It is also generally agreed that much of the land-use decision that presently drives forest change takes relatively little account of these values. The challenge for policy makers is, therefore, to bring these values into the markets, cross-sectoral decisions, macro-economic policy making, and into the development of economy in general.

A CASE STUDY

Sardar Sarovar Dam

A dam is located on Narmada River and is extended over the States of Madhya Pradesh, Gujarat and Maharashtra. The project was designed for irrigation, drinking water and hydro-electricity to these three States, but the environmental impacts of the project have raised certain questions.

A total of 1,44,731 ha of land will be submerged by the dam, out of which 56,547 ha is forest land. A total of 573 villages are to be submerged by Narmada Dam.

Submergence of about 40,000 ha of forest land under Narmada Sagar, 13,800 ha under Sardar Sarovar and 2,500 ha under Omkareshwar would create more strain on remaining forest areas in neighbouring areas. Submergence area is very rich in wildlife e.g. tigers, panthers, bears, wolves, pangolins, hyenas, jackals, flying squirrels, antelopes, black bucks, chinkara, marsh crocodiles, turtles etc. Many of these species are listed in Schedule I & II of Wild Life Protection Act, 1972.

As per the estimates of the Institute of Urban Affairs, New Delhi, the Narmada Valley Project will lead to eventual displacement of more than one million people, which is probably the largest rehabilitation issue ever encountered as per the World Bank.

Displacement will effect the tribal culture, their beliefs, myths, rituals, festivals, songs and dances, all closely associated with the hills, forests and streams. The displaced persons have to undergo hardship and distress for the sake of development and prosperity of a large section of the society. It is, therefore, the duty of government to pay maximum thought for proper rehabilitation of the displaced tribes as well as the wildlife.

➢ Forest Research and Education in India

In order to strengthen the system of forestry research in India, the Indian Council of Forestry Research and Education (ICFRE), an autonomous umbrella organization, was established in 1986 in Dehradun. ICFRE has the mandate to undertake aid, promote and coordinate forestry research and its application; function as a clearing house for research results and information; and disseminate technology. It works through its network of ten institutes and centres. There are a number of research facilities outside the ICFRE network under the auspices of different agencies such as the Kerala Forest Research Institute (Peechi), the Indian Plywood Industries Research and Training Institute (Bangalore), and forestry faculties of the State Agriculture Universities. In addition, State Forest Departments have research divisions to address their practical problems. An increasing number of private companies and non-government organizations (NGOs) are funding their own research in areas such as tree breeding, medicinal plants and NWFPs.

A comprehensive national forestry research plan has been developed by ICFRE after working out due priorities. Regional research priorities were worked out in consultation with stakeholders by holding seminars/workshops in different States followed by a national workshop for deciding projects and resource allotment, Research Advisory Committees have been constituted on which all the State Forest Departments have been duly represented.

(e) Forest Conservation

Forest conservation is development and management of forests. The first instance of forest administration is found in 300 BC during the period of Chandra Gupt Maurya. The main ways in which forest can be conserved is summarized as follows.

- ☞ *Afforestation* : It is the planting of forests on the areas where they did not exist in the past. NAEB (National Afforestation and Eco-development Board) takes care of afforestation, tree plantation, their restoration and development of fragile areas. Indian Forest Policy (1988) aim at raising forests in 60 per cent of hills and 20 per cent areas in plains.
- ☞ *Reforestation* : It is development of the forests on the land where they had been destroyed previously.
- ☞ *Reserve Forests* : They are grown over slopes, water sheds and ecologically fragile areas.
- ☞ *Sacred Grooves* : They are the patches of vegetation around religious places where felling of vegetation is not allowed.
- ☞ *Van Mahotsav* : Since 1950, every year in July and February a large number of trees are planted in India.
- ☞ *Urban Forestry* : It is plantation of multipurpose fruits, shade and flower bearing trees in urban areas along road side and rail tracks.
- ☞ *Forest Protection* : Protecting forest by natural hazards like pests and fires.

IV. Water Resources

When Neil Armstrong saw the Earth from the Moon, it appeared blue ! This is because water covers more than two-thirds of the Earth's surface. But fresh water

CASE STUDY

Regenerating Forest through Community Action in Orissa

By September 1987, the five villages had formalized their commitment to protect Dhani Forest. They formed a forest protection committee called the Dhani Panch Mauza Jungle Surakhya Committee. Out of lengthy discussions on the causes of the forest's poor condition and the possible ways to relieve pressures on the forest came a plan to restrict human uses of the forest.

From the beginning, the effort to protect and rejuvenate Dhani Forest was a true community affair. The elders of all households in each of the villages sat on the general body of the forest protection committee, which made all policy and budgetary decisions. A smaller executive committee included two members from each village to help implement the general committee's decisions. Community members were also required to take turns serving on the 25-person patrol squad that kept a daily vigil at the forest, restricting public access and preventing further degradation.

At first, the protection plan was simple: keep people and cattle out except for very restricted uses. Gradually, as the community's experience with protection evolved, so did the protection plan. The forest protection committee drew up an elaborate set of regulations and a schedule of fines. Cutting a valuable timber species like teak, for example, drew a fine of rupees 1,001. In essence, the committee forbade any unsupervised cutting or collection of forest materials and set strict limits on those goods that could be harvested. The committee banned anyone entering the forest from carrying an axe or other sharp implement that could be used to cut woody material. It also banned grazing during the rainy season (July–September) to encourage regrowth of ground vegetation and restricted human access during the summer months to prevent fires. To help restore the lower slopes of the forest, the committee negotiated with local farmers to end the practice of periodically cultivating these areas.

It did not take long for Dhani Forest to rebound. Although they had lost much of their foliage, many of the trees and shrubs still had intact root systems and a number of these species were naturally fast growing; simple protection from defoliation allowed them to spring back. Still, Dhani is not the forest it once was. Some valuable species that were once abundant, like Sissoo, mango, Kendu, and Harida, are now scarce. The original forest species composition has been altered further with the planting of non-native species like eucalyptus.

Dhani Forest boasted more than 250 plant species and 40 bird species. Other wildlife had begun to return as well. Soil erosion had diminished and stream volumes had increased, benefiting the agricultural fields that border the forest.

represents less than 0.5 per cent of the total water on Earth. The rest is either in the form of seawater or locked up in icecaps or the soil, which is why one often hears of water scarcity in many areas.

Water is continuously moving around the earth and constantly changing its form. It evaporates from land and water bodies and is also produced by all forms of life on Earth. This water vapour moves through the atmosphere, condenses to form clouds and precipitates as rain and snow. In time, the water returns to where it came from, and the process begins all over again. Although water is constantly moving, its total quantity on Earth's surface is constant.

(a) Forms of Water

Water is found in three different forms — liquid, solid or gas, depending on the temperature but it constantly changes from one form to another.

Liquid : Water is usually encountered in the liquid state, because this is its natural state when temperatures are between 0° C and 100° C.

Solid : It occurs when temperatures are below 0° C (32° F). For a given mass, ice occupies 9 per cent more volume than water. Being less dense than water, ice floats. This property of ice is vital to aquatic life in cold regions. As the temperature drops, ice forms a protective, insulating layer on the surfaces of streams, pools and other water bodies, allowing water to remain liquid in the layers beneath and life to survive. Glaciers, icebergs, and ice caps are all frozen water.

Gas : Water is found in the atmosphere in its gaseous form as water vapour. Steam is nothing but vaporized water.

'Fresh' or drinking water is found as groundwater in underground aquifers, and on the surface in ponds, lakes, and rivers.

In regions of young volcanic activity, hot water emerges from the earth in hot springs (examples are *Garampani* in Assam and Badrinath in Uttarakhand). Surface water percolates downward through the rocks below the Earth's surface to high temperature regions surrounding a magma reservoir, either active, or recently solidified but still hot. There the water is heated, becomes less dense, and rises back to the surface through fissures and cracks. In certain regions hot water springs called geysers, jets of steam and hot water rise one hundred feet or more from the ground. Geysers are found in Iceland, the North Island of New Zealand and in USA's Yellowstone National Park.

(b) Importance of Water

Because of overpopulation, mass consumption, misuse, and water pollution, the availability of drinking water per capita is inadequate and shrinking.

Worldwide, the consumption of water is doubling every 20 years or more than twice the rate of increase in population. For this reason, water is a strategic resource in the globe and an important element in many political conflicts. Some have predicted that clean water will become the "next oil". There is a long history of conflict over water. UNESCO's World Water Development Report (WWDR, 2003) from its World Water Assessment Programme indicates that, in the next 20 years, the quantity of water available to everyone is predicted to decrease by 30 per cent.

40 per cent of the world's inhabitants currently have insufficient fresh water for minimal hygiene. More than 2.2 million people died in 2000 from diseases related to the consumption of contaminated water or drought. In 2004, the UK Charity Water Aid reported that a child dies every 15 seconds from easily preventable water-related diseases.

Utilisation of water in different sectors are as follows:

⅄ Human Uses

About 70 per cent of the fat free mass of the human body is made of water. To function properly, the body requires between one and seven litres of water per day to avoid dehydration; the precise amount depends on the level of activity, temperature, humidity, and other factors. Most of this is ingested through foods or beverages other than drinking straight water. It is not clear how much water intake is needed by healthy people, though most experts agree that 8-10 glasses of water (approximately 2 litres) daily is the minimum to maintain proper hydration. For those who do not have kidney problems, it is rather difficult to drink too much water, but (especially in warm humid weather and while exercising) it is dangerous to drink too little. People can drink far more water than necessary while exercising.

⅄ As a Solvent

Dissolving is used to wash everyday items such as the human body, clothes, floors, cars, food, and pets. Sometimes, water is not enough, and many chemicals can be added in order to improve the solvating power of water. These chemicals include saliva, soap, shampoo, alcohol, vinegar and various surfactants; these are all examples of emulsifying agents.

⅄ As a Thermal Transfer Agent

Boiling, steaming, and simmering are popular cooking methods that often require immersing food in water or its gaseous state, steam. Water is also used in industrial contexts as a coolant, and in almost all power-stations as a coolant and to drive steam turbines to generate electricity. In the nuclear industry, water can also be used as a neutron moderator.

⅄ Recreation

Humans use water for many recreational purposes, as well as for exercising and for sports. Some of these include swimming, waterskiing, boating, fishing, and diving. In addition, some sports, like ice hockey and ice skating, are played on ice.

Lakesides and beaches are popular places for people to go to relax and enjoy recreation. Many find the sound of flowing water to be calming, too. Some keep fish and other life in water tanks or ponds for show, fun, and companionship. People may also use water for play fighting such as with snowballs, water guns or water balloons.

⅄ Industrial Applications

Pressurized water is used in water blasting and water jet cutters. Also, very high pressure water guns are used for precise cutting. It works very well, is relatively safe, and is not harmful to the environment.

⅄ Food Processing

Water plays many critical roles within the field of food science. It is important for a food scientist to understand the roles that water plays within food processing to ensure the success of their products.

Solutes such as salts and sugars found in water affect the physical properties of water. The boiling and freezing points of water is affected by solutes. One mole of sucrose (sugar) raises the boiling point of water by 0.52° C, and one mole of salt raises the boiling point by 1.04 degrees while lowering the freezing point of water in a similar way. Solutes in water also affect water activity which affects many chemical reactions and the growth of microbes in food.

Water hardness is also a critical factor in food processing. It can dramatically affect the quality of a product as well as playing a role in sanitation. Water hardness is classified based on the amounts of removable calcium carbonate salt it contains per gallon. Water hardness is measured in grains; 0.064 g calcium carbonate is equivalent to one grain of hardness. Water is classified as soft if it contains 1 to 4 grains, medium if it contains 5 to 10 grains and hard if it contains 11 to 20 grains. The hardness of water may be altered or treated by using a chemical ion exchange system. The hardness of water also affects its pH balance which plays a critical role in food processing. For example, hard water prevents successful production of clear beverages.

⅄ Power Generation

Hydroelectricity is electricity obtained from hydropower. Hydroelectric power comes from water driving a water turbine connected to a generator. Hydroelectricity is a low-cost, non-polluting, renewable energy source.

Fresh water is now more precious than ever in our history for its extensive use in agriculture, high-tech manufacturing, and energy production, it is increasingly receiving attention as a resource requiring better management and sustainable use.

A large amount of water is wasted in agriculture, industry, and urban areas. It has been estimated that with available technologies and better operational practices, agricultural water demand could be cut by about 50 per cent and that in urban areas by about 33 per cent without affecting the quality or economics of life. But most governments do not have adequate laws or regulations to protect their water systems

Irrigation

Approximately 70 per cent (2,800 km^3) of the 4,000 km^3 of water humans withdraw from freshwater systems each year is used for irrigation. This volume of water irrigates 271 million hectares of croplands. Although this number represents only 17 per cent of total cropland, it produces 40 per cent the world's crops. Of the water used for irrigation, 50-80 per cent is returned to the atmosphere or otherwise lost to downstream. As a consequence, irrigation can significantly decrease river flows and aquifer levels and can shrink lakes and inland seas. Both irrigated and rain-fed agriculture can pose threats to water quality from the leaching of fertilizer, pesticides, and animal manure into groundwater or surface water.

(c) Distribution of Water on the Earth

You can see how water is distributed by viewing following bar charts.

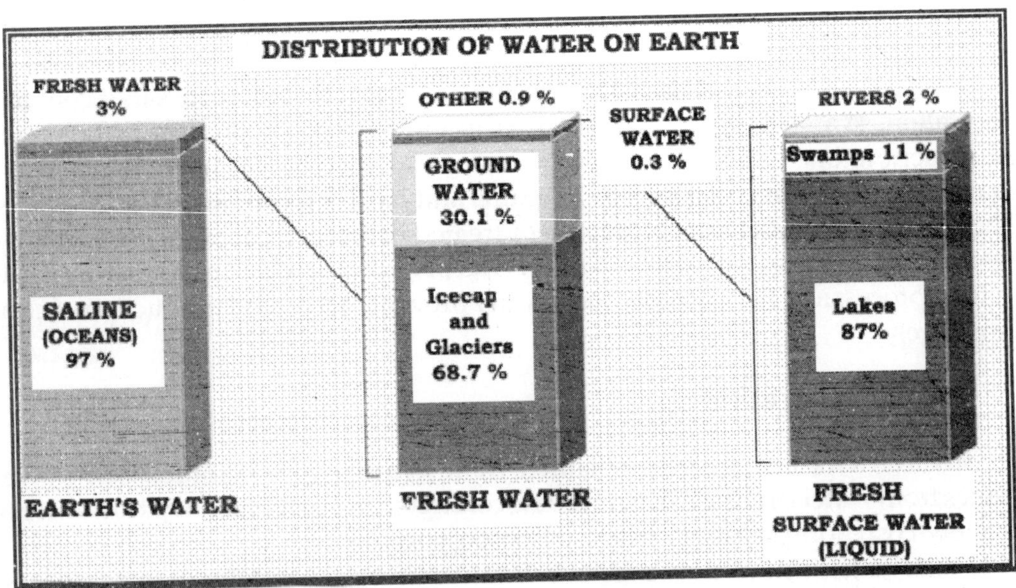

Source : Gleick, P. H., 1996: Water resources. In *Encyclopedia of Climate and Weather*, ed. by S. H. Schneider, Oxford University Press, New York, Vol. 2, pp.817-823.

The left-side bar shows where the water on Earth exists; about 97 per cent of all water is in the oceans. The middle bar shows the distribution of that three per cent of all Earth's water that is freshwater. The majority, about 69 per cent, is locked up in glaciers and icecaps, mainly in Greenland and Antarctica. You might be surprised that of the remaining freshwater, almost all of it is below your feet, as ground water. No matter where on Earth you are standing, chances are that, at some depth, the ground below you is saturated with water. Of all the freshwater on Earth, only about 0.3 per cent is contained in rivers and lakes, yet rivers and lakes are not only the water we are most familiar with, it is also where most of the water we use in our everyday lives exists.

(d) Water Resources in India

India's water resource is the most important natural endowments enabling its economy and its human settlement patterns. India is rich in water resources and it is endowed with a network of great rivers and vast alluvial basins to hold ground water. Conditions, however, vary widely from region to region.

- *Freshwater Resources :* Fresh water comprises surface water, groundwater and atmospheric water (rain/atmospheric moisture).

1. Surface Water

The surface water is found in ponds, tanks, rivers, streams and reservoirs. Rivers are major source of surface water in India. According to K.L. Rao, there are 10,360 rivers and their tributaries longer than 1.6 km each, spread over the whole country. The mean annual flow is estimated to be 1,869 billion cubic metres. However because of the topographical, hydrological and other constraints, only about 690 billion cubic metres (32 per cent) of the available surface water can be utilized. The Indus, the Ganga and the Brahmaputra carry nearly 60 per cent of the total. It is worth mentioning that the Brahmaputra and the Ganga are within the first ten major rivers of the world positioned at eighth and tenth ranks respectively. The total flow of all rivers of India is about 6 per cent of the discharge of all rivers in the world.

The effective water storage capacity built or under construction in India is about 147 billion cubic metres (bcm). It was about 18 bcm at the time of independence. It is 8.47 per cent of the total flow in the basins.

⅄ *Rivers*

All major rivers of India originate from one of the three main watersheds. They are as following :

1. The Himalaya and the Karakoram ranges.
2. Vindhya and Satpura range in central India.
3. Sahyadri or Western Ghat in western India.

The Himalayan river networks are snow fed and have continuous flow throughout the year. The other two networks are dependent on the monsoons and shrink into rivulets during the dry season.

On the basis of size, rivers of India can be classified under three categories :

Major Rivers : having a catchment's area over 20,000 sq km There are 14 such basins having high rainfall—Indus, Ganga, Brahamaputra, Sabarmati, Mahi, Narmada, Tapi, Subernarekha, Brahamni, Mahanadi, Godavari, Krishna, Pennar, and Cauvery.

Medium Rivers : having a catchment's area of 2000 - 20,000 sq km each; 44 rivers fall in this category. Like Baitarani, Purna, Mandavi, Sharswati, Peryar, Sarda, etc.

Minor River : having a catchment's area less than 2000 sq km.

India's rivers carry 90 per cent of the water during the period from June-November. Thus, only 10 per cent of the river flow is available during the other six months.

National level statistics for water availability mask huge disparities from basin-to-basin and region to region. Spatially Rajasthan, for instance, with 8 per cent of the country's population has only 1 per cent of the country's water resources while Bihar with 10 per cent of population has just 5 per cent of the water resources. Thus, while India is considered rich in terms of annual rainfall and total water resources, its uneven geographical distribution causes severe regional and temporal shortages.

Problems with Rivers

According to the Third Assessment Report of the Intergovernmental Panel on Climate Change (IPCC, 2001) almost 67 per cent of the glaciers in the Himalayan mountain range have retreated in the past decade. Available records suggest that the Gangotri glacier is retreating by about 30 metres per year. Elevated global mean temperature may increase net melting rates resulting in glacial retreat and consequent adverse impact on flows in major rivers.

They are also subject to significant net water withdrawals along their course, due to agricultural, industrial, and municipal use; as well as pollution from human and animal waste, agricultural run-offs, and industrial effluents.

Although the rivers possess significant natural capacity to assimilate and render harmless many pollutants, the existing pollution inflows in many cases substantially exceed such natural capacities.

India's rivers are inextricably linked with the history and religious beliefs of its peoples, and the degradation of important river systems accordingly offends their spiritual, aesthetic, and cultural sensibilities.

Wetlands

Wetlands, natural and manmade, freshwater or brackish, provide numerous ecological services. They provide habitat to aquatic flora and fauna, as well as numerous species of birds, including migratory species. The density of birds, in particular, is an accurate indication of the ecological health of a particular wetland.

India : State-wise Details of Inland Water Resources—1993 (lakh hec.)

S. No.	*States*	*Rivers & Canals (Length in km)*	*Reservoir*	*Tanks, Lakes & Ponds*	*Beels, Oxbow, Lakes & Derelict Water*	*Brackish Water*	*Total Water Bodies*
1.	Andhra Pradesh	11514	2.34	5.17	—	0.64	8.15
2.	Arunachal Pradesh	2000	—	0.01	0.03	—	0.04
3.	Assam	1820	0.55	0.21	1.10	—	1.86
4.	Bihar	3200	0.60	0.95	0.05	—	1.60
5.	Goa	250	0.03	0.03	—	—	0.06
6.	Gujarat	3865	2.43	0.71	—	0.95	4.09
7.	Haryana	5000	Neg.	0.10	0.10	—	0.20
8.	Himachal	3000	0.40	0.01	—	—	0.41
9.	Jammu & Kashmir	27781	0.07	0.17	0.06	—	0.30
10.	Karnataka	9000	2.11	3.52	—	0.08	5.71
11.	Kerala	3092	0.30	0.03	2.43	2.43	5.19
12.	Madhya Pradesh	20661	2.91	1.17	—	—	4.08
13.	Maharashtra	3200	2.79	0.32	—	0.10	3.21
14.	Manipur	3360	0.01	0.05	0.40	—	0.46
15.	Meghalaya	5600	0.08	0.02	Neg.	—	0.10
16.	Mizoram	1743	—	0.02	—	—	0.02
17.	Nagaland	1600	0.17	0.50	Neg.	—	0.67
18.	Orissa	4500	2.56	0.64	1.80	4.33	9.33
19.	Punjab	15270	Neg.	0.07	—	—	0.07
20.	Rajasthan	N.A.	1.20	1.80	—	—	3.00
21.	Sikkim	900	—	—	0.03	—	0.03
22.	Tamil Nadu	7420	0.53	2.24	5.24	0.56	8.57
23.	Tripura	1200	0.05	0.12	—	—	0.17
24.	Uttar Pradesh	31200	1.50	1.62	1.33	—	4.45
25.	West Bengal(P)	2526	0.17	2.76	0.42	2.10	5.45
26.	Delhi	150	0.04	—	—	—	0.04
	Total	170282	20.90	22.54	13.00	12.35	68.79

Source : Fisheries Div. Deptt.of Agriculture & Cooperation, Ministry of Agriculture, India.
N.A. : Not Available; (P) ; Provisional; Neg. Negligible.

Several wetlands have sufficiently unique ecological character as to merit international recognition as Ramsar Sites.

Wetlands also provide freshwater for agriculture, animal husbandry, and domestic use, drainage services, and provide livelihoods to fisherfolk. Larger wetlands may also comprise an important resource for sustainable tourism and recreation.

They may be employed as an alternative to power, technology, and capital intensive municipal sewage plants; however, if used for this purpose without proper reckoning of their assimilative capacity, or for dumping of solid and hazardous waste, they may become severely polluted, leading to adverse health impacts.

Wetlands are under threat from drainage and conversion for agriculture and human settlements, besides pollution. This happens because public authorities or individuals having jurisdiction over wetlands derive little revenues from them, while the alternative use may result in windfall financial gains to them.

However, in many cases, the economic values of wetlands' environmental services may significantly exceed the value from alternative use. On the other hand, the reduction in economic value of their environmental services due to pollution, as well as the health costs of the pollution itself, are not taken into account while using them as a waste dump. There also does not yet exist a formal system of wetland regulation outside the international commitments made in respect of Ramsar sites. A holistic view of wetlands is necessary, which looks at each identified wetland in terms of its causal linkages with other natural entities, human needs, and its own attributes.

2. *Groundwater*

The replenishable groundwater potential in India is estimated at 433.9 billion cubic metres. Water percolates easily in the alluvial soils and hence the potential of the groundwater development is high in the Great Plains of India. Uttar Pradesh alone accounts for 19.0 per cent of the estimated groundwater potential. More than 42 per cent of the potential is confined to States of the Great Plains of north India. Contrary to it, seepage of water in the rocky lands of peninsular India is slow, resulting in low groundwater potential. However, because of their size Maharashtra, Madhya Pradesh and Tamil Nadu also have large potential of groundwater resources.

Of the total groundwater resources one-fourth is used for domestic, industrial and related purposes and three-fourths for irrigation. Only 37.23 per cent of the total available groundwater resources have so far been developed in India. State-wise percentage of developed groundwater resources to total available potential ranges from 1.07 per cent in Jammu and Kashmir to 98.34 per cent in Punjab.

Those States and union territories where there is scarcity of surface water due to low and highly variable rainfall have developed their groundwater resources on large scale. Punjab, Haryana, western Uttar Pradesh, Rajasthan, Gujarat and Tamil Nadu are such States. There is need for the development of groundwater resources in Andhra Pradesh, Madhya Pradesh, Chhattisgarh, Karnataka and Maharashtra also where rainfall is comparatively insufficient and variable.

Overuse of Underground Water

The water table has been falling rapidly in many areas of the country in recent decades. This is largely due to withdrawal for agricultural, industrial, and urban use, in excess of annual recharge. In urban areas, apart from withdrawals for domestic and industrial use, housing and infrastructure such as roads prevent sufficient recharge. In addition, some pollution of groundwater occurs due to leaching of stored hazardous waste and use of agricultural chemicals, in particular, pesticides. Contamination of groundwater is also due to geogenic causes, such as leaching of arsenic and fluoride from natural deposits. Since groundwater is frequently a source of drinking water, its pollution and contamination leads to serious health impacts.

3. Rainfall in India

India receives an average annual rainfall equivalent to about 4,000 billion cubic metres (BCM). This source of water is unevenly distributed both spatially as well as temporally. Most of the rainfall is confined to the monsoon season, from June to September, and levels of precipitation vary from 100 mm a year in western Rajasthan to over 9,000 mm a year in the northeastern State of Meghalaya. With 3,000 BCM of rainfall concentrated over the four monsoon months and the other 1,000 BCM spread over the remaining eight months.

Water Use in India

Out of the total water withdrawn from various sources, 97 per cent is used for agriculture and livestock, the rest being accounted by withdrawal for domestic consumption, industrial use and power generation. However, not all the water abstracted is effectively used, there are sizeable losses in conveyance and application of irrigated water, a large part of water used by industry and domestic purposes is returned to the streams as effluent waste; and most of the water drawn by power station is used for cooling purposes and is available for reuse.

The water pollution in India comes from three main sources : domestic sewage, industrial effluents and run off from activities such as agriculture. Major industrial sources of pollution in India include the fertilizer plants, refineries, pulp and paper mills, leather tanneries, metal plating and other chemical industries.

(e) Floods

Flood Affected Area in India	
Year	*Area (Million ha.)*
1995	5.245
1996	8.049
1997	4.569
1998	9.133
1999	3.978
2000	5.166
2001	3.008
2002	2.808

Source: Rashtriya Barh Ayog, India.

Floods occur in almost all rivers basins of India. Heavy rainfall, inadequate capacity of rivers to carry the high flood discharge, inadequate drainage to carry away the rainwater quickly to streams/rivers are the main causes of floods. Ice jams or land slides blocking streams; typhoons and cyclones also cause floods. Excessive rainfall combined with inadequate carrying capacity of streams resulting in over spilling of banks is the cause for flooding in majority of cases. The annual average area affected is 7.181 million ha. The maximum was in 1978 when 17.50 million ha was affected.

➢ Flood Control

- Flood control in flood prone area involve building dams to store water.
- Planting trees on eroded slopes.
- Along coasts, engineers build dykes, floodwalls and hurricane barriers to keep sea water off the land.
- Sand bagging also controls floods.
- Floods losses can be minimized by insurance and relief aid.

(f) Drought

There are about 80 countries in the world, lying in the arid and semi arid regions that experience frequent spell of drought. When annual rainfall is below normal and less than evaporation, drought conditions created. Throughout the world, drought affect more people than does any other single type of disaster and it causes about 20 per cent of disaster related deaths. The continent most affected by drought is Africa.

Drought Prone Areas —State-wise (Area in Hectares)

S.No.	*State*	*Drought Prone Area*
1.	A.P.	12511303
2.	Bihar +Jharkhand	4338450
3.	Gujarat	12123890
4.	Haryana	1658785
5.	J&K	1599930
6.	Karnataka	15216333
7.	M.P.+ Chhatisgarh	8721952
8.	Maharashtra	12376705
9.	Orissa	2286241
10.	Rajasthan	21895045
11.	Tamil Nadu	8409114
12.	U.P.	4303310
13.	West Bengal	2672080
	Total	108113138

Source : National Commission on Agriculture, India.

In India, Irrigation Commi-ssion, 1972 has identified 67 drought prone districts located in 8 States having an area of 49.73 million ha. Subsequently, the National Commission on Agriculture, 1976 identified a few more drought prone areas with a slightly different criteria. The total geographical area of the drought districts is 108 million ha out of which 81 million ha is culturable (75%), gross sown area is 61.9 million ha (57.4%) and the gross irrigated area is 14.3 million ha. About 23.23 per cent of the total cropped area is irrigated in the drought districts.

➤ Drought Control

The systematic Government intervention to tackle drought started as early as during the Second Five Year Plan (1956-61) when the Dry Farming Projects were initiated. During 1970-71, the Rural Works Programme (RWP) was formulated with the object of creating assets designed to reduce the severity of drought, wherever it occurred and to provide employment in the drought affected areas. Later, the RWP was redesignated as Drought Prone Area Programme (DPAP) in 1973-74 and taken up as a centrally sponsored scheme. The burden of funding was borne both by the Central Government and the State Government on a 50 : 50 sharing basis. The major thrust of the programme was laid on the activities related to soil conservation and development, afforestation, pasture, fodder and grassland development, etc. These activities are harmoniously related to each other and their integrated implementation would have the capability to effectively combat drought.

Irrigation has proved to be the most effective drought proofing mechanism and single biggest factor in bringing about a large measure of stability in agricultural production.

To produce rain iodine crystals are scattered among clouds from the aircrafts (It works in the areas where rainfall readily occurs naturally). Afforestation and planting of trees around the ponds and water bodies helps in improving the quantity of water in an area.

(g) Conflicts over Water

Unequal distribution of water has often led to inter-State or international dispute. In India out of 18 major rivers, 17 are shared between different States. Some major water conflicts in India are as following :

The Indus Water Treaty

Under this treaty in 1960, Indus, Jhelum and Chenab were given to Pakistan and Sutlej, Ravi and Beas were allocated in India. India can construct barrage across its rivers as riparian State. But the treaty allows the non-consumptive use of rivers allocated to Pakistan i.e., its quality and flow should not be changed.

The Cauvery Water Dispute

The Cauvery river water is a bone of contention between Tamil Nadu and Karnataka since last 100 years. The river water is almost is fully utilized and both the States have increasing demands for agriculture and industry. The consumption is more in Tamil Nadu than Karnataka where the catchments area is rockier. On June 2, 1990, the Cauvery Water Dispute Tribunal was set up which through an interim award directed Karnataka to ensure that 205 TMCF of water was made available in Tamil Nadu's Mettur Dam every year till a settlement was reached. Proper selection of crop varieties, optimum use of water, better rationing, rational sharing patterns, and pricing of water are suggested as some measures to solve the problems.

The Sutluj -Yamuna Link (SYL) Canal Dispute

Eradi Tribunal (1985) allocated the waters of Ravi-Beas Rivers between Punjab and Haryana on the basis of the times inflow data of 20 years (1960-80). According to this 17.17 MAF (million acre feet) water was available. But now the Punjab's view is that in last 17 years quantity of water has declined. The Supreme Court on January 15, 2002 directed Punjab Government to complete and commission the SYL within a year failing, which Central Government has failed to complete it.

Punjab claims his riparian rights for Beas, Ravi and Sutlej. Haryana is facing acute shortage of water since 1966 and has completed the stretch of SYL falling within the boundaries of Haryana. Punjab has recently refused to follow. Eradi awards by passing legislation unanimously. The entire conflict is being observed by the centre.

(h) Interlinking of Rivers

Most of the years some part of the India like Bihar and Assam are flooded while some other parts like Rajasthan, Maharashtra, and Karnataka experience severe drought. To find a lasting solution to this age old problem and the related problem of drinking water and irrigation, the union government embarked on a mammoth project to link India's major rivers. It was given added weight by the Supreme Court of India, which on public interest litigation for water management passed an order requiring the project to be completed by 2016.

The project is estimated to cost Rs. 560,000 crore envisages creating 30 inter-basins links to transfer water from surplus to deficit basins, and to prevent surplus to deficit basins, and to prevent surplus water from flowing into the sea. Besides flood control in the Ganga and Brahamaputra Basins and drought - proofing in perennial drought-prone of 30,000 mega watts of cheap hydro-electric power as major benefits. The network of the river transport is expected to release the pressure on road and railway. There could also be 10 million new jobs a year.

Water from Brahmaputra will flow into Ganga, which will be connected to Mahanadi and Godavari. Godavari will be linked to Krishna, Pennar, and Cauveri. Narmada will flow into Tapti and Yamuna into Sabarmati. The eastern Indian tributaries of India will supply in western India, and Peninsular India is Mahanadi and Godavari rivers will supply water-deficit basin in Southern India's Karnataka, Tamil Nadu, Maharashtra States. Several major dams and canals are envisaged including powered schemes to "lift" the waters of the river Godavari in southern India.

Environmentalists say that the interlinking of the rivers will disrupt the hydrological cycle by stopping rivers from performing their ecological functions before reaching the ocean. They also warn about displacement of some 4.5 lakh people and submersion about 8,00,000 hectares of forests.

(i) Dams

Dam is a barrier placed a cross river to stop the flow of water. Dam very in size from small earth or rock barrier to concrete structure that rise as high as a sky- scrapper. Throughout the history, wherever people settled, an important first concern was locating an adequate, perennial water supply. Some Roman dams built in Italy, Spain and North America are still being used today.

➢ Benefits of Dams

- As a barrier across a river or stream, a dam stops the flow of water.
- It stores the water, creating a lake or reservoir and raises the level of the water almost as high as the dam itself. The stored water maintains steady availability of water throughout the year.
- The stored water also flows through the hydraulic turbines, producing electric power that is used in homes and industries.
- Water releases from the dam in uniform quantities guarantees water for fish and other wild life in the stream below the dam. Otherwise the stream would go dry there.
- River navigation.

- Flood can be held back.
- Dams provde attraction for tourists.
- They give refuge to wild life.

➢ Problems with Dams

Upstream Problems

- Dam caused swamps, which affect agriculture, forest and grassland areas.
- Disturbances of natural ecosystem.
- Large scale deforestation.
- Collapse of river food web, consequently flora and fauna will be disturbed.
- Displacement of tribal people.
- Siltation and sedimentation of reservoir.

Downstream Problems

- Waterlogging and salinity due to over irrigation Micro-climatic changes.
- Reduced water flow and silt deposition in river.
- Outbreak of vector-borne diseases like malaria.
- Flash floods.

Because of the certain severe effects of large dams, now there is a shift towards construction of small dams or mini- hydel projects.

(j) Conservation of Water Resources

The uneven distribution of water in space and season, growing demand and rapid degradation, it has become very important to conserve the water resources.

1. The first step in this way is to collect the rainwater and stop it from draining off.
2. Second step consists of scientifically managing the water resources of all the rivers.
3. Third step is keeping the water unpolluted.

Rainwater Harvesting : It is a technique of increasing the recharge of groundwater by capturing and storing rainwater locally in subsurface water reservoirs to meet the household needs.

Objectives of the rainwater harvesting are to :

* Reduce the run-off which chokes drains,
* Avoid the flooding of roads,
* Meet the ever increasing demand for water,
* Augment the groundwater storage and raise the water table,
* Reduce groundwater pollution,
* Improve the quality of groundwater,
* Reduce the soil erosion, and
* Supplement domestic water requirement during summer and drought.

Several low cost techniques are obtainable to recharge the groundwater aquifers. Among them mention may be made of roof water harvesting, refilling of dug wells, recharging of hand pumps, construction of percolation pits, trenches around fields, and bunds and stop dams on small rivulets.

These techniques are not new to the nation. Rainwater has been harvested in India since ancient times. There are evidences of sophisticated water harvesting systems like canals, tanks, embankments and wells. In hills and mountains, rainwater harvesting from rooftops and springs was carried over long distances. In arid and semiarid regions, structures like wells and step-wells were built to tap groundwater aquifers. Rainwater harvesting from rooftops used artificially created catchments, which drained water into artificial '*kunds*' in Rajasthan. Construction of tanks throughout the country has been very popular measure of conserving rainwater.

Watershed Development

Watershed is geographic area that drains to a common point, which makes it an ideal planning unit for conservation of soil and water. It may comprise one or several villages; contain both arable and non-arable lands, various categories of land holding and farmers. The watershed approach enables a holistic development of agriculture and allied activities, such as horticulture, agro-forestry and, silviculture (forests).

Watershed development programme in India is implemented by the Ministries of Agriculture, Rural development, Environment and Forests.

So watershed approach is an important means to conserve water resources to increase agricultural production, to stop ecological degradation in rain fed and resource-poor areas. At the same time it improves the level of living of the people.

CASE STUDY

Ganga Basin : Groundwater Resource Potential in India

It is bounded on the north by the Himalayas, on the west by the Aravallis as well as the ridge separating it from Indus basin, on the south by the Vindhyas and Chhotanagpur Plateau and on the east by the Brahmaputra ridge. Its catchment lies in the States of Uttar Pradesh (294,364 km^2), Madhya Pradesh (198,962 km^2), Bihar (143,961 km^2), Rajasthan (112,490 km^2), West Bengal (71,485 km^2), Haryana (34,341 km^2), Himachal Pradesh (4,317 km^2) and Delhi (1,484 km^2). The basin has a population of 356.8 million.

The Ganga originates as Bhagirathi from the Gangotri Glaciers in the Himalayas at an elevation of about 7010 metres above mean sea level, in the Uttarkashi district of Uttarakhand.

The Important tributaries are the Yamuna, the Ramaganga, the Gomti, the Ghagra, the Sone, the Gandak, the Burhi Gandak, the Kosi and the Mahananda. At Farakka in West Bengal the river divides into two arms namely the Padma which flows to Bangladesh and the Bhagirathi which flows through West Bengal.

The important cities and towns situated on the banks of the Ganga are Haridwar, Kanpur, Allahabad, Varanasi, Patna, Bhagalpur etc. The Ganga has a special place in the psyche of the Indian people as being the most sacred of all Indian rivers.

The annual surface water potential of the basin has been assessed as 525.0 km^3. Out of this, 250.0 km^3 is utilisable water. Culturable area of the basin is about 58.0 million.ha, which is 29.5 per cent of the total culturable area of the country. Live storage capacity in the basin has increased significantly since independence. From just about 4.2 km^3 in the pre-plan period, the total live storage capacity of the completed projects has increased to 37.8 km^3. In addition, a substantial storage capacity of over 17.0 km^3 would be created on completion of projects under construction. An additional storage to the tune of over 29.6 km^3 would become available on the execution of projects under consideration. The hydropower potential of the basin has been assessed as 10,715 MW at 60 per cent load factor.

The Upper Ganga Canal and the Eastern and Western Yamuna Canals built during the nineteenth century, are among the oldest major projects in the basin. Some of the other important projects constructed since independence are Gandhi Sager Dam, Rana Partap Sagar Dam, Narora Barrage, Rajghat Dam, Rihand Dam, Gandak Barrage, Tenughat Dam, Maithon Dam, Kangasabati Dam etc.

Large-scale urbanisation and industrial development brought in its wake the problem of pollution of river water. The Ganga Action Plan taken up in the mid-eighties together with enforcement of various legislative and administrative measures has considerably helped in reducing the pollution of the river especially at Haridwar, Kanpur, Allahabad and Varanasi.

A network of 352 hydrological observation stations is maintained by the Central Water Commission in the basin for various purposes like inflow/flood forecasting, water quality monitoring, assessment of hydrological parameters like discharge, water level, suspended sediment etc.

The water related issues of the basin are both due to high and low flow. Uttar Pradesh, Bihar and West Bengal are the States affected by floods. Many of the flood problems are caused by northern tributaries of Ganga such as Kosi and Mahananda. Besides these problems are also caused by southern tributaries. Ganga Flood Control Commission (GFCC) was set up in 1972 to prepare comprehensive flood control plan and monitoring of flood control projects in the basin.

V. Mineral Resources

Minerals are naturally occurring, inorganic, crystalline solids having a definite composition and characteristics physical properties.

(a) Classification of Minerals

Minerals may be classified according to their use in industries as follows :

Metallic minerals	Ferrous	Iron, Chromites manganese and nickel etc.
	Non-ferrous	Copper, lead, zinc, tungsten, al., etc.
Non-metallic minerals	Mica, steatite, asbestos, etc.	
Refractory minerals	They are used as heat resistance in furnaces and moulds such as chromites, magnesite, fireclays and graphite, etc.	
Fertilizer minerals	Gypsum, rock phosphate and pyrite.	
Mineral fuels:	Coal, petroleum, natural gas, and nuclear minerals.	

(b) *Uses and Exploitation of Major Minerals in the World*

The economic development of a country is influenced by the availability of minerals. Minerals form the base for several large scale industries.

Steps involved in mineral utilization are as follows :

1. Extraction of raw ore;
2. Process of raw ore;
3. Purification of mineral;
4. Conversion of mineral into bulk state;
5. Manufacture of utility goods; and
6. Return to environment as waste.

There are about 3,000 kinds of minerals but only about 100 of them are common, some of them are as follows :

Aluminium : Is the most abundant metal element in the Earth's crust. Bauxite is the main source of aluminium. Guinea and Australia have about one-half of the world's reserves. Other countries with major reserves include Brazil, Jamaica, and India.

Antimony : A native element, antimony metal is extracted from stibnite and other minerals. Antimony is used as a hardening alloy for lead, especially storage batteries and cable sheaths, also used in bearing metal, type metal, solder collapsible tubes and foil, sheet and pipes, and semiconductor technology.

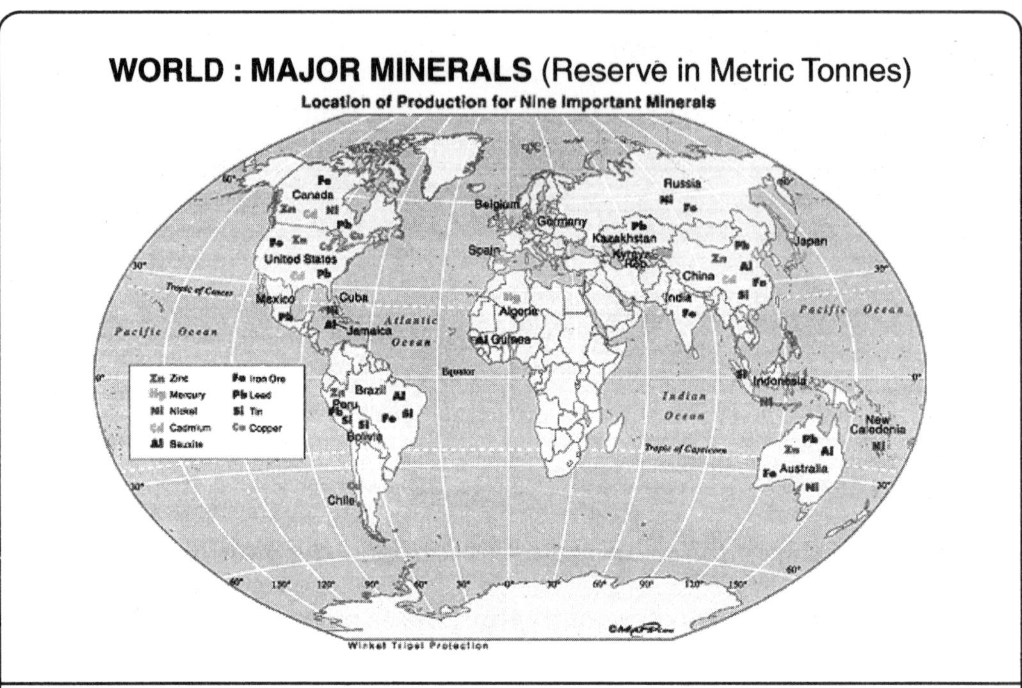

Mineral	Uses	Reserves	Major Countries
Bauxite	Ore of Aluminium	215,590,002	Australia, Jamaica, Brazil
Chromium	Alloys, Electroplating	418,900	India, S. Africa, Turkey
Copper	Alloys, Electric Wires	321,000	Chile, USA, Canada
Gold	Jewellery	42	South Africa, USA, Australia
Iron Ore	Iron and Steel	64,648,000	Brazil, Australia, China, Canada
Lead	Solder, Pipes	70,440	USA, Mexico, Canada
Manganese	Iron and Steel	812,800	South Africa, Gabon, Australia
Nickel	Stainless Steel	48,660	Canada, Norway
Silver	Jewellery	780	Mexico, USA, Peru, Canada
Tin	Tin Cans, Alloys	5,930	China, Brazil, Indonesia
Zinc	Iron and Steel	143,910	Canada, Australia, China, Peru

Source: World Resource Institute, Washington, DC, USA.

Asbestos : Because this group of silicate minerals can be readily separated into thin, strong fibres that are flexible, heat resistant, and chemically inert, asbestos minerals are suitable for use in fireproof fabrics, yarn, cloth, paper, paint filler, gaskets, roofing composition, reinforcing agent in rubber and plastics, brake linings, tiles, electrical and heat insulation, cement, and chemical filters.

Coal : One of the world's major sources of energy. It is a very complex and diverse energy resource that can vary greatly, even within the same deposit. In general, there are four basic varieties of coal, which are the result of geologic forces having altered plant material in different ways. On the basis of the amount of carbon, moisture and volatile matter, coal can be classified into anthracite, bituminous, lignite and peat (Anthracite is the best quality while peat is lowest).

Cobalt : Used in super alloys for jet engines, chemicals (paint driers, catalysts, magnetic coatings, pigments, rechargeable batteries), magnets, and cemented carbides for cutting tools. Principal cobalt producing countries include Democratic Republic of the Congo, Zambia, Canada, Cuba, Australia, and Russia. The United States uses about one-third of total world consumption.

Copper : Used in electric cables and wires, switches, plumbing, heating, roofing and building construction, chemical and pharmaceutical machinery, alloys (brass, and bronze), alloy castings, electroplated protective coatings and undercoats for nickel, chromium, zinc, etc., and cooking utensils. The leading producer is Chile, followed by the U.S., and Indonesia.

Feldspar : A rock-forming mineral, industrially important in glass and ceramic industries, pottery and enamelware, soaps, abrasives, bond for abrasive wheels, cements and concretes, insulating compositions, fertilizer, poultry grit, tarred roofing materials, and as a sizing (or filler) in textiles and paper. Albite is feldspar mineral and is a sodium aluminium silicate. This form of feldspar is used as a glaze in ceramics.

Gold : Used in dentistry and medicine, in jewellery and arts, in medallions and coins, in ingots as a store of value, for scientific and electronic instruments, as an electrolyte in the electroplating industry. South Africa has about half of the world's resources. Significant quantities are also present in the U.S., Australia, Brazil, Canada, China, and Russia.

Gypsum : Processed and used as prefabricated wallboard or as industrial or building plaster, used in cement manufacture, agriculture and other uses.

Iron Ore : About 98 per cent of iron ore is used to make steel—one of the greatest inventions and most useful materials ever created. While the other uses for iron ore and iron are only a very small amount of the consumption, they provide excellent examples of the ingenuity and the multitude of uses that man can create from our natural resources.

Kaolin : Also known as "china clay" is a white, aluminosilicate widely used in paints, refractories, plastics, sanitary wares, fibreglass, adhesives, ceramics, and rubber products.

Lead : Used in lead batteries, gasoline tanks, and solders, seals or bearings, used in electrical and electronic applications, TV tubes, TV glass, construction, communications, protective coatings, in ballast or weights, ceramics or crystal glass, tubes or containers, type metal, foil or wire, X-ray and gamma radiation shielding, soundproofing material in construction industry, and ammunition. The U.S. is the world's largest producer and consumer of refined lead metal. Major mine producers other than the U.S. include Australia, Canada, China, Peru, and Kazakhstan.

Limestone: A sedimentary rock composed mostly of the mineral calcite and comprising about 15 per cent of the Earth's sedimentary crust. Uses are numerous. Limestone is a basic building block of the construction industry (dimension stone) and the chief materials from which aggregate, cement, lime, and building stone are made. As a source for lime, it is used to make paper, plastics, glass, paint, steel, cement, carpets, used in water treatment and purification plants, in the processing of various foods and household items (including medicines).

Manganese : Essential to iron and steel production. The U.S., Japan, and Western Europe are all nearly deficient in economically mineable manganese. South Africa and the Ukraine have over 80 per cent of the world's reserves.

Mica : Mica commonly occurs as flakes, books, or sheets. Sheet muscovite (white) mica is used in electronic insulators (mainly in vacuum tubes), ground mica in paint, as joint cement, as a dusting agent, in well-drilling muds, and in plastics, roofing, rubber, and welding rods. India is the largest producer of Mica in the world.

Nickel : Vital as an alloying constituent of stainless steel, plays key role in the chemical and aerospace industries. Leading producers include Australia, Canada, Norway and Russia. Large reserves are found in Australia, Cuba, New Caledonia, Canada, Indonesia, the Philippines, and Russia.

Potash : Usually chloride of potassium. Used as a fertilizer, in medicine, in the chemical industry, and is used to produce decorative colour effects on brass, bronze, and nickel. Can also be potassium sulfate, potassium-magnesium sulfate, and potassium nitrate. It is an essential mineral for vegetable and animal life.

Quartz (Silica) : As a crystal, quartz is used as a semiprecious gem stone. Cryptocrystalline forms may also be gem stones: agate, jasper, onyx, carnelian, chalcedony, etc. Crystalline gem varieties include amethyst, citrine, rose quartz, smoky quartz, etc. Because of its piezoelectric properties quartz is used for pressure gauges, oscillators, resonators, and wave stabilizers; because of its ability to rotate the plane of polarization of light and its transparency in ultraviolet rays it is used in heat-ray lamps, prism, and spectrographic lenses. Used in the manufacture of glass, paints, abrasives, refractories, and precision instruments.

Silver : Used in photography, jewellery, in electronics because of its very high conductivity, as currency — generally in some form of an alloy, water distillation, catalyst in manufacture of ethylene, mirrors, electric conductors, batteries, silver plating, table cutlery, dental, medical, and scientific equipment, electrical contacts, bearing metal, magnet windings, brazing alloys, solder. Silver is mined in approximately 56 countries. Nevada produces over one-third of the U.S. silver. Largest silver reserves are found in the U.S., Canada, Mexico, Peru, and China.

Titanium : Titanium is a strong light weight metal often used in airplanes. When titanium combines with oxygen, it forms titanium dioxide (TiO_2), a brilliant white pigment used in paint, paper, and plastics. Major deposits of titanium minerals are found in Australia, Canada, India, Norway, South Africa, Ukraine, and the United States.

Tungsten : Used in metalworking, construction and electrical machinery and equipment, in transportation equipment, as filament in light bulbs, as a carbide in drilling equipment, in heat and radiation shielding, textile dyes, enamels, paints, and for colouring glass. Major producers are China, Korea, and Russia. Large reserves are also found in the U.S., Bolivia, Canada, and Germany.

Zinc : Used as protective coating on steel, as die casting, as an alloying metal with copper to make brass, and as chemical compounds in rubber and paints. Zinc is mined in about 40 countries with China the leading producer, followed by Australia, Peru, Canada, and the United States.

(c) Environmental Damages caused by Mining Activities

Environmental damages caused by mining activities are as following:

- *Devegetation and defacing of landscape* : The topmost fertile soil as well as vegetation is removed from the mining areas to get access to the deposits. Consequently ecology of the region badly affected.
- *Subsidence of land* : This is associated with underground mining. Consequently cracks in houses, buckling of roads, bending of rail tracks, etc. take place.
- *Water Pollution* : Underground as well as surface water pollute due to mining activities. Heavy metals get leached into the groundwater and contaminate it posing health hazards. The acid mine drainage often contaminates the nearby rivers.

- *Air Pollution* : The suspended particles matter (SPM), Sulphur dioxide, Arsenic particles, lead, etc. shoot up in the atmosphere near the smelters and several health problems arises.
- *Occupational Health hazards* : Most of the miners suffer from various respiratory diseases due to constant exposure to the SPM, and toxic substances.

(d) Minerals Resources in India

India has a large number of economically useful minerals and they constitute one-quarter of the world's known mineral resources. India is rich in 35 minerals like iron, aluminium (Bauxite), Manganese, Chromium, Limestone, Dolomite, Mica, etc. India is deficient in lead, copper phosphate, potassium, nickel, gold, and silver.

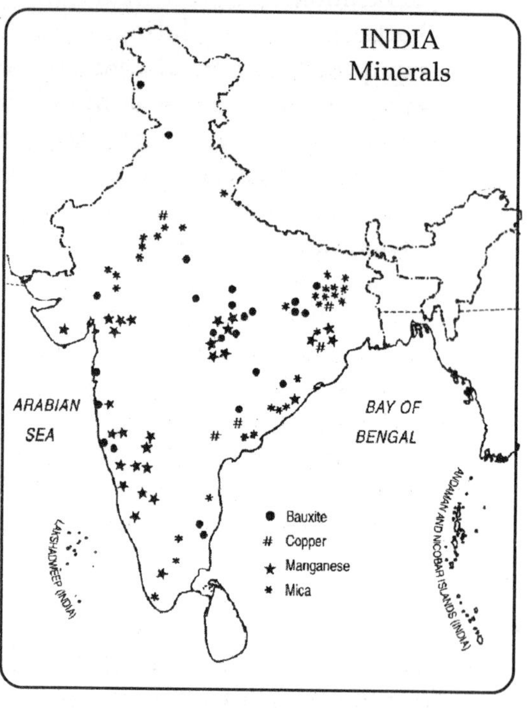

➢ Energy Generating Minerals

- *Petroleum :* Deposits are found in Maharashtra, Assam and Gujarat. The potential oil bearing areas are Assam, Tripura, Manipur, West Bengal, Punjab, Himachal, Kutch and the Andamans.
- *Coal :* India has the world's largest deposits of coal. Bituminous coal is found in Jharia and Bokaro in Bihar and Ranigunj in West Bengal. Lignite coals are found in Neyveli in Tamil Nadu.

India also possesses the all-too valuable nuclear uranium as well as some varieties of rare earths.

➢ Other Minerals for Industrial Development

- *Iron deposits :* About two-thirds of its Iron deposits lie in a belt along Orissa and Jharkhand border. Other hematite deposits are found in Chhattisgarh, Karnataka, Maharashtra and Goa. Magnetite iron-ore is found in Tamil Nadu, Bihar and Himachal Pradesh.
- *Manganese :* Next to Russia, India has the largest supply of manganese.

The manganese mining areas are Madhya Pradesh, Maharashtra and Jharkhand—Orissa area.

- *Chromites :* Its deposits are found in Bihar, Cuttack district in Orissa, Krishna district in Andhra and Mysore and Hassan in Karnataka.
- *Bauxite :* It is main ore of aluminium. The deposits are found in Jharkhand, southwest Kashmir, Central Tamil Nadu, and parts of Kerala, U.P., Maharashtra and Karnataka.
- *Mica :* India produces third quarters of the world's mica. Belts of high quality mica are in Jharkhand, Andhra and Rajasthan.
- *Gypsum :* Its reserves are in Tamil Nadu and Rajasthan.
  Nickel ore : It is found in Cuttack in Bihar and Mayurbhanj in Orissa.
- *Copper ore :* Copper ore bearing areas are Agnigundala in Andhra, Singhbhum in Jharkhand, Khetri and Dartiba in Rajasthan and parts of Sikkim and Karnataka.
- *Gold :* The Ramagiri field in Andhra Pradesh, Kolar and Hutti in Karnataka are the important gold mines.
- *Diamond :* The Panna diamond belt is the only diamond producing area in the country, which covers the districts of Panna, Chatarpur and Satna in Madhya Pradesh, as well as some parts of Banda in Uttar Pradesh.

➢ Major mines causing severe problems in India are as follows :

- *Jaduguda Uranium Mine, Jharkhand :* Exposing local people radioactive hazards.
- *Jharia Coal Mines, Jharkhand :* Underground firing leading to land subsidence.
- *Kudremukh Iron Ore Mine, Karnataka :* Causing river pollution.
- *North Eastern Coal Fields, Assam :* Very high sulphur contamination of groundwater.
- *Sukinda Chromites Mines, Orissa :* Seeping of hexavalent chromium into river posing serious health hazards.

(e) Conservation of Mineral Resources

Minerals are limited in quantity and are being depleted very fast. Following are the steps for the conservation of mineral resources :

- ☞ Application of eco friendly mining methods.
- ☞ Reuse and recycling of metals.
- ☞ Search for new deposits.
- ☞ Recovering all possible elements as co-product or by-products.
- ☞ Optimum and economic use of minerals.

☞ A complete data base of reserve, production and expected future demand of minerals.

VI. Food Resources

Food is a biological drive. Each organism needs food. All relations that exist among living organism are oriented towards food. Nature offers different source of food. Therefore, for food security, man has to be dependent on natural food resources.

(a) World Food Problems /Food Crises

The food and agriculture organization (FAO) of United Nations estimated that on an average the minimum caloric intake on a global scale is 2,500 calories/day. People receiving less than 90 per cent of these minimum dietary calories are called undernourished and if it is less than 80 per cent they are said to be seriously undernourished. Besides the minimum caloric intake we also need proteins, minerals etc.

Food security is an important issue that will be faced by policy makers in future, particularly in the world's poorest countries with potentially large population growth.

Food security depends on available supplies of food, the income of the designated population, accessibility to the available supplies, the consumption rate of food, and the amount that can be set aside for future use.

No one knows exactly how many of the world's people are undernourished today because there is a lack of reliable population counts from many countries. But, even in the absence of appropriate data collection and analysis, there is general agreement that the number of people who are severely affected by hunger and malnutrition is extremely large. According to a World Food Programme estimate, hunger affects one out of seven people on the planet. In 1996, the World Bank estimated that more than one billion of the world's people do not have enough food to lead healthy and productive lives. Furthermore, another 1.52 billion are at risk of falling into the ranks of the hungry and, if trends continue, the number is expected to grow dramatically (World Bank, 1996; Foster, 1992).

According to the Food and Agriculture Organization (FAO, 1997), 840 million of the world's 1.1 billion poors live in rural areas, whereas 15 million die each year from starvation and related diseases.

Global food supply has improved enormously since the early 1960s. Based on current trends and improved agricultural technology, world aggregate food production will be sufficient to meet demand in the decades ahead. This optimistic forecast, however, does not mean that in every country food security will improve. It is evident that there is more than enough food for every man, woman, and child on the planet, but all too often the poor do not have access to that food. Despite the availability of viable technologies to increase food and agricultural production, economic and social progress is not expected to occur at similar rates across countries. This is because many of the poorer countries are unable to be self-sufficient in food and agricultural production due to various economic, social, and political constraints.

➢ *Major Causes of World Food Problems*

Food insecurity is not just a problem related to food production; it is closely linked to poverty and economic stagnation. The persistence of widespread food insecurity underscores the futility of increasing production without addressing the underlying social, political, and economic structures that make or keep people poor and hungry. One obviously must look beyond farm size, arable land use, population growth, technology, international trade, and the environment in order to understand the long-term trends in food consumption, production, and distribution. National government policies have exacerbated domestic food shortages, poverty, and income disparities in developing countries.

Poverty alleviation and food security have long been recognized as among the most central challenges facing the human condition, today in an era of unprecedented plenitude, there are probably more human beings suffering from chronic deprivation than ever before in history. One of the problems of poor countries is lack of purchasing power among the poorest segments of the population. Purchasing power is made up of a combination of income and the price of goods and services purchased. Since income distribution in poor countries is skewed toward the high end of the scale, it is difficult for the poor to purchase adequate food supplies.

In addition, there has been relatively little motivation on the part of agricultural establishments and international organizations to examine fully the complex nexus of social situations and economic conditions that underlie the real needs of developing countries.

Economic development is more than economic growth. It entails meeting basic human needs food, shelter, clothing, education, and health services. The alleviation of poverty and ensuring of food security should be the criteria to alleviate hunger and malnutrition. Long-range solutions to food shortages and economic development in low-income countries, therefore, will require profound social, political, and economic changes.

In spite of the formidable difficulties of achieving such changes by deliberate government policy, particularly in market-type economies, evidence is accumulating to show what can be achieved, even in less developed countries. However, long range solutions to poverty are multifaceted, with appropriate strategies required for each country based on its unique situation and location-specific characteristics.

Moreover, alleviation of world food insecurity must come through such specific measures as (a) better distribution of control over food-producing resources, (b) instituting people-oriented public policies, and (c) sustainable and broad-based development at the grass-roots level which is socially just, economically efficient, and ecologically sound (Society for International Development, 1988).

We live in a world characterized by hunger, poverty, and increasing disparities. It is a world of disturbing contrasts with hunger in some lands and waste of food in others, and with the disparity between many of the rich and poor nations widening constantly. We also live in a world of interdependence. This global interdependence has inescapable political and economic dimensions because boosting agricultural production in developing countries can stimulate commercial trade for developed countries. Likewise, security and peace for developed countries also depend on peace and stability in the developing countries. This is one planet. It should therefore be acknowledged that poverty is no longer a problem contained within the borders of the developing world alone. The problem has substantial effects on domestic policies, international markets, and world peace.

It is also evident that the globalization of the world's economy and the deepening interdependence among nations can present challenges and opportunities for sustained economic growth and development, as well as risks and uncertainties for the future of the world economy. However, unless there are dramatic new and appropriate strategies for bringing about collaborations among all countries, rich and poor, on a much larger scale and through better approaches than have existed in the past, the global problems of food insecurity and resource degradation, particularly in poor countries, will be considerable and enduring.

(b) Sources of Food

Primitive societies obtained food through hunting and gathering. Today man obtains food from cultivated plants and domesticated animals. Although some food is obtained from ocean and fresh water, 95 per cent of the human population's protein demand is met from agricultural crops and animals.

➢ Plants

Most of Our Food Comes from three Plants

- About 7,000 plants have been used for food (3% of the total)
- 90 per cent of food comes from 20 species
- More than 50 per cent of food comes from 3 species : wheat, corn, rice

Although there are 2,50,000 species of plants, only 300 are grown as food and only 100 are used on large scale agricultural produce. Most of the world's food is provided by 20 crops species, e.g. wheat, rice, corn, potato, barley, sweet potatoes, cassavas, soyabeans, oats, sorghum, millet, sugarcane, sugar beets, rye, peanuts, field beans, chick peas, bananas and coconut.

Origin of Domestication

Centre	*Years Ago*	*Plants Domesticated*	*Animals Domesticated*
Fertile Crescent (Near East)	10,500	Wheat, pea, olive, rye, barley, oats, cantaloupe, lettuce, cabbage, cherry.	Sheep, goat, cow.
China	9,500	Rice, millet, peach, apricot, walnut, tea.	Pig, silkworm, water buffalo.
(Mexico & Central America)	5,500	Corn, beans, squash, sweet potato, cacao, papaya.	Turkey
Andes & Amazonia	5,500	Potato, manioc, peppers, tomatoes, pineapple.	Llama, guinea pig.
Eastern US	4,500	Sunflower, goosefoot.	
Ethiopia	11, 00	Coffee, sesame.	
New Guinea	9,000	Sugarcane, banana.	

Source : Jared Diamond, Kingsley Stern & E.O. Wilson, USA.

As a matter of fact 149 of the top 150 plant crops were developed by primitive peoples. We have improved the varieties selected by our ancient ancestors but have done little to discover new food plants, it is estimated that 80,000 plants are edible.

➢ *Animals*

Domestic animals are used as food such as cattle, sheep, and goats are the major food livestock. Out of 148 large grazing mammals only 14 were suitable for domestication such as dog, sheep, goat, pig, cow, horse, donkey, water buffalo, llama, Bactrian camel, Arabian camel, reindeer, yak, gaur, bunting. Several countries in the world grow food in water. This practice is called as aquaculture.

(c) Agriculture

The food, fibre, and animal feed that the world's agriculture produce is worth approximately $ 1.3 trillion per year. Agriculture is most important to the economies of low-income countries, accounting for 31 per cent of their GDP, and more than 50 per cent of GDP in many parts of Sub-Saharan Africa. In middle-income countries, agriculture accounts for 12 per cent of GDP. But in the high-income countries of Western Europe and North America, where other economic sectors dominate, the contribution of agriculture to GDP is just 1-3 per cent, even though the value of the agricultural output in these countries represents 79 per cent of the total market value of world agricultural products.

Conventional measures of agriculture's share of GDP actually understate agriculture's contribution to economies. For example, agricultural GDPs in the Philippines, Argentina, and the United States comprise 21 per cent, 11 per cent, and 1 per cent of those countries' total GDPs, respectively; yet the total value of agriculture, including manufacturing and services further along the marketing chain, comprises 71 per cent, 39 per cent, and 14 per cent of their respective total GDPs.

Beyond the economic value of the food produced, agro-ecosystems also provide employment for millions. Agricultural labour represents the livelihood, employment, income, and cultural heritage of a significant part of the world's population. In 1996, of the 3.1 billion people living in rural areas, 2.5 billion—44 per cent of the world population—were estimated to be living in households dependent on agriculture. The labour force directly engaged in agriculture is an estimated 1.3 billion people—about 46 per cent of the total labour force. In North America, only 2.4 per cent of the labour force is directly engaged in agriculture, while in East, South, and Southeast Asia as well as in Sub-Saharan Africa, agricultural labour accounts for 56–65 per cent of the labour force.

➢ *Human Nutrition*

Agriculture was developed for a simple but fundamental purpose to provide adequate human nutrition. Globally, agro-ecosystems produce enough food to provide every person on the planet with 2,757 kcal each day, which is sufficient to meet the minimum human requirement for nutrition (FAO 2000). However, many people do not have adequate access to that food, and an estimated 790 million people are chronically undernourished. In Sub-Saharan Africa, 33 per cent of the population is undernourished; in the Caribbean 31 per cent; and in South Asia 23 per cent.

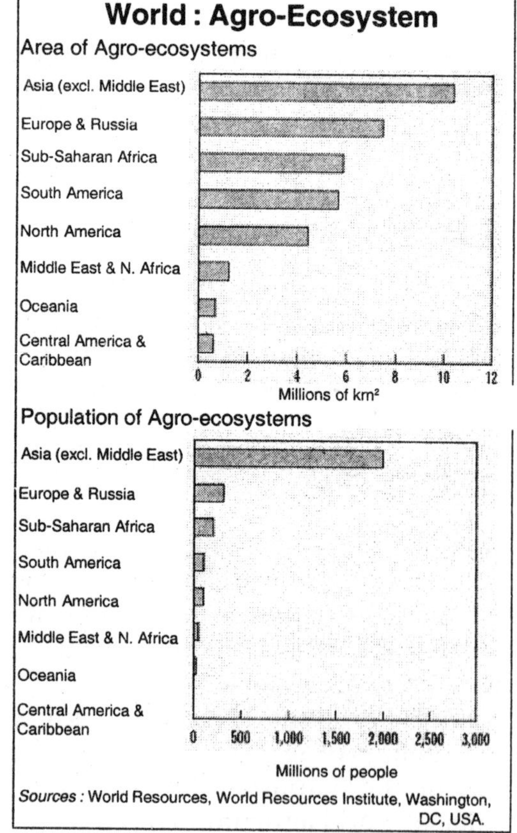

Sources : World Resources, World Resources Institute, Washington, DC, USA.

Global demand for food is still increasing significantly, driven by population growth, urbanization, and growth in per capita income. One of the most notable changes in demand is the dramatic increase in meat consumption, particularly in the developing world. This has been dubbed the "livestock revolution." Between 1982 and 1994, global meat consumption grew by 2.9 per cent per year, but it grew five times faster in developing countries than in developed countries, where meat consumption is already high.

➢ *World Food Demand*

Between 1995 and 2020, global population is expected to increase by one-third, totalling 7.5 billion people. Global demand for cereals is projected to increase by 40 per cent, with 85 per cent of the increase in demand coming from developing countries. Meat demand is projected to increase by 58 per cent, with approximately 85 per cent of the increase coming from developing countries. Demand for roots and tubers is expected to grow 37 per cent, with 97 per cent of this increase coming from the developing world. And, if significant progress is made in alleviating poverty during this period, there will be an additional increase in demand as the poor and malnourished use their increased income to buy food they previously could not afford.

➢ *The Global Extent of Agriculture*

Agricultural lands cover about 36 Mha, 28 per cent, of Earth's land area (excluding Greenland and Antarctica). Although agricultural area has increased worldwide in the past 30 years, it has decreased in many industrialized countries. Globally, about 31 per cent of agroecosystems are croplands and 69 per cent are pasture, but actual proportions of each vary widely among regions.

World : Composition of Agricultural Land, 2000

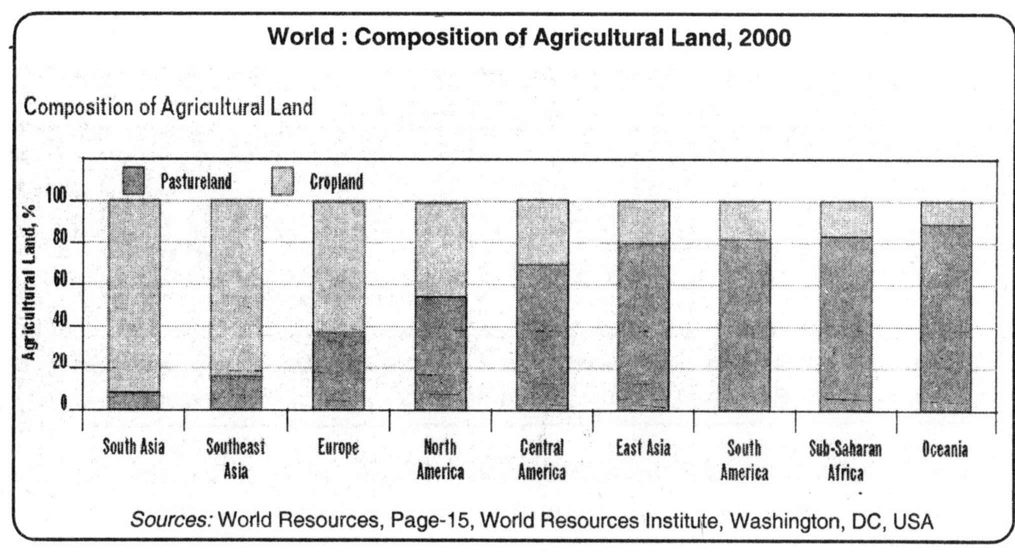

Sources: World Resources, Page-15, World Resources Institute, Washington, DC, USA

Agriculture faces an enormous challenge to meet the food needs of an additional 1.7 billion people over the next 20 years.

Agro-ecosystems cover more than one quarter of the global land area, but almost three-quarters of the land has poor soil fertility and about one-half has steep terrain, constraining production.

While the global expansion of agricultural area has been modest in recent decades, intensification has been rapid, as irrigated area increased, fallow time has decreased, and the use of purchased inputs and new technologies has grown and is producing more output per hectare. About two-thirds of agricultural land has been degraded in the past 50 years by erosion, salinization, compaction, nutrient depletion, biological degradation, or pollution. About 40 per cent of agricultural land has been strongly or very strongly degraded.

➢ *The Intensification of Agriculture*

As population has grown and good agricultural land has become scarcer, inputs such as water, fertilizer, pesticides, and labour have been applied more intensively to increase output. In Asia, where population pressures are greatest, virtually all of the cropland is harvested each year, sometimes two to three times a season, as the use of irrigation, new varieties of quick-growing seeds, and fertilizers has replaced traditional practices of leaving land fallow to restore fertility. Even marginal lands in Africa are in continuous use to meet demands for food, although water and fertilizer inputs are much lower there.

Wheat Yield in the World (1866-1996)

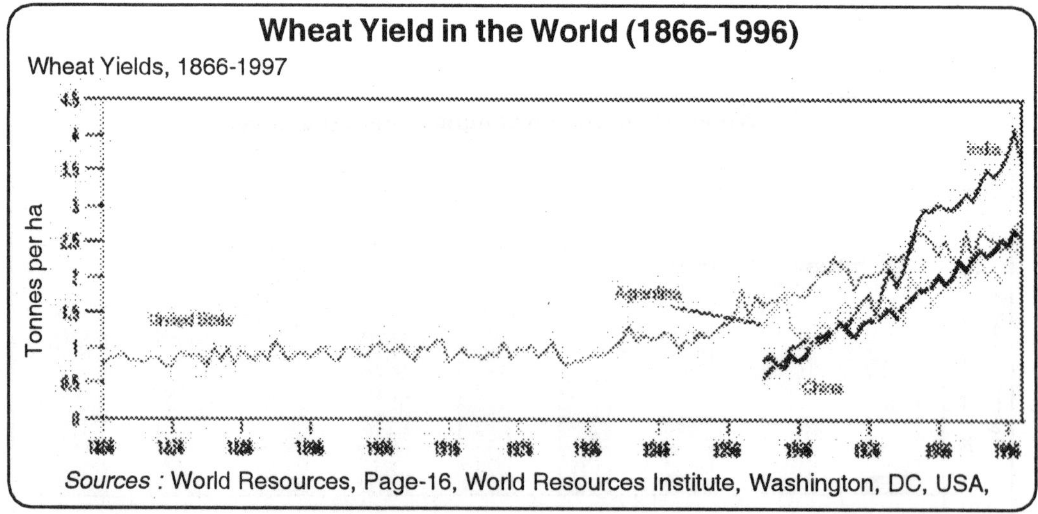

Sources : World Resources, Page-16, World Resources Institute, Washington, DC, USA,

Continued agricultural intensification need not lead inexorably to environmental degradation, however, farming communities in all parts of the world have responded to degradation, particularly when it affects their livelihoods, with measures such as planting trees to control erosion, regulating cultivation around local water sources, restricting pesticides and other pollutants, rehabilitating degraded soils, and adopting new technologies.

(d) Effects of Modern Agriculture

➢ Changes in Yield Growth

Rapid yield growth in most major crops has been instrumental in meeting the food needs of growing populations, particularly in the second half of twentieth century. Recently, however, the growth of cereal crop yields has been slowing, raising concerns that future production may not be able to keep pace with demand. Moreover, there is evidence from some parts of the world that maintaining the growth in yields, or even holding yields at current levels, requires proportionately greater amounts of fertilizer input, implying that the quality of the underlying soil resource may be deteriorating.

These trends must be interpreted cautiously. Even if yields continue to grow rapidly, this does not necessarily indicate that agroecosystems are in good shape, since increased inputs like fertilizer and pesticides could mask underlying depletion of soil nutrients. Nor does a slow down in the growth of crop yields prove agroecosystem conditions are worsening, since market factors such as falling commodity prices and high fertilizer prices may also account for slower production. Nonetheless, the declining rate of yield growth is worrisome in a world where the growth in food demand is not expected to slow.

➢ Soil Degradation

One measure of the long-term productive capacity of an agroecosystem is the condition of its soil. Natural weathering processes and human management practices can both affect soil quality. Sustaining soil productivity requires that soil-degrading pressures be balanced with soil conserving practices. The principal processes of soil degradation are erosion by water or wind, waterlogging and salinization (the buildup of salts in the soil), compaction and crusting, acidification, loss of soil organic matter and soil microorganisms, soil nutrient depletion, and accumulation of pollutants in the soil.

➢ Waterlogging

Waterlogging occurs in poorly drained soils where water can't penetrate deeply. For example, there may be an impermeable clay layer below the soil. It also occurs on areas that are poorly drained topographically. What happens is that the irrigation water (and/or seepage from canals) eventually raises the water table in the ground—the upper leyel of the groundwater—from beneath. Growers don't generally realize that waterlogging is happening until it is too late—tests for water in soil are apparently very expensive.

The raised water table results in the soils becoming waterlogged. When soils are waterlogged, air spaces in the soil are filled with water, and plant roots essentially suffocate — lack oxygen. Waterlogging also damages soil structure.

Worldwide, about 10 per cent of all irrigated land suffers from waterlogging. As a result, productivity has fallen about 20 per cent in this area of cropland.

➢ *Salinization*

Salinization refers to a build up of salts in soil, eventually to toxic levels for plants. 3,000—6,000 ppm salt results in trouble for most cultivated plants. Salt in soils decreases the osmotic potential of the soil so that plants can't take up water from it. When soils are salty, the soil has greater concentrations of solute than does the root, so plants cannot get water from soil. The salts can also be directly toxic, but plant troubles usually result primarily from inability to take up water from salty soils.

All irrigation water contains dissolved salts derived as it passed over and through the land, and rain water also contains some salts. These salts are generally in very low concentration in the water itself.

However, evaporation of water from the dry surface of the soil leaves the salts behind. Salinization is especially likely to become a problem on poorly drained soils when the groundwater is within 3 m or less of the surface (depending on the soil type). In such cases, water rises to the surface by capillary action, rather than percolating down through the entire soil profile, and then evaporates from the soil surface.

Salinization is a worldwide problem, particularly acute in semi-arid areas which use lots of irrigation water, are poorly drained, and never get well flushed.

Globally, something on the order of 20 per cent of the world's irrigated acreage is estimated to be affected by salinization, with salt concentrations high enough about 10 per cent of irrigated acreage to decrease yields significantly.

Both waterlogging and salinization could be reduced if the efficiency of irrigation systems could be improved, and more appropriate crops (less water hungry) could be grown in arid and semi-arid regions. The "treatment" for salinization is to flush the soil with lots of water. However, this results in salinization of the river and groundwater where the flush water goes. In extreme cases, when the salt crust is too thick, it cannot be flushed, as water just runs off the salty surface.

➢ *Food Crisis and Malthusian Theory*

The increase in human population is greater than the production of food. Thomus

Malthus in 1978 wrote an essay and concluded. "The power of population is indefinitely greater than the power of the Earth to produce subsistence for man. Population when unchecked increases in a geometrical ratio (1, 2, 4, 8, 16, 32......). Resources remain constant or increase in arithmetic ratio (1, 2, 3, 4, 5, 6......). Thus after some time an imbalance is created.

Anti-Malthusians argue that technology will save the human race whereas Malthusians believe that unless population growth is checked, man will face the problem of food crisis.

(e) *Food Demand in India*

India has been self-sufficient in foodgrain production but slow growth rate of agriculture production in recent years is a matter of consideration. The population has been increasing at 1.2 per cent annually while the average growth rate of total foodgrain production is about 0.8 per cent.

Production Trends in Indian Agriculture (unit in million tonnes)

Commodity Group	1962-63	1972-73	1982-83	1992-93	2003-04
Foodgrains	81.6	103.5	130.8	174.8	199.7
Cereals	69.6	92.6	119.5	161.7	186.5
Pulses	12.0	10.9	11.3	13.0	13.2
Oil seeds	7.2	8.6	10.5	19.1	20.3
Sugarcane	101.9	121.6	176.7	241.0	293.5
Potato	2.9	4.7	9.9	15.6	24.2
Milk	20.2	23.0	34.0	55.8	87.7
Eggs (billion nos.)	3.2	6.6	—	21.7	40.8
Fish (lakh tonnes)	12.2	18.3	24.1	41.2	61.8

Source : Survey of Indian Agriculture, 2006.

The food demand will be driven by income and population growth, urbanization, food prices and income distribution. Food demand projections have been made using the piece-wise linear expansion system (LES) model developed at Centre for Economic and Social Studies (CESS), Hyderabad.

The projections given below assume real expenditure growth of 5 per cent per annum between 2000 and 2020, increase of population to 1.343 billion in 2020, rate of urbanization and rural urban disparity consistent with the historical trends and the inequality in the income distribution and relative prices same as in 1998. Under these assumptions, the demand is projected to grow at 2.2 per cent for cereals during 2000-10 and 2.0 per cent during 2010-20, 3-4 per cent for edible oils and pulses, and 4-5 per cent for milk and milk products, meat, fish, eggs, fruits, vegetables, sugar and gur.

At the current cereal intake of 143 kgs./per capita/annum, cereal requirement for household consumption will be around 192 million tonnes in 2020. The requirement will be more if the increase in household demand due to income growth is also considered. At 5 per cent per annum growth in total expenditure and population of 1.343 billion, household cereal demand works out to 221 million tonnes in 2020 and for foodgrains 241 million tonnes. With a grossing factor of 1.14, the total (household plus non-household) demand for cereals may be around 253 million tonnes. The above cereal demand projections are made with the assumption of stability of tastes and preferences in food consumption. If the secular trend of foodgrain production as witnessed during the last two decades is sustained, the production of additional 57 million tonnes of cereals and 76 million tonnes of total foodgrains in the coming two decades may not be out of reach for India. The demand projections may turn 12 out to be on a higher side if the secular trend of change in consumer preferences away from cereal consumption persists. Demand for superior food items such as dairy and animal husbandry products, sugar, fruits and vegetables are expected to grow much faster during the coming decades. The estimated demand in 2020 for milk and milk products will be around 166 million tonnes, edible oils 11 million tonnes, meat, fish and eggs 11 million tonnes, sugar and gur 25 million tonnes and fruits and vegetables 113 million tonnes. However, there may be a significant growth of demand for foodgrains as milk consumption is likely to increase at a high rate. The balance of 35 million tonnes over and above the direct household cereal consumption can absorb any reasonable increase in foodgrain demand.

India: Projections of household food demand (million tonnes per annum)

Food Item		*2010*	*2020*
CEREALS	Rice	97.99	118.93
	Wheat	72.07	92.37
	Other Cereals	14.11	15.57
	All Cereals	181.12	221.11
Pulses		14.58	19.53
Foodgrains		195.69	240.64
Milk & Milk Prod.		106.43	165.84
Edible Oils		7.67	10.94
Meat and Fish		7.25	10.80
Sugar & Gur		17.23	25.07
Fruits & Vegetables		75.21	113.17

Source : CESS, Hyderabad, India.

A major challenge to food security comes from dietary diversification of the poor. If cereal pricing is left to the market forces, government playing the facilitating role, land will be released from rice and wheat cultivation to meet the growing demand for non-cereal crops such as oilseeds, fruits and vegetables in accordance with diet diversification. This policy would facilitate agricultural diversification in tune with emerging demand patterns. Long term food security demands that research in production technology of non-cereal food as well as technology access to the poor small producers should be promoted. Improvement in the quality of food items and reduction in transaction costs associated with their market access need to be policy priorities.

➤ Food insecurity in Urban India

In 1996, the Food and Agricultural Organisation (FAO) defined food security as a situation which "exists when all people, at all times, have physical and economic access to sufficient, safe and nutritious food to meet their dietary needs and food preferences for an active and healthy life"

Providing food security to the urban population has been made more vital by the fact that urbanization has been a dominating trend throughout the world in the last half century. According to the 1961 Census of India, 17.97 per cent of the country's population lived in urban areas. In 2001, that figure was 27.78 per cent, amounting to 285 million people. The United Nations estimates that India's urban population will reach 600 million by the year 2025.

A recent publication, Food Insecurity Atlas of Urban India, brought out by the M.S. Swaminathan Research Foundation (MSSRF) and the World Food Programme (WFP) indicates that more than 38 per cent of children under the age of three in India's cities and towns are underweight and more than 35 per cent of children in urban areas are stunted (shorter than they should be for their age).

Livelihood access is vital in achieving urban food security. Large sections of lower income groups depend on casual employment or are self-employed in petty businesses and these types of employment are usually accompanied by uncertain incomes. For the country as a whole, more than 14 per cent of the urban population is dependent on casual labour as a means of livelihood. For the lowest 10 per cent of the urban population in India, 37.49 per cent are engaged in casual labour and 41.34 per cent are self-employed, suggesting that a vast majority of the urban poor are vulnerable to uncertain incomes and, hence, vulnerable to under-nourishment.

More than 21 per cent of India's urban population lives in slums, 23 per cent of urban households do not have access to toilet facilities and nearly 8 per cent of urban households are unable to find safe drinking water. Wages and salaries are higher in urban areas; infrastructure is superior in cities and towns when compared with villages; schools and hospitals are more accessible; food availability is rarely a problem; and small signs of wealth such as radios and televisions are common, even in the slums.

The problem of hunger in India is definitely not one of scarce food production. At the start of December 2002, India had a surplus of 53.56 million tonnes of foodgrains. As with many other aspects of poverty, the problem of food insecurity is often one of governance.

CASE STUDY

Climax of Malnutrition in Udaipur, Rajasthan

What unfolds is a tale of growing unemployment, vanishing livelihoods, mounting debts, dwindling food resources and falling nutrition levels. This is the stark profile of poverty and hunger that you would come across anywhere in the southern and western parts of Rajasthan where acute famine conditions prevail as a result of three successive years of drought.

Veera (29) of Nakola village, mortgaged his only piece of land, which measured just one bigha (one bigha is an extent of one-third to two-thirds of an acre), when it stopped yielding anything. Early this year he could find no work in neighbouring Gujarat where he goes in search of work during what is for him the lean labour season every year. With no money for the return trip, Veera trekked 70 km to reach Nakola on February 2, only to see an empty barn and his wife and three children with empty stomachs. With no work in the village — or in the fields or at government relief sites, where relief work was yet to start — and not enough forests around to sustain the village, he was worried about his family.

For two days he and his family tried to live off kajari seeds which they gathered from the forests and sold to the local shopkeepers. Soon, there were no more of these seeds, from which oil is extracted to make soap. They were again left with no work and hence no food. The children kept crying for food. Unable to stand this agony, Veera committed suicide by consuming a pesticide. In accordance with the local tribal custom, beside his grave were kept for a few days two earthen cups, one filled with offerings of a little rice and another with milk, both luxuries for Veera when alive.

The story is taken from India's Frontline *magazine (April, 2001 edition). It is called "Drought and Deaths," written by Neelabh Mishra.*

VII. Energy Resources

Energy can be defined as the capacity to do work. Work is the product of force. The agent used for "pushing or pulling" an object is called force. Thus energy is an abstract concept. You cannot see it or feel it. It is an important factor for the development of an economy. The demand for energy has increased with the economic development of the world.

The sun is the ultimate source of energy on the earth. Coal, Petroleum, and Natural Gas are fossil fuels, and also known as non-renewable resources.

(a) Energy Consumption

☞ *World*

Energy consumption broadly tracks with gross national product, although there is a significant difference between the consumption levels of the United States with

11.4 kW per person and Japan and Germany with 6 kW per person. Canada has the highest energy consumption per person, whereas the lowest energy consumption takes place in the third world countries. In developing countries such as India the per person energy use is closer to 0.5 kW.

The most significant growth of energy consumption is currently taking place in China, which has been growing at 5.5 per cent per year over the last 25 years. Its population of 1.3 billion people is currently consuming energy at a rate of 2 kW per person.

World: Energy use by source, 2000	
Energy source	*% of total*
Non-Renewable	
Oil	32
Natural gas	23
Coal	21
Nuclear	6
Renewable	
Biomass	11
Solar, Wind, Hydropower	7
Total	100

Source: U.S. Department of Energy.

Industrial users (agriculture, mining, manufacturing and construction) consume about 37 per cent of the total 15 TW energy. Personal and commercial transportation consumes 20 per cent; residential heating, lighting, and appliances use 11 per cent; and commerical uses (lighting, heating and cooling of commercial buildings, and provision of water and sewer services) amount to 5 per cent of the total. The other 27 per cent of the world's energy is lost in energy transmission and generation.

In 2005, global electricity consumption equalled 2 TW. The energy used to generate 2 TW of electricity is approximately 5 TW, as the efficiency of a typical existing power plant is around 38 per cent. The new generation of gas-fired plants reaches a substantially higher efficiency of 55 per cent. Coal is the most popular fuel for the world's electricity plants.

India

India's energy consumption is increasing rapidly, from 4.16 quadrillion BTU (quads) in 1980 to 12.8 quads in 2001. This 208 per cent increase is largely the result of India's increasing population and the rapid urbanization of the country. Higher energy consumption in the industrial, transportation, and residential sectors continues to drive India's energy usage upwards at a faster rate even than China, which experienced a 130 per cent increase in energy consumption from 1980 to 2001.

Despite the rapid growth between 1980 and 2001, India's energy consumption is still below that of Germany (14.35 quads), Japan (21.92 quads), China (39.67 quads), and the United States (97.05 quads). In addition, India's per capita energy consumption, which stood at 12.6 million BTU in 2001, is well below most of the rest of Asia and is one of the lowest in the world (although this may be more the result of India's large population rather than a low level of energy consumption). The 103 per cent rise in India's per capita consumption between 1980, when per capita energy usage was just 6.2 million BTU, and 2001, is more problematic in the long-term, however.

WORLD : ENERGY CONSUMPTION (2004)

(*Source :* World Resources, World Resources Institute, Washington, DC, USA.)

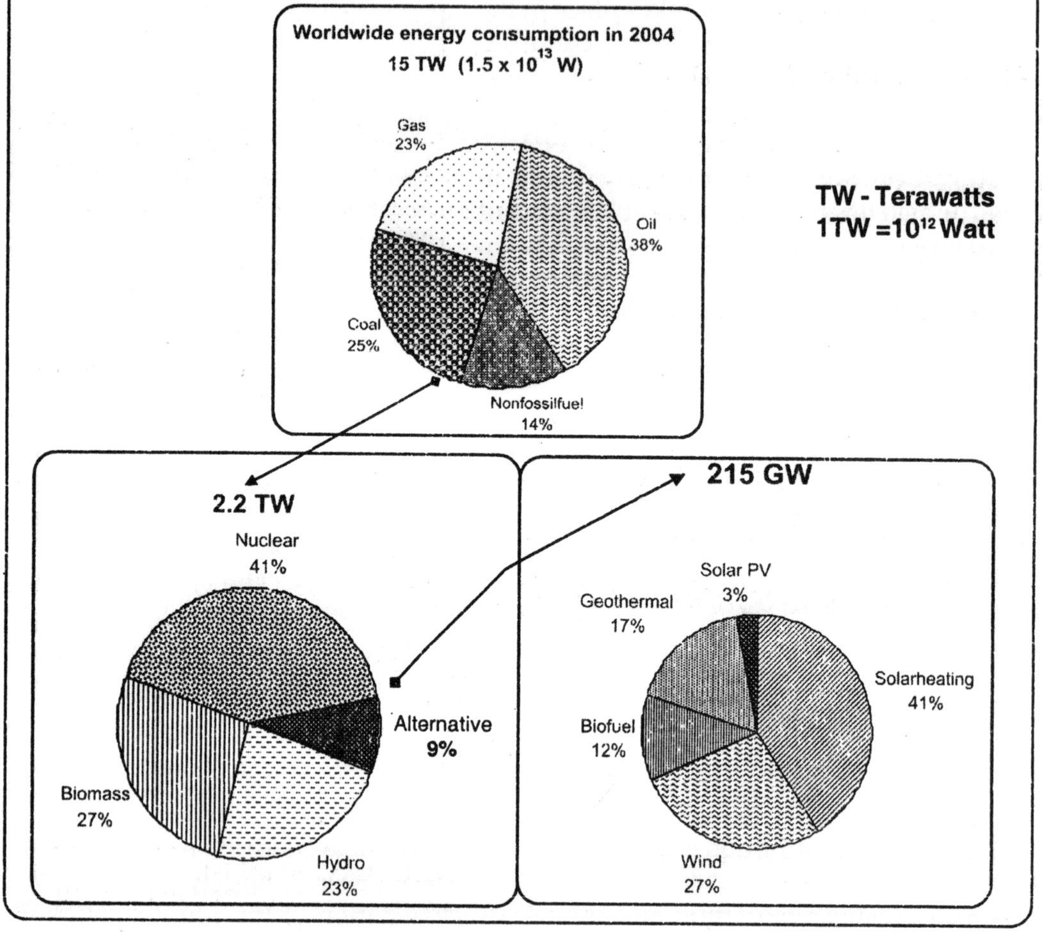

Worldwide energy consumption in 2004
15 TW (1.5 x 10^13 W)
Gas 23%
Oil 38%
Coal 25%
Nonfossilfuel 14%
TW - Terawatts
1TW =10^12 Watt
2.2 TW
Nuclear 41%
Alternative 9%
Biomass 27%
Hydro 23%
215 GW
Solar PV 3%
Geothermal 17%
Solarheating 41%
Biofuel 12%
Wind 27%

POWER IN INDIA:1999-2000
NUCLEAR POWER 2,680 MW
WIND ENERGY 1,154.71 MW
HYDRO POWER 23,816.01 MW
THERMAL POWER 70,186.16 MW

Coal accounts for just over 50 per cent (6.5 quads) of India's energy consumption. The power generation sector uses the majority of this coal, with heavy industry a distant second. Petroleum (4.4 quads) makes up 34.4 per cent of India's energy consumption, while natural gas (6.5%) and hydroelectricity (6.3%) account for much of the remainder. Natural gas is growing in importance, as its share of India's energy consumption has risen from just 1.4 per cent

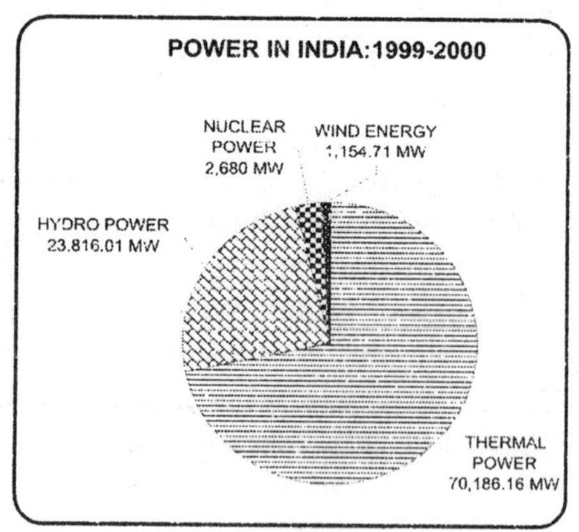

in 1980, while hydroelectricity—which made up 11.5 per cent of the country's energy usage in 1980 — has declined in relative importance. Nuclear (1.7%) and geothermal, wind, solar, and biomass (0.2%) made up a very small share of the country's energy consumption in 2001.

➢Power Generation in India

In India, the installed power generation capacity has increased from a meagre 1,400 MW in 1947 to 97,837 MW at the end of 1999-2000 comprising 23,816.01 hydro and 70,186.16 MW thermal (including gas and diesel), 1,154.71 MW wind and 2,680 MW nuclear.

(b) Types of Energy Resources

On the basis of renewability energy resources could be divided into two major types as follows :

- Non-Renewable Resources
- Renewable Resources

➢Non- Renewable Sources of Energy

A nón-renewable resource cannot be re-made or re-grown. Often fossil fuels, such as coal, petroleum and natural gas are considered non-renewable resources, as they do not naturally reform at a rate that makes the way we use them sustainable. With present rate of consumption petroleum is expected to run out in 35 years, coal in 200 years.

FOSSIL FUEL: RESERVE

Region	*Petroleum (billion barrel)*	*Natural gas (Trillion ft³)*	*Coal (billion tonnes)*
North America	75.7	291.4	285.2
S. & Central America	89.5	219.1	23.8
Western Europe	18.9	161.5	99.7
E. Europe and former USSR	58.9	1,999.4	288.4
Middle East	673.6	1,749.5	0.2
Africa	75.4	361.1	67.7
Far East and Oceania	43.0	359.6	322.3
Total	1,033.2	5,141.6	1,087.2

Source: U.S. Department of Energy.

1. Coal

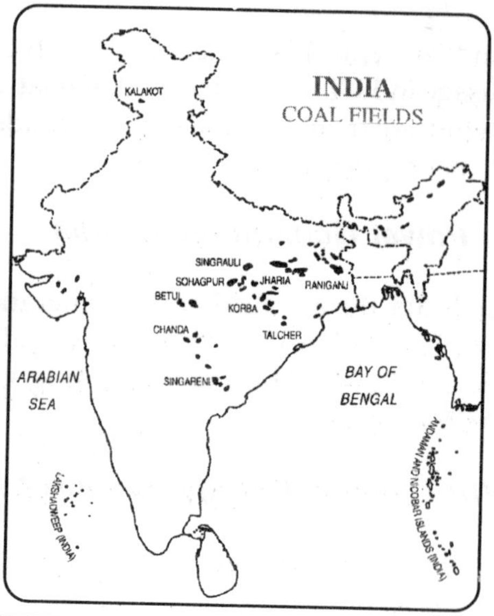

Coal is the major source of energy in the world. It was formed 255-350 million years ago in the hot, damp region of the earth during carboniferous period.

Coal constitutes carbon (60 to 90 %), hydrogen (1 to 12 %), oxygen (2 to 20 %), nitrogen (1 to 3%) and also small amount of phosphorous and sulphur.

Coal is especially abundant and by itself can sustain the current energy consumption of the entire planet for 600 years. This was the fuel that launched the industrial revolution. It is currently making a comeback; China is constructing a new coal fired power plant every week. Coal is the fastest growing fossil fuel and its large reserves would make it more popular to meet the energy demand of the global community, short of concerns of global warming. With the Fischer-Tropsch process it is possible to make liquid fuels such as diesel and jet fuel from coal.

In general, there are following four basic varieties of coal, which are the result of geologic forces having altered plant material in different ways.

INDIA
COAL FIELDS

KALAKOT
SINGRAULI
SOHAGPUR
JHARIA
RANIGANJ
BETUL
KORBA
CHANDA
TALCHER
SINGARENI
ARABIAN SEA
BAY OF BENGAL
LAKSHADWEEP (INDIA)
ANDAMAN AND NICOBAR ISLANDS (INDIA)

Consumption pattern of Coal in India (2004)

Sector	*Consumption*	*%*
Power	264.5 MMT	73.6
Steel	16.6 MMT	4.6
Railway	NIL	10.24
Cement	13.46 MMT	3.7
Fertilizer	2.30 MMT	0.6
Others	62.39 MMT	7.36
Total	—	100

1. *Anthracite :* Sometimes also called as "hard coal". It contains more than 80 per cent carbon. Anthracite has the highest energy content of all coals and is used for heating and generating electricity.
2. *Bituminous Coal :* It contains up to 80 per cent carbon. It has a higher heating value than either lignite or sub-bituminous, but less than that of anthracite. It is used to make coke.
3. *Lignite :* It contains 60 per cent carbon. Lignite is a brownish-black coal with generally high moisture and ash content and lower heating value.
4. *Peat :* It contains less than 60 per cent carbon.

India has about 5 per cent of world's coal and Indian coal is not very in terms of heat capacity. Major coal fields in India are Raniganj, Jharia, Bokaro, Singrauli, and Godavari valley. The coal States of India are Jharkhand, Orissa, West Bengal,

Madhya Pradesh, Andhra Pradesh and Maharashtra. Anthrasite coal occurs only in J&K.

At present rate of usage, the coal reserves are likely to last for about 200 years and if its use increases by 2 per cent per year, then it will last for another 65 years.

When coal is burnt it produces carbon dioxide. Which is a greenhouse gas responsible for causing enhanced global warming. Coal also contains impurities like sulphur and, therfore, as it burns the smoke contains toxic gases like oxides of sulphur and nitrogen.

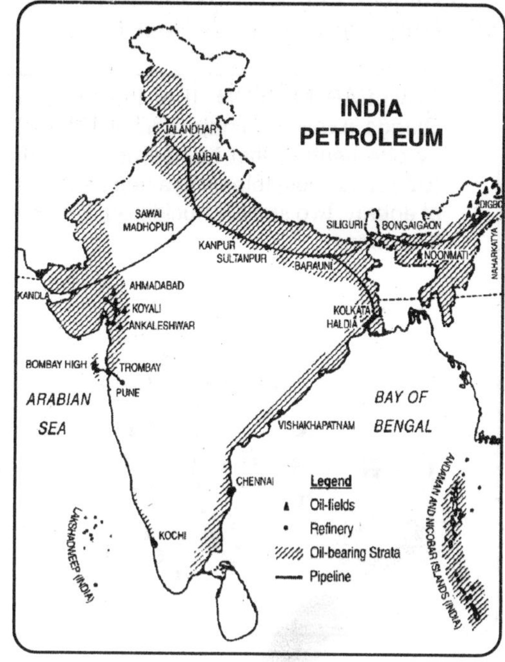

2. Petroleum

Petroleum means rock oil. It is a complex mixture of hydrocarbon compounds with minor amount of impurities like nitrogen, sulphur and oxygen.

There are 13 countries in the world having 67 per cent of the petroleum reserves which together form OPEC (Organisation of Petroleum Exporting Countries). About one-fourth of the oil reserves are in Saudi Arabia.

Petroleum is a cleaner fuel as compared to coal as it burns complitely and leave no residue. It is also easy to transport and use.

INDIA: PRODUCTION OF PETROLEUM (MMT)

Year	*1990*	*1993*	*1994*	*1995*	*1996*	*1997*	*1998*	*1999*	*2000*	*2001*
Production	34.09	26.96	27.02	32.24	34.5	32.9	33.8	32.7	31.9	32.4

INDIA : STATES PRODUCING OIL (2001)

RANK	*STATES*	*PRODUCTION (MMT)*
1.	Bombay High (Maharashtra)	20.1
2.	Gujrat	6.0
3.	Assam	5.1
4.	Tamil Nadu	0.44
5.	Andhra Pradesh	0.28
	Total	31.92

3. Nuclear Energy

Nuclear energy can be produced from minerals such as thorium, uranium, beryllium, zircon and ilmenite.

Nuclear energy can be generated by two types of reaction as given in the following Table as 1. Nuclear fission 2. Nuclear fusion.

1. NUCLEAR FISSION: It is the nuclear change in which, A chain reaction initiated by one neutron that bombards Uranium (U235) nucleus, releasing a huge amount of energy, two smaller nuclei (Ba, Kr) and 3 neutrons.	2. NUCLEAR FUSION: Between two hydrogen-2 nuclei, which take place at a very high temperature of 1 billion °C; one neutron and one fusion nucleus of helium-3 is formed with huge quantity of energy. It releases more energy than nuclear fission.
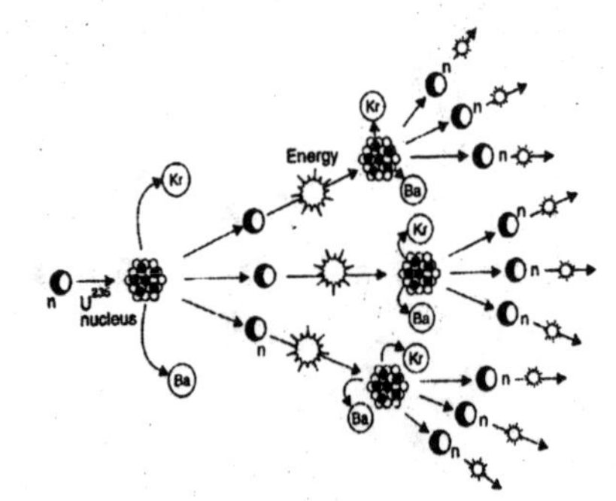	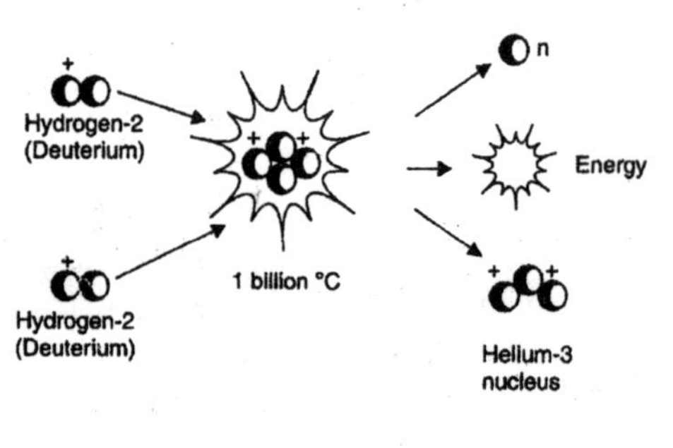

Worldwide, there are currently 435 operational nuclear power plants, with a further 30 under construction. Among the nations not currently using nuclear power are Iran, North Korea, Australia, Turkey, Indonesia, Vietnam, Egypt, Israel and Poland are building them, or are proposing to do so.

INDIA: ATOMIC POWER STATIONS		
Sl.No.	*Place*	*State*
1.	Tarapur	Maharashtra
2.	Kalpakkam	Chennai,T.N.
3.	Rawat Bhata	Kota, Rajasthan
4.	Naraura	Uttar Prades
5.	Kakrapara	Gujrat
6.	Kaiga	Karnataka

India is very rich in nuclear energy minerals such as thorium (500 tonnes) and uranium (30,000 tonnes). In terms of energy, these reserves are equivalent to more than 30 times of our reserve of coal. Hence, India has ample of potential for the development of nuclear energy.

Jharkhand, Rajasthan and Andhra Pradesh are well known uranium possesing States of India. The nuclear power programme in India envisages installing a total capacity of 20,000 MW by the year 2020.

★ *Renewable Energy Resources*

Renewable energy sources capture their energy from existing flows of energy, from *on-going natural processes,* such as sunshine, wind, wave power , flowing water (hydropower), biological processes such as anaerobic digestion, and geothermal heat flow.

In 2004, renewable energy supplied around 7 per cent of the world's energy consumption. The renewables sector has been growing significantly since the last years of the twentieth century, and in 2005 the total new investment was estimated to have been 38 billion US dollars. Germany and China lead with investments of about 7 billion US dollars each, followed by the United States, Spain, Japan, and India.

1. Solar Energy

Solar energy refers to energy that is directly collected from sunlight. However, most fossil and renewable energy sources are ultimately derived from "solar energy,".

Solar energy can be applied in many ways, including :

- ☞ to generate electricity using photovoltaic solar cells.
- ☞ to generate electricity using concentrated solar power.
- ☞ to generate electricity by heating trapped air which rotates turbines in a Solar updraft tower.
- ☞ to heat buildings, directly. Careful positioning of windows and use of brises *soleil* can maximise inflow of light at the times it is most needed, heating the building while preventing overheating during midday and summer.
- ☞ to heat foodstuffs, through solar ovens.
- ☞ to heat water for domestic consumption and heating using rooftop solar panels.
- ☞ to heat and cool air through use of solar chimneys.

Solar energy used worldwide during 2005 was approximately 93.4 GW, however the available resources are 3.8 YJ/yr (120,000 TW). Only a small fraction of available resources are sufficient to entirely replace fossil fuels and nuclear power as an energy source, however, it is likely that at least biodiesel will always be used in certain types of transport.

Portugal has opened the world's most powerful solar power plant. The 11 megawatt solar power plant, comprising 52,000 photovoltaic modules is based in southern Portugal which is one of the sunniest places in Europe.

Obviously the sun does not provide constant energy to any spot on the Earth, so its uninterrupted use requires a means for energy storage. This is typically accomplished by battery storage. However, battery storage implies energy losses. Some home owners use a grid-connected solar system that feeds energy to the grid during the day and draw energy from the grid at night; this way no energy is expended for storage.

Advantages from solar energy sources include the inexhaustible supply of energy and zero emissions of greenhouse gas and air pollutants.

❖ Technology used for Solar Energy

The use of solar energy for thermal applications is well known in the country. The applications include water heating, cooking, drying, space heating, distillation and power generation.

➢ *Solar Photovoltaic (SPV) Cells*

Solar photovoltaic is a technology that directly converts the radiation from the sun into electricity based on the physical process that requires no moving parts. SPV is a proven technology. It is possible to generate about 120 watts of electricity from a 10 sq.ft. area of SPV panel on a sunny day. It is reliable on different scale applications.

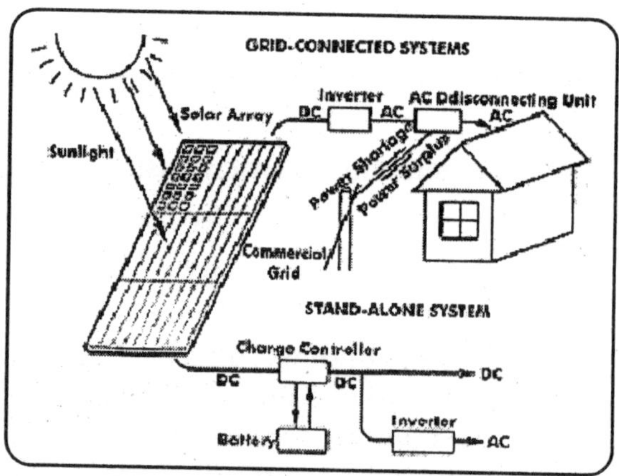

Solar photovoltaic technology has the following possible functions/ applications :

- Lighting (streets, residences, public places, etc.);
- Running or operating electro-mechanical equipment (radio and other systems, TV and video players, fans, pump sets to supply drinking or irrigation water, etc.); and
- Supplying electrical power to operate poultry incubators, rice mills telecommunications' equipment in remote areas, charge NiCd batteries for use in torches, radios, and so on.

Solar Photovoltaic modules provide an independent, reliable power source at the point of use, making it suitable for remote or inaccessible places such as hills and mountains. The majority of the population living in dispersed communities in rural areas away from the main power grid could be supplied with electricity without difficulty.

Environmental and Efficiency Implications

- SPV systems could provide national economic benefits as it would reduce reliance on imported fossil fuels.
- SPV systems are economically viable. Taking into consideration the high reliability of SPV, many small-scale applications can be more economically powered by this system than with diesel or other small power systems.
- SPV systems are environmentally friendly. Their use protects the ecology and environment from degradation through the conservation of forests and reduction in the emission of harmful gases. A SPV system is a carbon dioxide free and clean energy converter.

➢ Solar Lantern

This is a portable lighting device (fluorescent lamp) powered by solar radiation or a PV (photo volatic) array :

- It can supply a few hours of bright light a day (suitable for reading) without using any conventional fuels or AC main grid power connections.
- The lantern can be used in remote areas without electricity.
- The solar lantern is ideal for campers, researchers, remote classrooms, rural park offices, and military and police use.

The SOLANT 7 model of solar lanterns (with a 7 watt fluorescent lamp) is a durable and rugged product that can give three to four hours of bright light per day, with optional DC output. (It can be set at from 1.5 - 12 Volts DC). It can also supply power to other appliances such as radios, LCD TV, small computers, and so on.

➢ Solar Passive Space Heating System

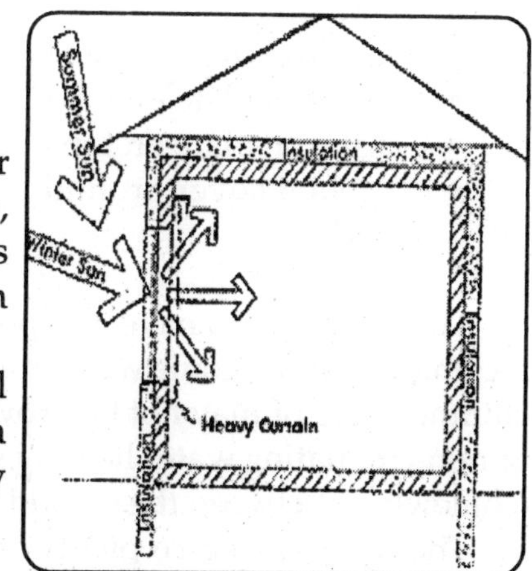

Solar heat can be used for space heating in order to provide adequate warmth inside houses, lodges, restaurants, and other facilities in the hills and mountains. A solar space heating system can be :

An active system which requires conventional energy to operate it, or a passive system which operates entirely on the renewable energy available in the immediate environment.

The passive heating of buildings through solar energy involves the integration of the system into the structure of the building itself. The system works in three ways :

- collection of sun rays,
- storage of the heat collected, and
- release of the heat in a useful way.

Passive heating of buildings is achieved by understanding and using the knowledge of heat and its effects on different building materials. Operation of the passive heating system takes advantage of the natural characteristics of materials such as those given below :

- The convective flow of air and water;
- The absorption qualities of dark colours and dense materials;
- The heat storing properties of dense materials and water; and
- The poor heat conductivity of insulating materials.

The buildings are designed in such a way that the heating needs of the occupants are performed with the sun as a heat source and the night sky as a heat sink. The various passive solar space heating systems need very little maintenance.

❖ Cooking / Heating Stoves

Stoves for cooking and heating rooms/water can be found in different shapes and sizes. The stoves are generally improved versions of the traditional cooking stoves. Ceramics, straw, mud, cast iron, mild steel, and sheet steel are used to make these stoves. The whole body of the stove can be made of :

- mud and ceramics,
- cast iron (KTS model based on a western design),
- cast iron plate on top of a mud and stone body,
- cast iron plate on top of a mild steel body, or
- a metal cover around a stone/mud body to protect the stove from the cold.

The stoves could have 2 - 3 pot holes of different sizes; the shape can be oval or rectangular; it can come with or without a baffle made of mud or other materials; a chimney may or may not be provided with a damper fuel control; and circulating or non-circulating water heating systems (back boiler) may or may not be attached (somewhere between the second pot hole and chimney).

The stoves produce plenty of heat in the room. The cast iron stoves produce more heat while ones with a stone/mud body and cast iron plate produce moderate heat.

❖ Solar Dryer for Agricultural Produce

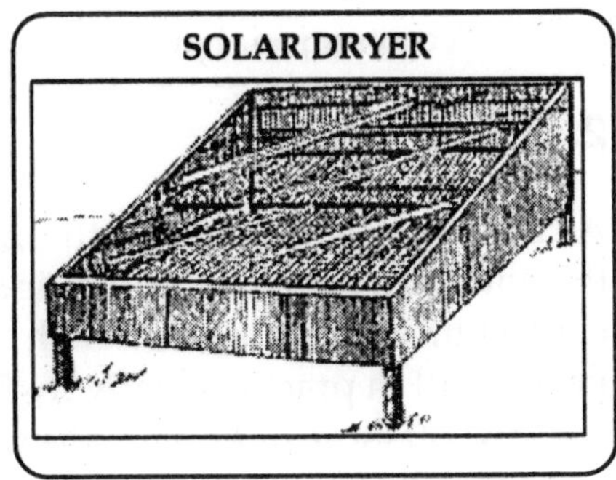
SOLAR DRYER

Any food or agricultural product with high moisture contents is easily attacked by insects and rots quite quickly. To guard against such possibilities and to preserve food for longer periods, the food needs to be dried.

The traditional method of drying is to spread the food openly in the sun. In this drying method, the food is often contaminated by dust and birds. A per centage is lost or damaged due to insects/birds.

A solar dryer is an enclosed unit, so the food is safe from damage, birds, and insects. The food is dried using solar thermal energy in a cleaner and healthier way. This is a passive system of heating using only solar and wind energy in its operation.

Solar dryers can be made in different sizes and shapes based on the quantity and type of food to be dried. The size and shape also depend on domestic or commercial use. There is quite a variety of solar dryers.

Some solar dryers can be made out of locally available materials in the hills and mountains. These are the :

- cabinet solar dryer,
- flat solar dryer, and
- tent solar dryer.

A solar dryer can be used to dry a variety of agricultural products and foodstuffs such as :

- fruits (grapes, bananas),
- vegetables (potatoes, onions),
- grains (paddy, wheat, maize, millet),
- spices (ginger, garlic, chillies),
- cash crops (coffee, herbs, flowers), and
- fish.

Solar dryer works as following :

- Solar rays entering the cabinet through the solar collector are converted into heat energy raising the temperature inside.

- The heat energy is transferred to the food to be dried.
- The heated food gives out water vapour and dries up gradually.
- The heated moist air leaves the cabinet and dry air enters in a natural and conventional process.

2. Wind Energy

As the sun heats up the Earth unevenly, winds are formed. The kinetic energy in the wind can be used to run wind turbines. The power output is a function of the cube of the wind speed, so such turbines generally require a wind in the range 20 km/h, and in practice relatively few land areas have significant prevailing winds. Luckily, offshore or at high altitudes, the winds are much more constant.

According to the Global Wind Energy Council, the installed capacity of wind power increased by 25.6 per cent from the end of 2005 to end of 2006 to total 74 GW with over half the increase in the United States, Germany, India and Spain. Doubling of capacity took about three and half years. The total installed capacity is approximately three times that of the actual average power produced as the nominal capacity represents peak output; actual capacity is generally from 25-40 per cent of the nominal capacity.

The wind power potential of India is estimated to be about 20,000 MW, while at present we are gathering about 1020 MW. India has the fifth largest wind power installed capacity in the world. The largest wind farm of our country is near Kanyakumari in Tamil Nadu generating 380 MW of electricity.

New wind farms and offshore wind parks are being planned and built all over the world.

Wind power is renewable and is one of the few energy sources that contributes to greenhouse gas mitigation because it removes energy directly from the atmosphere without producing net emissions of greenhouse gases such as carbon dioxide and methane (others greenhouse gas mitigating energy sources include solar thermal and ocean thermal).

3. Water Power

Energy in water can be harnessed and used in the form of motive energy or temperature differences. Since water is about a thousand times heavier than air, even a slow flowing stream of water, or moderate sea swell, can yield great amount of energy.

There are many forms of water power :

- Hydroelectric energy is a term usually reserved for hydroelectric dams.
- Tidal power captures energy from the tides in vertical direction. Tides come in, raise water levels in a basin, and tides roll out. The water must pass

through a turbine to get out of the basin. If the basin is a river delta then silt will block the turbine.

- Tidal stream power captures a stream of water as it is pushed horizontally around the world by tides.
- Wave power uses the energy in waves. The waves will usually make large pontoons go up and down in the water, leaving an area with no waves in the "shadow".
- Ocean thermal energy conversion (OTEC) uses the temperature difference between the warmer surface of the ocean and the cool (or cold) lower recesses. To this end, it employs a cyclic heat engine.
- Deep lake water cooling, although not technically an energy generation method, can save a lot of energy in summer. It uses submerged pipes as a heat sink for climate control systems. Lake-bottom water is a year-round local constant of about 4° C.
- Blue energy is the reverse of desalination. A difference in salt concentration exists between sea water and river water. This gradient can be utilized to generate electricity by separating positive and negative ions by ion specific membranes. This form of energy is in research; costs are not the issue, and tests on pollution of the membrane are in progress. At this moment it is predicted that if everything works out, one-third of the electricity needs in the Netherlands can be covered with this system.

Hydropower

The water flow in a river is collected by constructing a dam where it is stored and allowed to fall from a height. The blades of the turbine located at the bottom of the dam move with fast moving water which in turn rotate the generator and produce electricity. We can also costruct mini or micro hydel power plants on the rivers in the hilly regions for harnessing the hydroenergy on a small scale, but the minimum height of the water falls should be 10 metres. Worldwide hydroelectricity consumption reached 816 GW in 2005, consisting of 750 GW of large plants, and 66 GW of small hydro installations. Large hydro capacity totalling 10.9 GW was added by China, Brazil and India during the year, but there was a much faster growth (8%) in small hydro, with 5 GW added, mostly in China where some 58 per cent of the world's small hydro plants are now located.

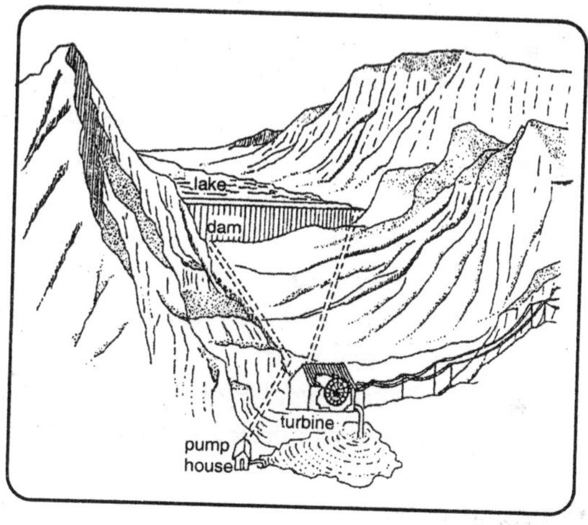

In the western world although Canada is the largest producer of hydroelectricity in the world, the construction of large hydro plants has stagnated due to environmental concerns.

The hydropower potential of the country is estimated to be about 4 × 1011 kW-hour. Till now we have utlised only a little more than 11 per cent of this potential. Hydro power does not cause any pollution, it is renewable and normally the hydropower projects are multi-purpose projects helping in controlling floods, used for irrigation, navigation, etc.

India has witnessed considerable progress in the field of hydro-electicity since independence. Besides various multipurpose river valley projects such as Bhakra-Nagal, Dmodar Valley, Hirakund and Chambal, there has been construction of a few exclusive hydel power projects as follows :

- *The Rihand Project*—Located on the border of U.P. and M.P. on river Rihand. The capacity of this project is 300 MW every year.
- *The Konya Project*—The project is on river Konya tributary of river Krishna. The capacity of project is 880 MW every year. It supplies power to Mumbai-Pune industrial region.
- *The Kundoh Project*—Located in Tamil Nadu. The capacity of this project is 535 MW every year.
- *The Balimela Project*—Located in Orissa. The capacity of this project is 360 MW every year.
- *The Ukai Project*—Located in Gujarat. The capacity of this project is 300 MW every year.
- *The Sharavathy Project*—Located at Jog fall in Karnataka. The capacity of this project is 891 MW every year. It supplies power to Bangalore industrial region and also to the State of Goa and T.N.
- *The Kalinadi Project*—Located in Karnataka. The capacity of this project is 200 MW every year.
- *The Sabarigiri Project*—Located in Kerala. The capacity of this project is 300 MW every year.
- *The Idduki Project*—Located in Kerala. The capacity of this project is 370 MW every year.
- *The Tehri Hydel Power Project*—Located in Uttarakhand .The goal of this project is to generate 2,400 MW power every year.

Wave Energy

Waves are caused by the unequal pressure exherted by the atmosphere over large water columns. The energy of waves, generated in their continuous upward and downward motion, is harnessed to activate a water operated or air operated turbine to generate electricity. The wave energy potential of India's vast coastline is estimated at 40,000MW as the trade wind belts of the Arabian sea and the Bay of Bengal are considered ideal sites for trapping wave energy. Earlier, a very modest beginning was made in the form of 150 KW capacity wave energy plant at Vizhinjam Harbour, Kerala.

Tidal Energy

At the end of 2005, 0.3 GW of electricity was produced by tidal power. Thanks to the gravitational pull of the moon (68%) and the sun (32%) there is 3 TW of tidal energy available of which approximately 1 per cent is practical to exploit.

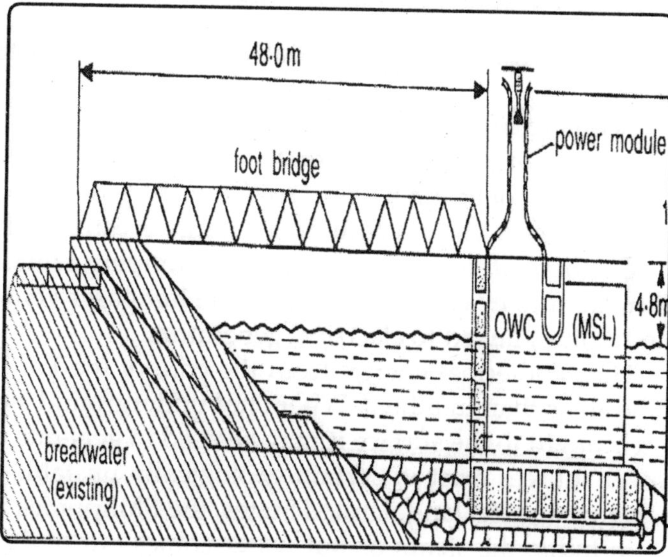

As in the case of wave energy, the regular feature of alternate rise and fall in the ocean water - produced by the gravitational pull of the moon and the sun over vast water column, can produce electricity. It operates on the principle of Oscillating water column.

In India the potential sites have been identified at the Gulf of Cambay, the Gulf of Kutch and the Sunderbuns. India's tidal energy potential is estimated at about 9000 MW.

Ocean Thermal Energy Conservation (OTEC)

It involves making use of the temperature difference between the sun-warmed surface water of the ocean and the cold deep water at a depth of 1000 m or more. This temperature difference is used to cause evaporation of volatile substances like ammonia or propane, which in turn use to drive turbine.

India has a large potential of OTEC which could even of the order of 50,000 MW as some of the best OTEC sites in the world are situated off the Tamil Nadu, Lakshadeep and Andaman coasts.The groundwork for future expansion of plans in this field is going on.

4. Geothermal Energy

Geothermal energy is the energy obtained by tapping the heat of the earth itself, usually from kilometres deep into the Earth's crust. Ultimately, this energy derives from the radioactive decay in the core of the Earth, which heats the Earth from the inside out. This energy can be used in three ways :

- Geothermal electricity;
- Geothermal heating, through deep Earth pipes; and
- Geothermal heating, through a heat pump.

Usually, the term 'geothermal' is reserved for thermal energy from within the Earth.

Geothermal energy is used commercially in over 70 countries. By the end of 2005 worldwide use for electricity had reached 9.3 GW, with an additional 28 GW used directly for heating. If heat recovered by ground source heat pumps is included, the non-electric use of geothermal energy is estimated at more than 100 GW.

Geothermal electricity is created by pumping a fluid (oil or water) into the Earth, allowing it to evaporate and using the hot gases vented from the earth's crust to run turbines linked to electrical generators.

The geothermal energy from the core of the Earth is closer to the surface in some areas than in others. Where hot underground steam or water can be tapped and brought to the surface it may be used to generate electricity. Such geothermal power sources exist in certain geologically unstable parts of the world such as Iceland, New Zealand, United States, the Philippines and Italy.

In India, the steam or hot water comes out of the ground naturally through crakes in the form of natural geysers in Manikaran, Kullu and Sohana, Haryana.

Although geothermal sites are capable of providing heat for many decades, eventually specific locations cool down. Some interpret this as meaning a specific geothermal location can undergo depletion, and question whether geothermal energy is truly renewable.

5. Biogas

Many organic materials can release gases, due to metabolisation of organic matter by bacteria (anaerobic digestion, or fermentation). Landfills actually need to vent this gas (called landfill gas) to prevent dangerous explosions. Animal faeces releases methane under the influence of anaerobic bacteria.

Under high pressure, high temperature, anaerobic conditions many organic materials such as wood can be gasified to produce gas. This is often found to be more efficient than direct burning. The gas can then be used to generate electricity and/or heat.

Biogas can easily be produced from current waste streams, such as paper production, sugar production, sewage, animal waste and so forth. These various waste streams have to be slurried together and allowed to naturally ferment, producing methane gas. This can be done by converting current sewage plants into biogas plants. When a biogas plant has extracted all the methane it can then the remains are sometimes better suitable as fertilizer than the original biomass.

Biogas is a non-polluting, clean and low cost fuel which is very useful for rural areas where a lot of animal waste and agriculture waste is available. India has the largest cattle population in the world (240 million) and has tremendous potential for biogas production . From cattle dung alone, we can produce biogas of magnitude of 22,500 Mm3 annually. A sixty cubic feet gobar gas plant can serve the need of one average family.

Biogas plants used in our country are basically of two types :

1. Floating gas-holder type and 2. Fixed dome type.

1. *Floating gas-holder type biogas plants*: This type has well shaped digester tank which is placed under the ground and made up of bricks. In the digester tank, over the dung slurry an inverted steel drum floats to hold the biogas produced. The gas holder can move which is controlled by a pipe and the gas outlet is regulated by the valve. The digest tank has partition wall and one side of it receives the dungwater mixture through inlet pipe while the other side discharges the spent slurry through outlet pipe. Sometimes corrosion of steel gas-holder leads to the leakage of biogas. The tank has to be painted time and again for maintenance which increases the cost.

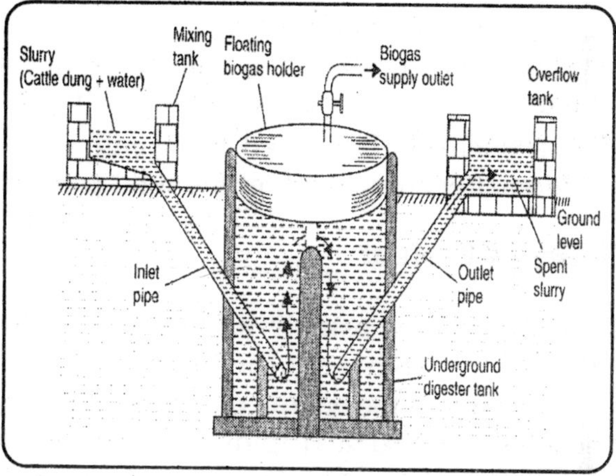

2. *Fixed dome type biogas plants :* The structure is almost similar to that of the previous type. However, instead of a steel gas holder there is dome shaped roof made of cement and bricks. Instead of partitioning, here there is a single unit in the main digester but it has inlet and outlet chambers.

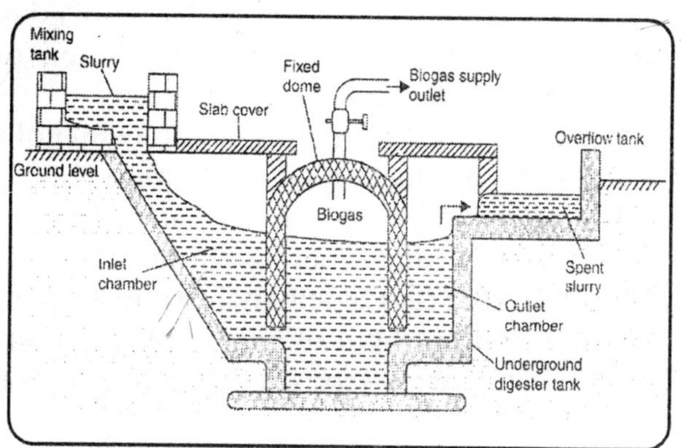

6. Biofuel

Plants use photosynthesis to store solar energy in the form of chemical energy. Biofuel is any fuel that derives from biomass, including living organisms or their metabolic byproducts, such as cow manure.

Typically biofuel is burned to release its stored chemical energy. Research into more efficient methods of converting biofuels and other fuels into electricity utilizing fuel cells is an area of very active work. Biomass, also known as biomatter, can be used directly as fuel or to produce liquid biofuel. Agriculturally produced biomass fuels, such as biodiesel, ethanol and bagasse (often a by-product of sugarcane cultivation) can be burned in internal combustion engines or boilers.

A drawback is that all biomass needs to go through some of these steps: it needs to be grown, collected, dried, fermented and burned. All of these steps require resources and an infrastructure. However, the United States government passed legislation that requires the integration of 7.5 billion U.S. gallons (28,000,000 m^3) of ethanol into the gasoline supply. Experts estimate that six billion dollars of investment will be created, along with 200,000 additional jobs in the United States.

Biomatter energy, under the right conditions, is considered to be renewable.

7. Liquid Biofuel

Liquid biofuel is usually bioalcohol such as ethanol and biodiesel and virgin vegetable oils. Biodiesel can be used in modern diesel vehicles with little or no modification to the engine and can be obtained from waste and virgin vegetable and animal oil and fats (lipids). Virgin vegetable oils can be used in modified diesel engines. In fact the Diesel engine was originally designed to run on vegetable oil rather than fossil fuel. A major benefit of biodiesel is lower emissions. The use of biodiesel reduces emission of carbon monoxide and other hydrocarbons by 20 to 40 per cent. In some areas corn, sugarbeets, cane and grasses are grown specifically to produce ethanol (also known as alcohol) a liquid which can be used in internal combustion engines and fuel cells. Ethanol is being phased into the current energy infrastructure. E85 is a fuel composed of 85 per cent ethanol and 15 per cent gasoline that is currently being sold to consumers

The EU plans to add 5 per cent bioethanol to Europe's petrol by 2010. For the UK alone the production would require 12,000 square kilometres of the country's 65,000 square kilometres of arable land assuming that no biofuels are created using waste produces from other agriculture. The supermarket chain Tesco has started adding the 5 per cent bioethanol to the petrol it sells as on January 2006.

In the future, there might be bio-synthetic liquid fuel available. It can be produced by Fischer-Tropsch processes, also called Biomass-To-Liquids (BTL).

8. Solid Biomass

Direct use is usually in the form of combustible solids, either wood, the biogenic portion of municipal solid waste or combustible field crops. Field crops may be grown specifically for combustion or may be used for other purposes, and the processed plant waste then used for combustion. Most sorts of biomatter, including dried manure, can actually be burnt to heat water and to drive turbines.

Sugarcane residue, wheat chaff, corn cobs and other plant matter can be, and is, burnt quite successfully.

Until the end of the nineteenth century biomass was the predominant fuel, today it has only a small share of the overall energy supply. Electricity produced from biomass sources was estimated at 44 GW for 2005. Biomass electricity generation increased by over 100 per cent in Germany, Hungary, the Netherlands, Poland and Spain. A further 220 GW was used for heating (in 2004), bringing the total energy consumed from biomass to around 264 GW. The use of biomass fires for cooking is excluded.

9. Hydrogen as a Biofuel

As hydrogen burns in air, it combines with oxygen to form water and a large amount of energy (150 kilojoules per gram). Due to its high calorific value, hydrogen can serve as as an excellent fuel. Moreover, it is non-polluting and can be eaily produced. Production of hydrogen is possible by thermal dissociation, photolysis or electrolysis of water :

- By thermal dissociation of water (at 30,000 K or above) hydrogen is produced.
- Thermochemically, hydrogen is produced by chemical reaction of water with some other chemicals in 2-3 cycles so that we do not need the high temperature as in direct thermal method and ultimately hydrogen is produced.
- Electrolytic method dissociates water into hydrogen and oxygen by making a current flow through it.
- Photolysis of water involves breakdown of water in the presence of sunlight to release hydrogen. Green plants also have photolysis of water during photosynthesis. Efforts are underway to trap hydrogen molecule which is produced during photosynthesis.

However, hydrogen is highly inflammable and explosive in nature. Hence, safe handling is required for using hydrogen as a fuel. Also, it is difficult to store and transport; and being very light, it would have to be stored in bulk.Presently, hydrogen is used in the form of liquid as a fuel in spaceship.

INDIA : NON- CONVENTIONAL ENERGY POTENTIAL AND ACHIEVEMENTS

Sl.No.	*Source/ System*	*Approximate Potential*	*Status (as on March 2000)*
1.	Biogas plants (No.)	120 lakh	30 lakh
2.	Improved chulha (No.)	1,200 lakh	320 lakh
3.	Solar water-heating system	—	Over 5,00,000 m^2 - collector area.
4.	Solar photovoltaic systems	20 MW/sq. km.	57 MW
5.	Biomass power	19,500 MW	
	i. Biomass gasifiers		34 MW
	ii. Biomass combustion/ gasifiers		39 MW
	iii. Biogas based cogeneration		183 MW
6.	Wind Power	20,000 MW	1,167 MW
7.	Small hydropower	10,000 MW	217 MW
8.	Solar photovoltaic power		1.16 MW grid connected 884 KW non- grid connected
9.	Integrated rural energy programme		860 blocks
10.	Energy Parks		180 Nos.
11.	Wind pumps		637 Nos.
12.	Solar cookers		4,90,000 Nos.
13.	Energy recovery from wastes	1,700 MW (e)	15.21 MW (e)

Discussion : Use of Alternative Source of Energy

Whether a significant investment in alternative energy is wise is currently the subject of much discussion. The debate rages between two very entrenched views. The renewable energy camp believes that the risk of global warming and the dependence on sources, such as those in the Middle East, justify a move away from fossil fuels. The other side of the debate believes, equally sincerely, that a government led switch to renewable energy will force economic dislocation, stifle and reverse economic growth and deny the developing world a path to prosperity.

Japan and Germany have started to make some investments in solar energy. They are now the largest consumers of photovoltaic cells in the world despite their unfavourable geographic locations. Denmark and Germany have installed 3 GW and 17 GW of wind power respectively. In 2005, wind generated 18.5 per cent of all the electricity in Denmark. Brazil invests in ethanol production from sugarcane which is now a significant part of the transportation fuel in that country. Starting in 1965, France made large investments in nuclear power and to this date three quarters of its electricity comes from nuclear reactors. Switzerland is planning to cut its energy consumption by more than half to become a 2000 Watt society by 2050 and the United Kingdom is working towards a zero energy building standard for all new housing by 2016.

VIII. Land Resources

"Land is a delineable area of the earth's terrestrial surface, encompassing all attributes of the biosphere immediately above or below this surface including those of the near-surface climate the soil and terrain forms, the surface hydrology (including shallow lakes, rivers, marshes, and swamps), the near-surface sedimentary layers and associated groundwater reserve, the plant and animal populations, the human settlement pattern and physical results of past and present human activity (terracing, water storage or drainage structures, roads, buildings, etc.)." (UN, 1994)

Earth's one-fourth area is covered by land which is largely covered with natural forests, grasslands, wetlands, and man-made urban and rural settlements along with agriculture. Out of total land surface 11 per cent is cultivated, 52 per cent is under forest cover, meadows and pastures, 20 per cent deserts, 2.6 per cent is occupied by human settlements, while rest is covered by ice, glaciers etc. Nearly 80 per cent land is covered by soil. In India, agriculture occupies 43 per cent land, forest 23 per cent, pastures 4 per cent and human habitation 8 per cent. Land availability in India is 0.34 per cent hectare per person. To prevent land degradation judicious land use is a must.

(a) Land as a Resource

Land is the basic natural resource that provides habitat and sustenance for living organisms, as well as being a major focus of economic activities.

The land has the following functions :

1. *The production function :* It is the basis for many life support systems, through the production of biomass that provides food, fodder, fibre, fuel, timber and other biotic materials for human use, either directly or through animal husbandry including aquaculture and inland and coastal fishery.
2. *The biotic environmental function :* Land is the basis of terrestrial biodiversity by providing the biological habitats and gene reserves for plants, animals and micro-organisms, above and below ground.
3. *The climate regulative function :* Land and its use are a source and sink of greenhouse gases and form a co-determinant of the global energy balance as reflection, absorption and transformation of radioactive energy of the sun, and of the global hydrological cycle.
4. *The hydrologic function :* Land regulates the storage and flow of surface and groundwater resources, and influences their quality.
5. *The storage function :* Land is a storehouse of raw materials and minerals for human use.
6. *The waste and pollution control function :* Land has a receptive, filtering, buffering and transforming function of hazardous compounds.

7. *The living space function :* Land provides the physical basis for human settlements, industrial plants and social activities such as sports and recreation.
8. *The archive or heritage function :* Land is a medium to store and protect the evidence of the cultural history of mankind, and a source of information on past climatic conditions and past land uses.
9. *The connective space function :* Land provides space for the transport of people, inputs and produce, and for the movement of plants and animals between discrete areas of natural ecosystems.

The suitability of the land for these functions varies greatly over the world. Landscape units, as natural resources units, have dynamism of their own, but human influences affect this dynamism to a great extent, in space and time. The qualities of the land for one or more functions may be improved (for instance, through erosion control measures), but more often than not the land has been or is being degraded by human action.

(b) Land Degradation

➢ Causes

Land degradation is a human induced or natural process which impairs the capacity of land to function.

A large portion of the fertile land is degraded due to the following reasons :

- *Unplanned cultivation :* Due to excessive use of agrochemicals and over cropping.
- *Overgrazing :* It makes soil prone to erosion and soil loses its fertility.
- *Mining :* It destroys the vegetation and causes soil erosion and land slide.
- *Desertification :* Fertile agriculturable soil convert into barren land.
- *Water logging :* Due to over irrigation, dam construction land degrades.
- *Salinity and alkalinity :* These makes fertile land uncultivated.
- *Brick Kilns :* It removes topmost fertile soil and leave it barren and uncultivated.
- *Urbanisation :* Urban sprawl changes land use pattern.
- *Soil erosion :* Leads deforestation and land degradation.
- *Floods :* floods impair the fertility of the soil.
- *Pollution :* Land pollution and dumping of the waste play a vital role in the land degradation.

➢ *Global Situation of Degradation*

The 1990 Global Assessment of Soil Degradation (GLASOD), based on a structured survey of regional experts, provides the only continental and global-scale estimates of soil degradation . The GLASOD study suggested that 1.97 Bha had been degraded between the mid-1940s and 1990. This represents 15 per cent of terrestrial area (excluding ice covered Greenland and Antarctica).

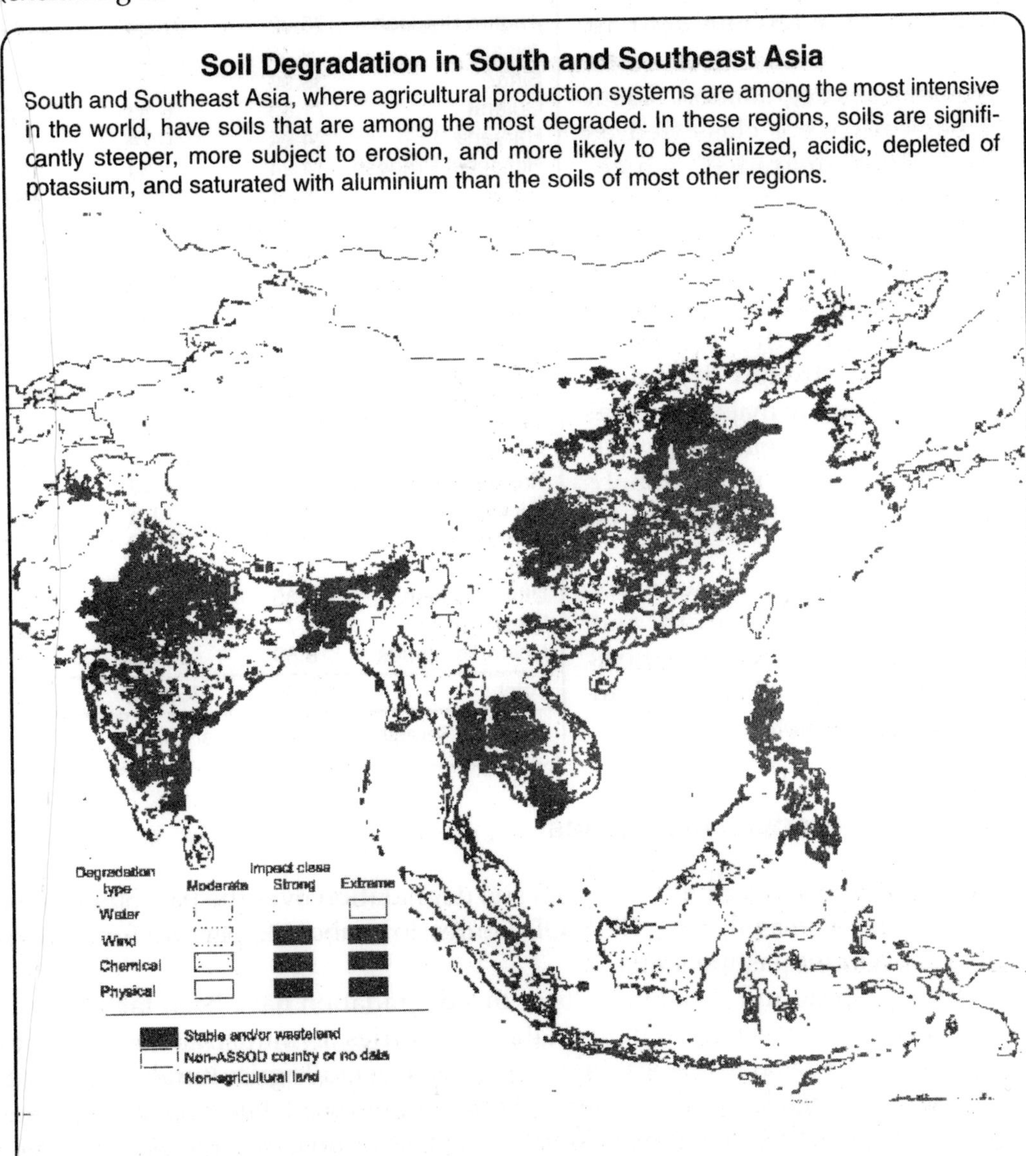

Sources: Wood *et al.*, [Page] 2000. The map is based on Van Lynden and Oldeman (1997), USA.

To assess the extent and severity of soil degradation on agricultural lands in particular, researchers overlaid the GLASOD data on the map of agricultural land (land with more than 30 per cent agricultural use). This revealed that 65 per cent of agricultural lands have some amount of soil degradation. About 24 per cent were classified as "moderately degraded" which, according to GLASOD, signifies that their agricultural productivity has been greatly reduced. A further 40 per cent of agricultural land fell into the GLASOD categories of "strongly degraded" (lands that require major financial investments and engineering work to rehabilitate) or "very strongly degraded" (lands that cannot be rehabilitated at all).

Among the most severely affected areas are South and Southeast Asia,where populations are among the densest and agriculture the most extensive.

LAND DEGRADATION IN INDIA, 1999
(Area in Thousand sq. km)

States/ Union Territories	*Non Forest Degraded Area*	*Forest Degraded Area*	*Total*
Andhra Pradesh	76.82	37.34	114.16
Assam	9.35	7.95	17.30
Bihar	38.96	15.62	54.58
Gujarat	71.53	6.83	78.36
Haryana	24.04	0.74	24.78
Himachal Pradesh	14.24	5.34	19.58
J & K	5.31	10.34	15.65
Karnataka	71.22	20.43	91.65
Kerala	10.53	2.26	12.79
Madhya Pradesh	129.47	71.95	201.42
Maharashtra	115.6	28.41	144.01
Manipur	0.14	14.24	14.38
Meghalaya	8.15	11.03	19.18
Nagaland	5.08	8.78	13.86
Orissa	31.57	32.27	63.84
Punjab	11.51	0.79	12.30
Rajasthan	180.01	19.33	199.34
Sikkim	1.31	1.5	2.81
Tamilnadu	33.92	10.09	44.01
Tripura	1.08	8.65	9.73
Uttar Pradesh	66.35	14.26	80.61
West Bengal	21.77	3.59	25.36
Union Territories	8.89	27.15	36.04
Total	936.85	358.89	1295.74

Source: Forestry Statistics, India 1999.

Agriculture Productivity Losses

The cumulative productivity loss from soil degradation over the past 50 years has been roughly estimated, using GLASOD figures, to be about 13 per cent for cropland and 4 per cent for pasture lands.

The economic and social impacts of this degradation have been far greater in developing countries than in industrialized countries. In industrialized countries, soil quality plays a relatively less important role in overall agricultural productivity because of the high level of fertilizer and other inputs used. Furthermore, the most important grain-producing areas in industrialized countries typically have deep, geologically "new" soils that can withstand considerable degradation without having yields affected.

Soil degradation has more immediate impacts on the food supply in developing countries. Agricultural productivity is estimated to have declined significantly on approximately 16 per cent of agricultural land, especially on cropland in Africa and Central America, pastures in Africa, and forests in Central America. The GLASOD study estimates that almost 74 per cent of Central America's agricultural land (defined by GLASOD as cropland and planted pastures) is degraded, as is 65 per cent of Africa's and 38 per cent of Asia's . Detailed studies based on predictive models for Argentina, Uruguay, and Kenya calculated yield reductions between 25 and 50 per cent over the next 20 years .

Subregional studies have documented significant aggregate declines in crop yields due to degradation in many parts of Africa, China, South Asia, and Central America. Crop yield losses in Africa from 1970 to 1990 due to water erosion alone are estimated to be 8 per cent. Estimates of the economic losses associated with soil degradation in eight African countries range from 1 to 9 per cent of agricultural GDP. Total annual economic loss from degradation in South and Southeast Asia is estimated to be 7 per cent of the region's agricultural GDP. Economic losses from erosion in different regions of Mexico vary from 3 to 13 per cent of agricultural GDP.

(c) Soil

Soil forms the uppermost layer of the earth's crust and is made up of inorganic and organic matter. The inorganic components are weathered rock, air, water and minerals. The organic components are the decomposing (rotting or decaying) fragments of plants and animals. The spaces between the small particles that make up the soil are filled with air or water.

Living plants (e.g. algae, lichen) and animals (e.g. earthworms, moles, termites) live in the soil and improve aeration and drainage. Some organisms, such as bacteria, play an important role in converting plant foods or nutrients, e.g. nitrogen, into a form that plants can use to grow.

Some important plant foods or nutrients in the soil are as follows :

Nitrogen—helps leaves and stems to grow;
Phosphate—helps roots and fruits to develop; and
Potassium—stimulates overall plant health.

As plants and animals die and decompose, humus is formed from their remains. Humus fertilizes and enriches the soil as it contains nutrients and improves the soil's ability to hold water and air. Thus, nutrients in the soil are used by plants and animals and are returned to the soil when they die and rot. In this way soil plays an important role in the recycling of nutrients.

➢ Formation of Soil

Soil takes thousands of years to develop from parent rock—10 mm of soil takes between 100 and 1000 years to form. The exact amount of time taken depends upon the speed at which the parent rock weathers, i.e. is broken down into small particles. Weathering occurs through chemical, physical and biological processes. Weathering is known as mechanical disintegration and chemical disintegration of the rocks.

- *Chemical weathering* is caused by the chemical action of water, oxygen, carbon dioxide and organic acids (secreted by lichens). Chemical weathering is very active in the humid tropics as it is accelerated by high temperatures and rainfall.
- *Physical weathering* is caused by frost, temperature changes and salt crystallization. For example in places where the temperature variation in one day is great, repeated cooling and heating of a rock surface will weaken it and layers sometimes peel off.
- *Biological weathering* is caused by plants and animals. For example, tree roots in rock crevices grow and widen the crack. Burrowing animals such as rabbits, worms and ants bring soil and rock to the surface where they can be weathered by chemical and physical processes.

Pioneer plants such as grasses, lichens and moss grow on the loose, weathered particles of rock and add organic material to the developing soil. These plants also trap water and wind-blown soil, contributing to more plant growth and soil formation.

➢ The Soil Profile

As soil is formed it develops layers or horizons which make up the soil profile. There are generally three horizons in soil.

- *Topsoil :* The upper layer, about 100 - 200 mm deep is where plants get their nutrients so that they are able to grow. Topsoil is often darker than the other layers as it is rich in humus. In addition to releasing nutrients for plants, humus improves the crumbly nature of the soil. When soil is crumbly it allows air to move through it, soaks up water, reduces runoff and erosion, and promotes plant growth. For topsoil to remain productive, humus must be constantly added to soil.
- *Sub-soil :* Generally more clay-like, this layer acts as a reservoir (water store) for plants growing in the topsoil. When the sub-soil is exposed it erodes fairly easily.

- *Bedrock or parent rock :* This is the underlying layer from which the first-two horizons are formed.

➢ *Soils in India*

Soil-types in India can be classified into three groups.

- *The first group* comprises of the *alluvial, black* and *red soils,* which are basically fertile and are arable and cultivable.
- *The second group* consists of the peaty and marshy, the *saline* and *alkaline* soils which are potentially arable.
- *The third group* is the *laterite* and *forest* and *hill soils,* which are not at all suitable for cultivation.

The main alluvial area is found in the Indo-Gangetic plain and the Peninsular regions. The main crops are rice, sugarcane and wheat. Black soil is found in the northwestern regions and in the Deccan lava areas and Tamil Nadu.

Black soil is especially suited for cotton. Red soil is particularly rich in potash and is found in northern and central India. The peaty and marshy soils are found in the Bengal deltas, Saline and alkaline soils in the semi-arid regions of Bihar, U.P, Gujarat, Punjab and Rajasthan. Desert soils are found in the minimum rain receiving areas of Gujarat, Punjab and Rajasthan. Laterite soil is common in the low hills of Andhra, Karnataka, Kerala, Madhya Pradesh, Orissa and Assam.

Soils are the critical component in land degradation when it involves the following problems :

(1) Soil Erosion;
(2) Desertification; and
(3) Landslides.

1. Soil Erosion

Erosion is displacement of solids (soil, mud, rock and other particles) by the agents of water, wind, ocean currents or ice by downward or down-slope movement in response to gravity or by living organisms (in the case of bioerosion).

Erosion is an intrinsic natural process but in many places it is increased by human land use. Poor land use practices include deforestation, overgrazing, unmanaged construction activity and road or trail building. However, improved land use practices can limit erosion, using techniques like terrace-building and tree planting.

❖ Causes of Soil Erosion

What causes erosion to be severe in some areas and minor elsewhere is a combination of many different things, including :

- ☞ The amount and intensity of precipitation (Rain),
- ☞ The texture of the soil,
- ☞ The gradient of the slope, and
- ☞ Ground cover (from vegetation, rocks, land use, and possibility of erosion from speed of a stream.

The first factor, rain, is the agent for erosion, but the degree of erosion is governed by other factors.

The first three factors can remain fairly constant over time. In general, given the same kind of vegetative cover, you expect areas with high-intensity precipitation, sandy or silty soils and steep slopes to be the most erosive. Soils with a greater proportion of clay that receive less intense precipitation and are on gentle slopes tend to erode less. But here, the impact of atmospheric sodium on erodibility of clay should be considered.

The factor that is most subject to change is the amount and type of ground cover. When fires burn an area or when vegetation is removed as part of timber operations or building a house or a road, the susceptibility of the soil to erosion is greatly increased.

Understandably, many human activities remove vegetation from an area, making the soil easily eroded. Logging and heavy grazing can reduce vegetation enough to increase erosion. Changes in the kind of vegetation in an area can also affect erosion rates. Different kinds of vegetation affect infiltration rates of rain into the soil. Forested areas have higher infiltration rates, so precipitation will result in less surface runoff, which erodes. Instead much of the water will go in subsurface flows, which are generally less erosive. Leaf litter and low shrubs are an important part of the high infiltration rates of forested systems, the removal of which can increase erosion rates. Leaf litter also shelters the soil from the impact of falling raindrops, which is a significant agent of erosion. Vegetation can also change the speed of surface runoff flows, so grasses and shrubs can also be instrumental in this aspect.

One of the main causes of erosive soil loss in the year 2006 is the result of slash and burn treatment of tropical forest. When the total ground surface is stripped of vegetation and then seared of all living organisms, the upper soils are vulnerable to both wind and water erosion. In a number of regions of the earth, entire sectors of a country have been rendered unproductive.

When land is overused by animal activities (including humans), there can be mechanical erosion and also removal of vegetation leading to erosion. In the case of the animal kingdom, this effect would become material primarily with very large animal herds stampeding such as the Blue wilder beast on the Serengeti plain. Even in this case there are broader material benefits to the ecosystem, such as continuing the survival of grasslands, that are indigenous to this region. This effect may be viewed as anomalous or a problem only when there is a significant imbalance or overpopulation of one species.

In the case of human use, the effects are also generally linked to overpopulation. For when large numbers of hikers use trails or extensive off road vehicle use occurs, erosive effects often follow, arising from vegetation removal and furrowing of foot traffic and off road vehicle tires. These effects can also accumulate from a variety of outdoor human activities, again simply arising from too many people using a finite land resource.

❖ Erosion Processes

(1) Gravity Erosion

Mass wasting is the down-slope movement of rock and sediments, mainly due to the force of gravity. Mass wasting is an important part of the erosional process, as it moves material from higher elevations to lower elevations where transporting agents like streams and glaciers can then pick up the material and move it to even lower elevations. Mass-wasting processes are occurring continuously on all slopes; some mass-wasting processes act very slowly, others occur very suddenly, often with disastrous results. Any perceptible down-slope movement of rock or sediment is often referred to in general terms as a landslide.

Slumping happens on steep hillsides, occurring along distinct fracture zones, often within materials like clay that, once released, may move quite rapidly downhill. They will often show a spoon-shaped depression, within which the material has begun to slide downhill. In some cases, the slump is caused by water beneath the slope weakening it. In many cases it is simply the result of poor engineering along highways where it is a regular occurrence.

Surface creep is the slow movement of soil and rock debris by gravity which is usually not perceptible except through extended observation. However, the term can also describe the rolling of dislodged soil particles 0.5 to 1.0 mm in diameter by wind along the soil surface.

(2) Water Erosion

Splash erosion is the detachment and airborne movement of small soil particles caused by the impact of raindrops on soil.

Sheet erosion is the result of heavy rain on bare soil where water flows as a sheet down any gradient, carrying soil particles.

Where precipitation rates exceed soil infiltration rates, runoff occurs. Surface runoff turbulence can often cause more erosion than the initial raindrop impact.

Gully erosion results where water flows along a linear depression eroding a trench or gully. This is particularly noticeable in the formation of hollow ways, where prior to being tarmacked, an old rural road has over many years become significantly lower than the surrounding fields.

Valley or stream erosion occurs with continued water flow along a linear feature. The erosion is both downward, deepening the valley, and headward, extending the valley into the hillside. In the earliest stage of stream erosion, the erosive activity is dominantly vertical, the valleys have a typical V-shaped cross-section and the stream gradient is relatively steep. When some base level is reached the erosive activity switches to lateral erosion which widens the valley floor and creates a narrow floodplain. The stream gradient becomes nearly flat and lateral deposition of sediments becomes important as the stream meanders across the valley floor. In all stages of stream erosion by far the most erosion occurs during times of flood, when more and faster-moving water is available to carry a larger sediment load. In such processes, it is not the water alone that erodes, suspended abrasive particles, pebbles and boulders can also act erosively, as they traverse a surface.

At extremely high flows, kolks, or vortices are formed by large volumes of rapidly rushing water. Kolks cause extreme local erosion, plucking bedrock and creating pothole-type geographical features.

(3) Shoreline Erosion

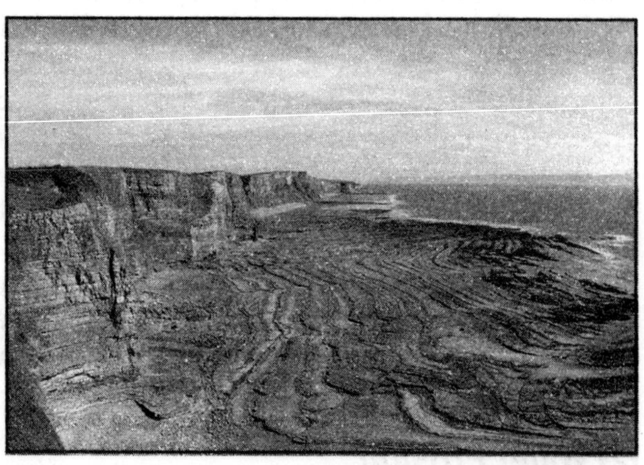

Shoreline erosion, which occurred on both exposed and sheltered coasts, primarily occurs through the action of currents and waves but sea level (tidal) change can also play a role.

Hydraulic action takes place when air in a joint is suddenly compressed by a wave closing the entrance of the joint. This then cracks it. Wave pounding is when the sheer energy of the wave hitting the cliff or rock breaks pieces off. *Abrasion* or *corrosion* is caused by waves launching seaload at the cliff. It is the most effective and rapid form of shoreline erosion (not to be confused with corrosion).

Corrosion is the dissolving of rock by carbonic acid in sea water. Limestone cliffs are particularly vulnerable to this kind of erosion.

Finally, *Attrition* is where particles/seaload carried by the waves are worn down as they hit each other and the cliffs. This then makes the material easier to wash away. The material ends up as shingle and sand.

Sediment is transported along the coast in the direction of the prevailing current (longshore drift). When the upcurrent amount of sediment is less than the amount being carried away, erosion occurs. When the upcurrent amount of sediment is greater, sand or gravel banks will tend to form. These banks may slowly migrate along the coast in the direction of the longshore drift, alternately protecting and exposing parts of the coastline. Where there is a bend in the coastline, quite often a build up of eroded material occurs forming a long narrow bank (a spit). Underwater sandbanks offshore may also protect parts of a coastline from erosion. Over the years, as the sandbanks gradually shift, the erosion may be redirected to attack different parts of the shore.

(4) Ice Erosion

Ice erosion is caused by movement of ice, typically as glaciers. Glaciers can scrape down a slope and break up rock and then transport it, leaving moraines, drumlins and glacial erratics in their wake, typically at the terminus or during glacier retreat. Ice wedging is the weathering process in which water trapped in tiny rock cracks freezes and expands, breaking the rock. This can lead to gravity erosion on steep slopes. The scree which forms at the bottom of a steep mountain side is mostly formed from pieces of rock broken away by this means. It is a common engineering problem, wherever rock cliffs are alongside roads, because morning thaws can drop hazardous rock pieces onto the road. In some places cold enough, water seeps into rocks during the daytime, then freezes at night. Ice expands, thus, creating a wedge in the rock. Over time, the repetition in the forming and melting of the ice causes fissures, which eventually breaks the rock down.

(5) Wind Erosion

Wind erosion is the result of material movement by the wind. There are two main effects. First, wind causes small particles to be lifted and, therefore, moved to another region. Second, these suspended particles may impact on solid objects causing erosion by abrasion.

Wind erosion generally occurs in areas with little or no vegetation, often in areas where there is insufficient rainfall to support vegetation. An example is the formation of sand dunes, on a beach or in a desert. Windbreaks are often planted by farmers to reduce wind erosion. This includes the planting of trees, shrubs, or other vegetation, usually perpendicular or nearly so to the principal wind direction.

❖ Erosion Control

Erosion control is the practice of preventing or controlling wind or water erosion in agriculture, land development and construction. This usually involves the creation of some sort of physical barrier, such as vegetation or rock, to absorb some of the energy of the wind or water that is causing the erosion.

Examples of some erosion control methods include :

- No-till farming
- Contour ploughing
- Cover crops
- Reforestation
- Riparian strip
- Riprap
- Strip farming
- Vegetated waterways
- Terracing
- Windbreaks

No-till farming, also known as *conservation tillage* or *zero tillage* is a way of growing crops from year to year without disturbing the soil through tillage. Once called chemical farming, the reference was subdued in order to promote the idea of no-till being more natural. It is becoming more common as researchers study its effects and farmers uncover its economic benefits.

Contour ploughing or contour farming is the farming practice of ploughing across a slope following its contours. In contour ploughing, the ploughman ploughs perpendicular rather than parallel to slopes, generally resulting in furrows that curve around the land and are level.

Cover crops is any annual, biennial, or perennial plant grown as a monoculture (one crop type grown together) or polyculture (multiple crop types grown together), to improve any number of conditions associated with sustainable agriculture. Cover crops are fundamental, sustainable tools used to manage soil fertility, soil quality, water, weeds (unwanted plants that limit crop production potential), pests (unwanted animals, usually insects, that limit crop production potential), diseases, and diversity and wildlife, in agroecosystems.

Strip farming is a method of farming used when a slope is too steep or too long, or when other types of farming may not prevent soil erosion. Strip farming alternates strips of closely sown crops such as hay, wheat, or other small grains with strips of row crops, such as corn, soybeans, cotton, or sugar beets. It is also known as strip cropping.

Strip Farming helps to stop soil erosion by creating natural dams for water, helping to preserve the strength of the soil. Certain layers of plants will absorb minerals and water from the soil more effectively than others. When water reaches the weaker soil that lacks the minerals needed to make it stronger, it normally washes it away. When strips of soil are strong enough to slow down water from moving through them, the weaker soil cannot wash away like it normally would. Because of this, farmland stays fertile much longer.

Reforestation is the restocking of existing forests and woodlands which have been depleted, with native tree stock. The term reforestation can also refer to afforestation, the process of restoring and recreating areas of woodlands or forest that once existed but were deforested or otherwise removed or destroyed at some point in the past. The resulting forest can provide both ecosystem and resource benefits and has the potential to become a major carbon sink.

Reforestation can occur naturally if the area is left largely undisturbed. Native forests are often resilient and can often re-establish themselves quickly.

Reforestation, if native several species are used can provide other benefits in addition to the financial returns, including restoration of the soil, rejuvenation of local flora and fauna, and the capturing and sequestering of 38 tonnes of carbon dioxide per hectare per year.

Riprap (also known as *rip rap, revetment, shot rock or rock armour)* is rock or other material used to stabilize shore. Riprap reduces water erosion by resisting the hydraulic attack and dissipating the energy of flowing water or waves. The shape of rock is important. Coarse, angular rock, usually made by crushing or blasting, or from scree, is more effective at ground reinforcement than round river rock. A correct mixture of aggregate size can also aid riprap's ability to create an interlocking structure.

In agriculture, a *terrace* is a levelled section of a hilly cultivated area, designed as a method of soil conservation to slow or prevent the rapid surface runoff of irrigation water. Often such land is formed into multiple terraces, giving a stepped appearance. The human landscapes of rice cultivation in terraces that follow the natural contours of the escarpments like contour plowing is a classic feature.

This form of land use is prevalent in many countries, and is used for crops requiring a lot of water, such as rice. Terraces are also easier for both mechanical and manual sowing and harvesting than a steep slope would be.

A windbreak, or *shelterbelt,* is usually made up of one or more rows of trees or shrubs planted in such a manner as to provide shelter from the wind and to prevent soil from erosion. They are commonly planted around the edges of fields on farms. If designed properly, windbreaks around a home can reduce the cost of heating and cooling and save energy.

2. Desertification

Desertification is the degradation of land in arid, semi-arid, and dry sub-humid areas. It is caused primarily by human activities and climatic variations.

Desertification does not refer to the expansion of existing deserts. It occurs because dry land ecosystems, which cover over one-third of the world's land area, are extremely vulnerable to over-exploitation and inappropriate land use.

Poverty, political instability, deforestation, overgrazing, and bad irrigation practices can all undermine the land's fertility. Over 250 million people are directly affected by desertification. In addition, some one thousand million (or one billion) people in over one hundred countries are at risk. These people include many of the world's poorest, most marginalized, and politically weak citizens.

❖ Causes of Desertification

Overgrazing is the major cause of desertification worldwide. Plants of semi-arid areas are adapted to being eaten by sparsely scattered, large, grazing mammals which move in response to the patchy rainfall common to these regions. Early human pastoralists living in semi-arid areas copied this natural system. They moved their small groups of domestic animals in response to food and water availability. Such regular stock movement prevented overgrazing of the fragile plant cover.

Destruction of vegetation in arid regions, often for fuel wood.

Poor grazing management after accidental burning of semi-arid vegetation.

Incorrect irrigation practices in arid areas can cause salinization, (the build up of salts in the soil) which can prevent plant growth.

When the practices described above coincide with drought, the rate of desertification increases dramatically.

Increasing human population and poverty contribute to desertification as poor people may be forced to overuse their environment in the short-term, without the ability to plan for the long-term effects of their actions. Where livestock has a social importance beyond food, people might be reluctant to reduce their stock numbers.

❒ Effects and Extent of Desertification

Desertification reduces the ability of land to support life, affecting wild species, domestic animals, agricultural crops and people. The reduction in plant cover that accompanies desertification leads to accelerated soil erosion by wind and water. Water is lost off the land instead of soaking into the soil to provide moisture for plants. Even long-lived plants that would normally survive droughts die.

A reduction in plant cover also results in a reduction in the quantity of humus and plant nutrients in the soil, and plant production drops further. As protective plant cover disappears, floods become more frequent and more severe. Desertification is self-reinforcing, i.e. once the process has started, and conditions are set for continual deterioration.

About one-third of the world's land surface is arid or semi-arid. It is predicted that global warming will increase the area of desert climates by 17 per cent in the next century. The area at risk to desertification is thus large and likely to increase.

Worldwide, desertification is making approximately 12 million hectares useless for cultivation every year. This is equal to 10 per cent of the total area of South Africa or 87 per cent of the area of cultivated lands in our country.

In the early 1980s it was estimated that, worldwide, 61 per cent of the 3257 million hectares of all productive dry lands (lands where stock are grazed and crops grown, without irrigation) were moderately to very severely desertified. The problem is clearly enormous.

South Africa losing approximately 300-400 million tonnes of topsoil every year. As vegetation cover and soil layer are reduced, rain drop impact and run-off increases.

★ Desertification Control

To halt desertification the number of animals on the land must be reduced, allowing plants to regrow. Soil conditions must be made favourable for plant growth by, for example, mulching. Mulch (a layer of straw, leaves or sawdust covering the soil) reduces evaporation, suppresses weed growth, enriches soil as it rots, and prevents runoff and hence erosion. Reseeding may be necessary in badly degraded areas. Mulching and reseeding are expensive practices.

However, the only realistic large scale approach is to prevent desertification through good land management in semi-arid areas.

3. Landslides *

(d) Management of Soil

One indicator of soil condition and productive capacity is soil nutrient balance. One of the most common management techniques used to maintain the condition of agroecosystems, particularly intensively cultivated systems, is to replenish soil nutrients with organic manures or inorganic fertilizers containing nitrogen, phosphorous, and potassium. Too little replenishment can lead to soil nutrient mining—the progressive loss of nutrients as crops draw on them for growth. Too much replenishment (over fertilization) can lead to leaching of excess nutrients and the consequent soil and water pollution problems as these unused nutrients find their way into surrounding soils and freshwater systems.

An estimate of the nutrient balance of an agroecosystem can be obtained by measuring the nutrient inputs (inorganic and organic fertilizers, nutrients from crop residues, and nitrogen fixation by soybeans and other legumes) and outputs (nutrient uptake in the main crop products and the crop residue). PAGE researchers calculated these nutrient balances at the national level for individual crops in Latin

* Landslides Description is given at page 207 in Unit 5.

America and the Caribbean and found that for most of the crops and cropping systems, the nutrient balance is significantly negative—in other words, soil fertility is declining. The observed increases in production in recent decades must, therefore, be due to a combination of area expansion, improved varieties, and other factors that mask or offset the effects of soil degradation. By overlaying nutrient balance with trends in yields, it is possible to identify potential degradation "hot spots" where yield growth is slowing and soil fertility is declining. Areas where the capacity of agroecosystems to produce food appears most threatened include northeast Brazil and sections of Argentina, Bolivia, Colombia, and Paraguay.

IX. Role of an Individual in Conservation of Natural Resources

Natural resources like water, soil, air, minerals, forests etc. are very important for the development of any country. But, overuse of these resources at present causing their depletion and several related problems. For the welfare of mankind conservation of these resources is must, which of course should be initiated by man himself.

Water Conservation

- Farmers should use drip irrigation and springing irrigation to improve irrigation efficiency and reduce evaporation.
- Check the water leaks from the pipes. A small pin-hole sized leak will lead to the wastage of 640 litres of water in a month.
- Don't keep water taps running.
- Install water saving toilets.
- Reuse the soapy water.
- Install a system to capture rain water.
- Keeping the water unpolluted.

Energy Conservation

- Don't misuse the electric power.
- For cooking, heating and drying try to use solar energy.
- Practice plantation for cooling effects because a big tree is estimated to have a cooling effect equivalent to five air conditioners.
- Prefer bicycling, public transportations instead of private vehicles.
- Wear adequate woollens instead of using heat convectors.

Protect the Soil

- Try to cover the ground from grasses, trees and haze to prevent soil erosion.
- Use green manures in the garden, it will not pollute the soil.
- Practice mixed farming so that some specific soil nutrients will not go depleted.
- Don't over irrigate agricultural field without proper drainage to prevent waterlogging and Salinization

Promote Sustainable Agriculture

- Don't waste food and take as per your requirements.
- Reduce the use of pesticide, chemical fertilizer.
- Control Pests by a combination of cultivation and biological control method.

X. Equitable Use of Resources for Sustainable Life Styles

A big gap exist in the world as North (more developed countries, MDC's) and South (less developed countries, LDC's).

More developed nations such as USA, Canada, Australia, Japan, Newzeland and the countries of Western Europe. With less than one fourth of world's population (22%), they utilise 88 per cent of natural resources and 73 per cent of the energy and contribute 85 per cent of total income. On the other hand, less developed nations; share 78 per cent of world population but use 27 per cent of energy, 12 per cent of natural resources and generate15 per cent of the total global income.

The Unequal Geography of Consumption

While consumption has risen steadily worldwide; there remains a profound disparity between consumption levels in wealthy nations and those in middle- and low-income nations.

- On average, someone living in a developed nation consumes twice as much grain, twice as much fish, three times as much meat, nine times as much paper, and eleven times as much gasoline as someone living in a developing nation.
- Consumers in high-income countries accounted for 80 per cent of the money spent on private consumption in 1997 was $14.5 trillion of the $18 trillion total. By contrast, purchases by consumers in low-income nations—the poorest 35 per cent of the world's population-represented less than

Disparities in Consumption : Annual per Capita Consumption in Selected High-, Medium-, and Low-Income Nations

Country	*Total Value of Private Consumption* (1997)*	*Fish (kg) (1997)*	*Meat (kg) 1998*	*Cereals (kg) (1997)*	*Paper (kg) (1998)*	*Fossil Fuels (kg of oil equivalent) (1997)*	*Passenger Cars (per 1,000 people) (1996)*
U.S.A.	$ 21,680	21.0	122.0	975.0	293.0	6,902	489.0
Singapore	$ 16,340	34.0	77.0	159.0	168.0	7,825	120.0
Japan	$ 15,554	66.0	42.0	334.0	239.0	3,277	373.0
Germany	$ 15,229	13.0	87.0	496.0	205.0	3,625	500.0
Turkey	$ 4,377	7.2	19.0	502.0	32.0	952	55.0
Indonesia	$ 1,808	18.0	9.0	311.0	17.0	450	12.2
China	$ 1,410	26.0	47.0	360.0	30.0	700	3.2
India	$ 1,166	4.7	4.3	234.0	3.7	268	4.4
Bangladesh	$ 780	11.0	3.4	250.0	1.3	67	0.5
Nigeria	$ 692	5.8	12.0	228.0	1.9	186	6.7

* Adjusted to reflect actual purchasing power, accounting for currency and cost of living differences (the "purchasing power parity" approach).

Source: World Bank, 1999.

2 per cent of all private consumption. The money spent on private consumption worldwide (all goods and services consumed by individuals except real estate) nearly tripled between 1980 and 1997 (World Bank 1999:44, 226).

The developmental efforts of developed and fast growing developing countries are causing huge amount of pollution. And are posing a great threat to the sustainability of the earth's system. The poor nations, on the other hand, are struggling hard with their large population and poverty problems. Their share of resources is too little leading to unsustainability.

As the rich nations continue to grow, they will reach a limit. If they have a growth rate of 10 per cent every year, they will show 1024 times increase in the next 70 years. Consequently, there will be more gap between haves and have not which will naturally lead unsustainability.

Thus the solution of this problem is to have more equitable distribution of resources and wealth. A global consensus has to be reached for more balanced distribution of the basic resources like safe drinking water, food, fuel, etc. So the poors of less developed countries could get the basic necessities of the life. Without the basic requirements of life, it is difficult to imagine the rooting out the problems related to dirty, unhygienic, polluted, disease infested settlements of the people.

Thus, the two basic causes of unsustainability are over population in poor countries who have under consumption of resources and over consumption of resources by rich countries, which generate wastes. In order to achieve sustainable lifestyle it is desirable to achieve a more balanced and equitable distribution of global resources.

Questions

Long answer type of questions

1. Define Resources. Defferentiate between renewable and non-renewable resources.
2. Write down the importance of forest resources.
3. What is the present status of forest resources in India?
4. Write down about causes and consequences of deforestation.
5. What are the utilities of water resources?
6. Discuss the water potential of India with special reference of Ganga Basin in India.
7. Discuss droughts and floods with respect of their occurrence and impacts.
8. What are the mineral resources? Discuss mineral resources in India.
9. What are the uses of various types of minerals?
10. What are the environmental damages caused by mining activities?
11. What are the causes of food problems in the world?
12. What are the impacts of modern agriculture on natural environment?
13. What is the trend of energy consumption in the world?
14. Discuss the merits of renewable energy.
15. Write the technology used for solar energy.
16. Discuss the food insecurity in urban India.
17. What are the major types of energy resources?
18. Write down the causes of soil erosion.
19. What are methods to control soil erosion?
20. Write down the role of an individual in conservation of natural resources?

Write short notes on the following

Deforestation, Interlinking of rivers, Solar energy, Wind energy, Tidal energy, Biogas, Geothermal energy, Salinization, Waterlogging, Drought, Floods, Land degradation, Desertification.

Fill in the blanks

1. The term "resources" was introduced to a broad audience by E.F. Schumacher in his 1970s book ....
2. Non-renewable resources have a high ....content.
3. Dense forests are defined as those with a canopy cover of more than ....

4. Degraded forest is described as a forest where the vegetative (crown) density is less than ....of the canopy covers.
5. Forests cover about ....of the world's land surface, excluding Greenland and Antarctica.
6. Forests provide habitats to about ....of all species on earth.
7. Since 1950, every year in July and February a large number of trees are planted on................in India.
8. The wind power potential of India is estimated to be about.....................
9. ....is the major cause of desertification worldwide.

Keys : - 1. Small Is Beautiful. 2. carbon. 3. 70 per cent. 4. 40 per cent. 5. 25 per cent. 6. Two-thirds. 7. Van Mahotsav. 8. 20,000 MW. 9. Overgrazing.

Tick the right answer

1. Which one is not the source of renewable energy?
   (a) sunshine
   (b) wind
   (c) wave power
   (d) coal
2. Forests worldwide cover some :
   (a) 3.9 billion hectares
   (b) 1.5 billion hectares
   (c) .9 billion hectares
   (d) 5.6 billion hectares
3. Indian Council of Forestry Research and Education (ICFRE), an autonomous umbrella organization, was established in 1986 in :
   (a) Bangalore
   (b) Delhi
   (c) Dehradun
   (d) Pune
4. How much of the earth's surface is covered with water :
   (a) 50%
   (b) 38%
   (c) 81%
   (d) 75%
5. Major Rivers are having a catchment's area over :
   (a) 20,000 sq. km.
   (b) 30,000 sq. km.
   (c) 40,000 sq. km.
   (d) 50,000 sq. km.

6. The continent most affected by drought is Africa :
   (a) Asia
   (b) Africa
   (c) Europe
   (d) America
7. Essential to iron and steel production
   (a) Zinc
   (b) Aluminium
   (c) Copper
   (d) Manganese
8. The most significant growth of energy consumption is currently taking place in :
   (a) China
   (b) Nepal
   (c) Bhutan
   (d) USA
9. Which of the following coal type contains more than 80 per cent carbon :
   (a) Anthracite
   (b) Bituminous
   (c) Lignite
   (d) Peat
10. Solar energy used worldwide during 2005 was approximately :
   (a) 102 GW
   (b) 93.4 GW
   (c) 75 GW
   (d) 50.20 GW

   Keys : - 1. d, 2. a, 3. c, 4. d, 5. a, 6. b, 7. d, 8. a, 9. a, 10. b

True / False types of questions

1. Degraded forest is described as a forest where the vegetative (crown) density is less than 10 per cent of the canopy cover. (f)
2. Forests act as a major carbon store because carbon dioxide (CO_2) is taken up from the atmosphere. (t)
3. The world's average rainfall is about 850 mm. (t)
4. About 70 per cent of the fat free mass of the human body is made of water. (t)
5. About 77 per cent of all water is in the oceans. (f)
6. There are about 80 countries in the world, lying in the arid and semi arid regions that experience frequent spell of drought. (t)
7. There about 3000 kinds of minerals but only about 100 of them are common. (t)

8. The food and agriculture organization (FAO) of United Nations estimated that on an average the minimum caloric intake on a global scale is 2,500 calories/ day.
9. The effective water storage capacity built or under construction in India is about 147 billion cubic metres.
10. India produces third quarters of the world's mica
11. In India, the current cereal intake is 143 kgs./per capita/annum.

    Keys : - 1. false, 2. true, 3. true, 4. true, 5. false, 6. true, 7. true, 8. true, 9. true, 10. true

Unit - 3

Ecosystems

Ecosystems sustain us. They are Earth's primary producers, solar-powered factories that yield the most basic necessities such as food, fibre, water. Ecosystems also provide essential services such as air and water purification, climate control, nutrient cycling, and soil production, these services we can't replace at any reasonable price.

I. Concept of Ecosystems

An *Ecosystem* is a combination of all the living and non-living elements of an area. Ecosystems are not just assemblages of species, they are systems combined of organic and inorganic matter and natural forces that interact and change. The energy that runs the system comes from the sun; solar energy is absorbed and turned into food by plants and other photosynthesizing organisms at the base of food chains. Water is the crucial element flowing through the system. The amount of water available, along with the temperature extremes and the sunlight the site receives, largely determine what types of plants, insects, and animals live there, and how the ecosystem is categorized.

Ecosystems are dynamic, constantly remaking themselves, reacting to natural disturbances and the competition among and between species. It is the complex, local interaction of the physical environment and the biological community that gives rise to the particular package of services and products that each ecosystem yields; it also is what makes each ecosystem unique and vulnerable.

Scale is also important. A small bog, a single sand dune, or a tiny patch of forest may be viewed as an ecosystem, unique in its mix of species and microclimate—a micro-environment. On a much larger scale, an ecosystem refers to more extensive communities, 100 or 1,000 km^2 forest, or a major river system, each having many such micro-environments.

The term *Ecology* was coined by Earnst Haeckel in 1869. It is derived from the Greek words *Oikos*- home+ *logos*-study. So ecology deals with the study of organism in their natural home interacting with their surroundings. The term ecosystem first appeared in a 1935 publication by the British ecologist Arthur Tansley (1935). However, the term had been coined already in 1930 by Tansley's colleague Roy Clapham, who was asked if he could think of a suitable word to denote the physical and biological components of an environment as a single unit. Tansley expanded on the term in his later work, adding the ecotope concept to define the spatial context of ecosystems.

II. Structure of Ecosystems

Ecosystems have two basic components :

(a) The abiotic (non-living) components; and
(b) The biotic (living) components.

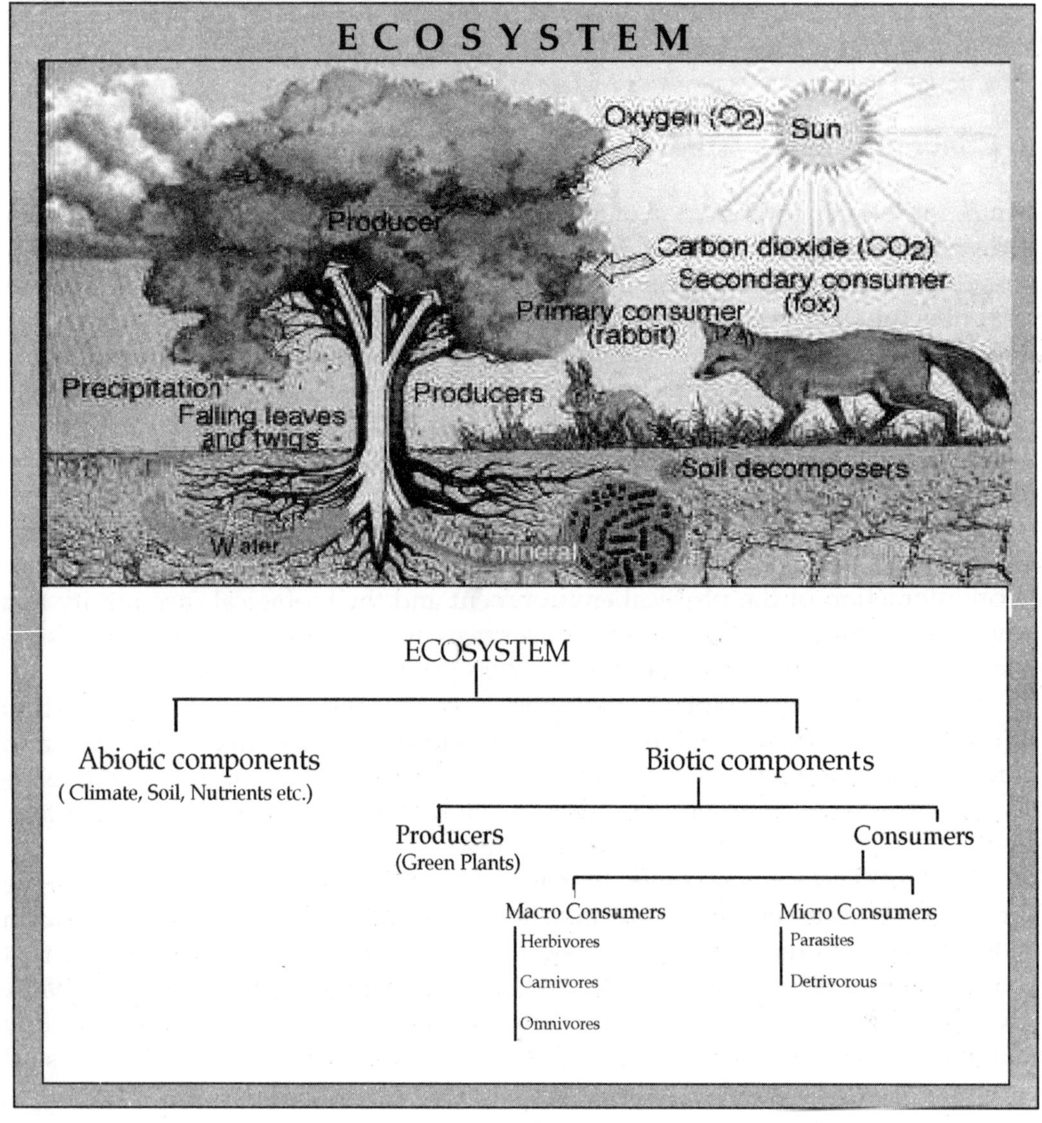

(a) The Abiotic Components

The physical and chemical components of an ecosystem constitute its abiotic structure. It includes climatic factors, edaphic (soil) factors, geographical factors, energy, nutrients and toxic substances.

1. *Physical Factors* : The sunlight and shade, intensity of solar flux, duration of sun hours, average temperature, maximum-minimum temperature, annual rainfall, wind, latitude and altitude, soil type, water availability, water current etc. are some of the important physical features which have a strong influence on the ecosystem.
2. *Chemical Factors :* Availability of major essential nutrients like carbon, nitrogen, phosphorous, potassium, hydrogen, oxygen and sulphur, level of toxic *substance,* salt causing salinity and various organic *substances* present in the soil or water largely influence the functioning of the ecosystem.

All the components of the ecosystem are influenced by the abiotic components and *vice versa,* and they are linked together through energy flow and matter cycling.

(b) The Biotic Components

The living components of an ecosystem constitute its biotic structure as following :

1. *Producers (autotrophs) :* They utilize energy from the sun and nutrients from the abiotic environment (carbon dioxide from the air or water, other nutrients from the soil or water) to perform photosynthesis and grow. Producers are generally green plants.
   Primary / Biomass production : Primary production is generation of biomass through photosynthesis. The highest producers of biomass are as follows :

   - ☞ Tropical rain forests, 2000 $g/m^2/yr$ of biomass
   - ☞ Swamps and marshes, 2500 $g/m^2/yr$ of biomass
   - ☞ Algal beds and reefs, 2000 $g/m^2/yr$ of biomass
   - ☞ River estuaries, 1800 $g/m^2/yr$ of biomass
   - ☞ Temperate forests, 1200 $g/m^2/yr$ of biomass
   - ☞ Cultivated lands; 600 $g/m^2/yr$ of biomass

While lowest producers are deserts and frozen areas (less than 200 $g/m^2/year$ of biomass).

2. Consumers

All the organisms that cannot make their own food (and need producers) are called consumers or heterotrophic components. They obtain food by eating other organisms. There are different levels of consumers.

On the basis of their size, they are categorized as follows :

- Macro consumers
- Micro consumers

Macro Consumers

Macro Consumers are also classified depending on what they eat. (*See* food chain fig. at page 113)

- *Herbivores* are those that eat only plants or plant products. Examples are grasshoppers, mice, rabbits, deer, beavers, moose, cows, sheep, goats and groundhogs.
- *Carnivores,* on the other hand, are those that eat only other animals. Examples of carnivores are foxes, frogs, snakes, hawks, and spiders.
- *Omnivores* are the last type and eat both plants (acting primary consumers) and meat (acting as secondary or tertiary consumers). Examples of omnivores are as follows :

  - Bears — They eat insects, fish, moose, elk, deer, sheep as well as honey, grass, and sedges.
  - Turtles — They eat snails, crayfish, crickets, earthworms, but also lettuce, small plants, and algae.
  - Monkeys— They eat frogs and lizards as well as fruits, flowers, and leaves.
  - Squirrels — They eat insects, moths, bird eggs and nestling birds and also seeds, fruits, acorns, and nuts.

Micro Consumers

Micro consumers decompose the dead and decaying organism and are known as decomposers e.g. fungi, bacteria, etc. Decomposers are essential for the long term survival of ecosystem. Without them, enormous wastes of plant litter, dead animal bodies, animal excreta and garbage will be deposited on the mother planet. Also important elements like nitrogen, phosphorous, and potassium woud remain indefinitely in dead matter. Then the producers would not get them and this would make life impossible.

Micro consumers are of two types :

- *Parasites :* Parasites derive their food from the living organism. The parasites may be microscopic bacteria, fungi, viruses, or macroscopic like angiosperms, nematodes, tapeworm, flatworms, and roundworms. They check the population of the host.
- *Detritivores and scanvengers:* The dead organic matter of an organism (both plants and animals) is known as detritus. Organisms depend upon detritus are known as Detrivorous e.g. protozoans, insects, and snails. They are known as reducers. They claen the environment by eating up dead organisms. Hence, they are also clead, scavengers.

III. Functions of Ecosystems

Every ecosystem performs under natural conditions in a systematic way. It reserves energy from the sun and passes it on through various biotic components and in fact, all life depends upon this flow of energy. Besides energy, various nutrients and water are also required for life processes which are exchanged by the biotic components within themselves and with their abiotic components within or outside the ecosystem. The biotic components also regulate themselves in a very systematic manner and show mechanism to encounter some degree of environmental stress. The major functional attributes of an ecosystem are as follows :

- ★ Trophic levels, food chain, and food webs;
- ★ Energy flow;
- ★ Cycling of nutrients (Biogeochemical cycle);
- ★ Primary and secondary production; and
- ★ Ecosystem development and regulation.

(a) *Trophic Levels*

In ecology, the trophic level is the position that an organism occupies in a food chain—what it eats, and what eats it.

In the *ocean,* phytoplankton is the primary producer (the first level in the food chain or the first trophic level). Phytoplankton converts inorganic carbon into protoplasm. Phytoplankton is consumed by microscopic animals called zooplankton (these are the second level in the food chain). Zooplankton is consumed by Crustaceans (the third level in the food chain). Fish that eat crustaceans could constitute the fourth trophic level, while seals consuming the fishes are the fifth.

Trophic levels are very similar on *land*, with plants being the first trophic level, goats eating the grass being the second, and humans eating the goats being the third.

The amount of biomass produced for a given amount of solar energy is highest at the first level. Less biomass is produced at the second level, for some energy is lost during the conversion. The more trophic levels there are, the more energy is lost through conversion.

Humans are generally primary and secondary consumers, and thus represent usually second and third trophic levels. Most humans are omnivores, which means they consume both plants and animals. Less energy is required to support vegetarian humans than omnivorous ones, for there is a significant energy loss during the conversion of grain and vegetables in animal matter.

(b) *Food Chain*

A food chain describes a single pathway that energy and nutrients may follow in an ecosystem. There is one organism per trophic level. They usually start with a primary producer and end with a top predator. Food chains are overly simplistic as representatives of what typically happens in nature. The food chain shows only one pathway of energy and material transfer. Most consumers feed on multiple species and are, in turn, fed upon by multiple other species. The loss of energy through the levels causes the species at the top to be less numerous. On average 10 per cent of the organism's energy is passed on to its predator. Trophic levels are different steps in the passage of food.

Types of Food Chains

1. *Predator or Grazing food chain:* It always starts with green plants and culminates in top carnivorous. It may be of two types as follows :

   ☞ Terrestrial grazing food chain; and

   ☞ Aquatic grazing food chain.

★ *Terrestrial grazing food chain :* It begins from producer (terrestrial green plants e.g. grasses) and then proceeds to herbivores, carnivores and then to top carnivores as given in the followin figure :

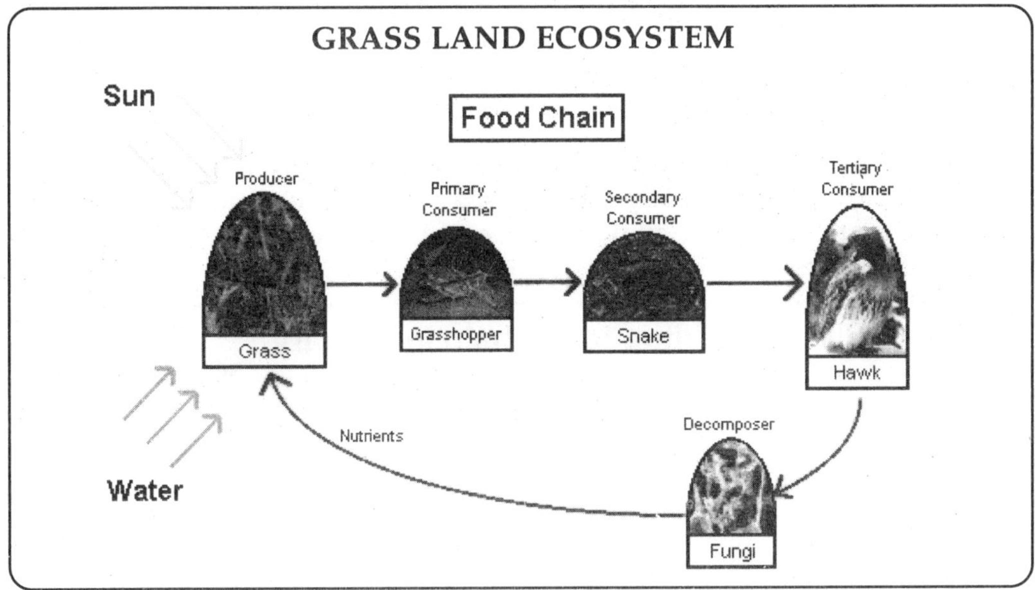

* *Aquatic grazing food chain :* It begins from aquatic green plants e.g. phytoplankton, then proceed to herbivores, carnivores and then to top carnivores as given in the followin figure :

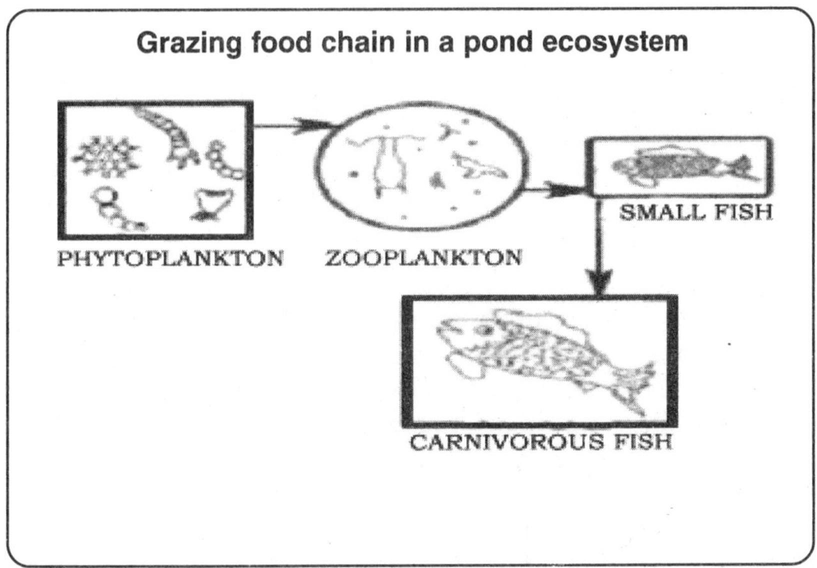

2. *Parasitic or Auxillary food chain* : This food chain starts from producers which prepare organic food through the process of photosynthesis. From here,

the food goes to herbivores and then to parasites and finally to hyperparasites. Thus here food proceeds from larger to smaller organisms. This chain is terminated by a parasite. Parasite is an organism that feeds on another living organism called host e.g. Green Plants > Sheep > Liver fluke.

Detritus food chain : It start with dead organic matter which the detrivorous and decomposers consume. Partially decomposed dead organic matter and even the decomposers are consumed by detrivorous and their pedators. Following is an example of the detritus food chain seen in mangroove (Estuary).

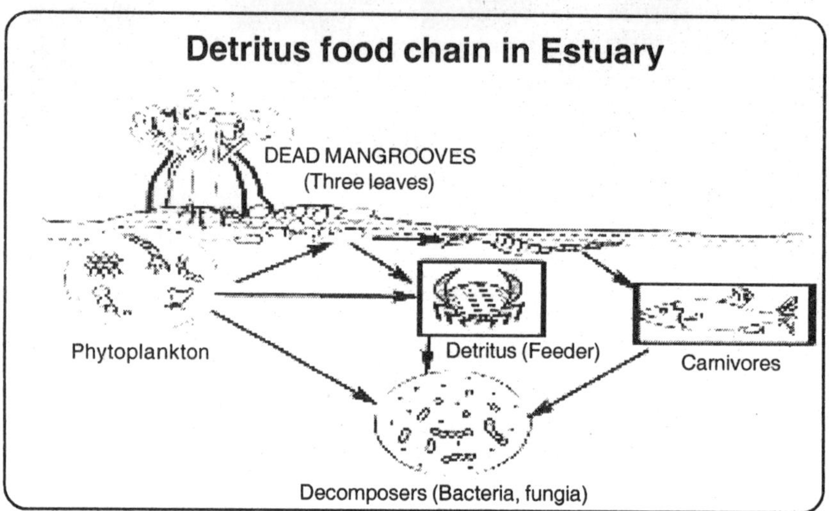

(c) *Food Web*

Interlinking of the food chains form a food web. The concept of food chain looks very simple, but in reality it is more complex. Think about it. How many different animals eat grass? And how many different foods does the hawk eat? One does not find simple independent food chains in an ecosystem, but many interdependent and complex food chains that look more like a web and are, therefore, called food webs. A food web that shows the energy transformations in an ecosystem looks like as follows :

Significance of Food Chain and Food Web

- Energy flow and nutrient cycling take place through food chain or food web.
- They check the overpopulation of different animals, thus maintain the ecological balance.

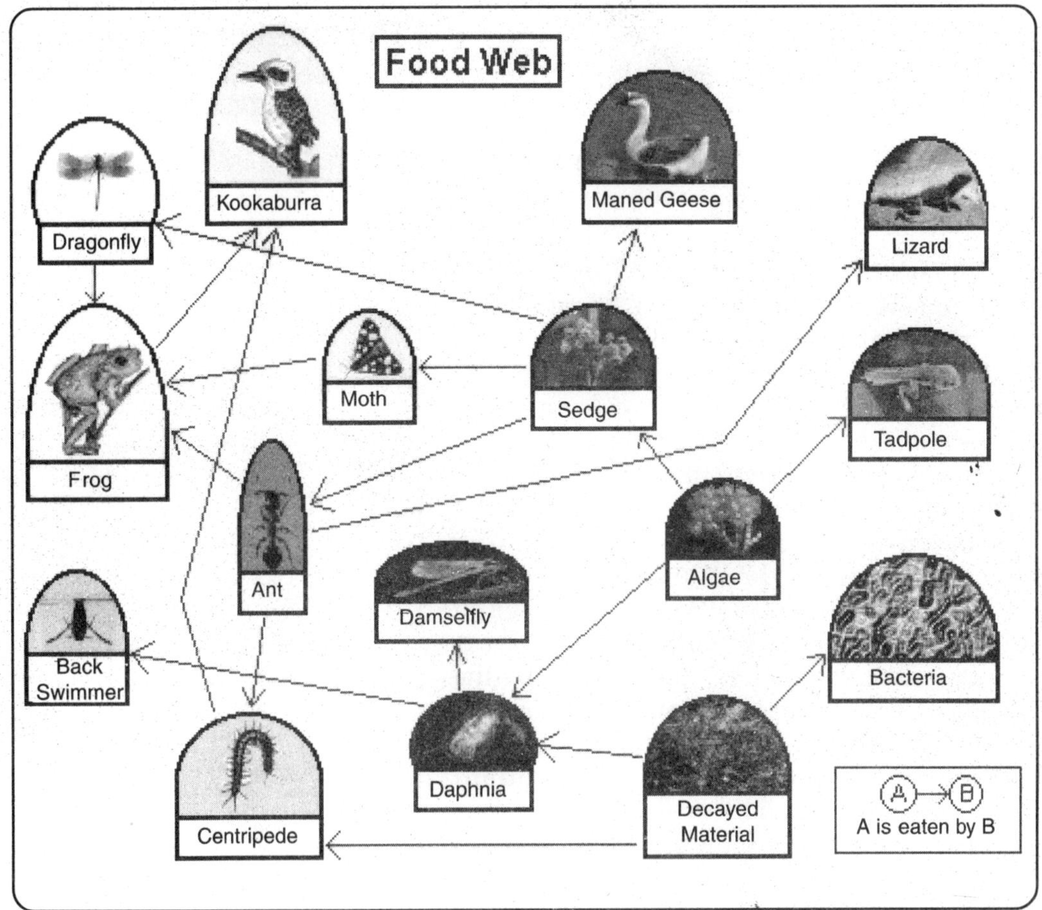

☞ Food chain have a unique property of biological magnification of some chemicals. There are several pesticides, heavy metals and other chemicals which are non-biodegradable in nature. Such chemicals are not decomposed by micro organism and they keep on passing from one trophic level to another. And, each successive trophic level, they keep on increasing in concentration. This phenomena is known as biomagnification or biological magnification.

☞ Food web helps in maintaining the stability in the ecosystem. The larger the number of alternative pathways occurring in a food web, the more stable is the ecosystem.

(d) *Ecological Pyramid*

Graphic representation of the relationship between the various trophic levels of a food chain is known as ecological pyramid.

Ecological pyramid are of three types :

1. Pyramid of numbers;
2. Pyramid of biomass; and
3. Pyramid of energy.

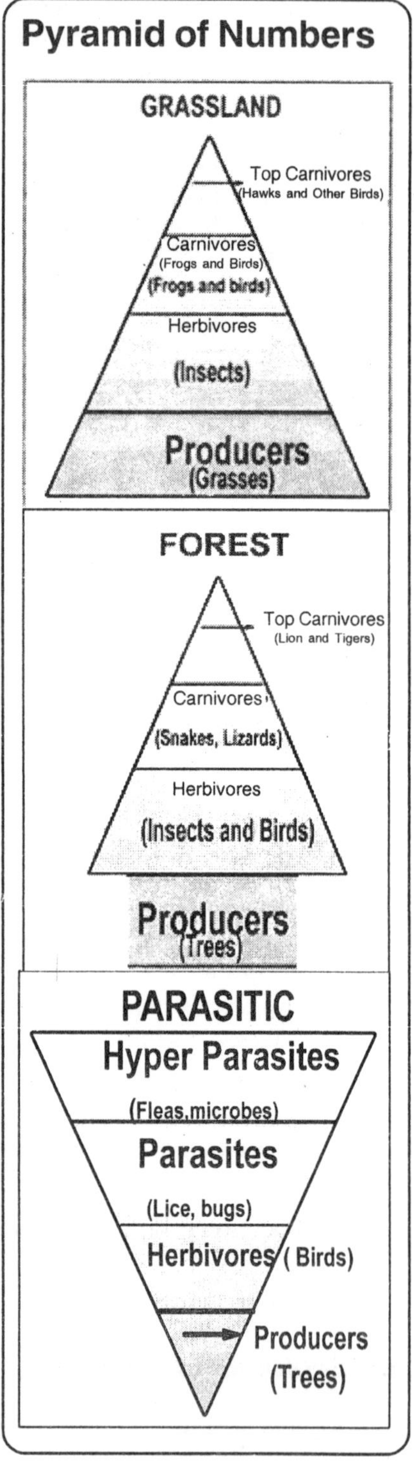

1. Pyramid of Numbers

It represents the number of individual organisms at each trophic level. So pyramids may be upright or inverted, depending upon the type of the ecosystem and food chain as shown in the figure.

Grassland Ecosystem : Here, the biomass of producer (grasses) is more than the dependent herbivores (insects) and that of the herbivores more than the dependent carnivores (frogs). Top carnivores (hawks) exhibits minimum biomass and thus shape of the pyramid is as given in the figure of grassland pyramid.

Forest Ecosystem : Here, the big trees are the producers, which are less than the dependent herbivores (birds, insects) and that of the herbivores are more than the dependent carnivores (snakes and lizards). Top carnivores (lion and tigers) exhibits minimum biomass and thus shape of the pyramid is as given in the figure of forest pyramid.

Parasitic Food Chain : It shows an inverted pyramid of number. The producers like a few big trees harbour fruit eating birds acting like herbivorous which are larger in number. A much higher number of lice, bugs, etc. grow as parasites on these birds while a still greater number of hyperparasites like bugs, fleas and microbes feed upon them, thus making an inverted pyramid.

2. Pyramid of Biomass

The amount of living material is known as biomass. Such types of pyramids are based on the total biomass at each trophic level in a food chain. Pyramids may be upright or inverted.

The pyramid of biomass in a forest is upright in contrast to its pyramid of numbers. This is because the producers (trees) accumulate huge biomass while the consumers' total biomass feeding on them declines at higher trophic level, resulting in broader base and narrowing top.

The Pond ecosystem shows an inverted pyramid of biomass. The total biomass of the Phytoplankton (Producers) is much less as compared to Zooplankton (herbivorous), Small fish (Carnivorous) and big fish (Tertiary Carnivorous). Thus the pyramid takes an inverted shape with narrow base and broader apex.

3. Pyramid of Energy

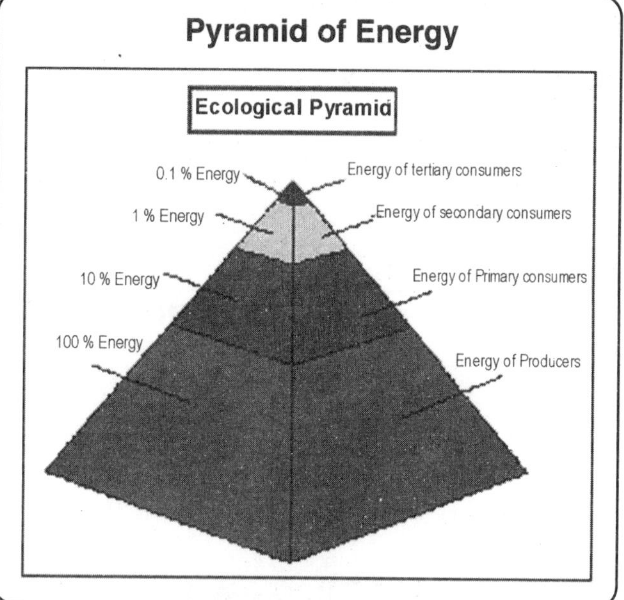

It is always upright in all ecosystems because as energy passes to a higher tropic level, approximately 90 per cent of the useful energy is lost. High tropic levels contain less energy and fewer organisms than lower levels.

In moving to the next tropic level, only 10 per cent of the original energy is available. By the third tropic level only 1 per cent of the energy is available.

(e) *Energy Flow*

In ecology, energy flow (calorific flow) refers to the flow of energy through a food chain. The sole source of the energy in an ecosystem is the light received from the sun. According to Geiger, 42 per cent of incoming solar radiation are reflected, (33% by clouds and 9 per cent by dust particles), about 10 per cent are absorbed by ozone, oxygen and water vapour. Finally only 48 per cent reach the surface of the earth. A portion of this radient energy is used by producers (green plants) and converted into chemical energy. This chemical energy is partially transferred to consumers through food. The concept of the energy flow in the ecosystem is governed by the first law of thermo-dynamics i.e. Energy can neither be created nor destroyed and every transfer of the energy is accompanied by some loss of energy in the form of heat.

A general energy flow scenario follows :

☞ Energy is taken up from the sun by the autotrophs, the so called *primary producers*, like green plants which transform it to glucose and ATP by photosynthesis.

- The primary consumers eating these autotrophs are herbivorous. They extract most of the energy stored in the plant through digestion, and transform it into the form of energy they need. A part of the energy received by the herbivore is converted to bodily heat, which is radiated away and lost from the system.
- Carnivores feed on the herbivores, recovering their energy for themselves. Again some energy is lost from the system.
- Other carnivores prey on those carnivores, and most of the energy is passed along, while some is again lost.

The energy is passed on from trophic level to trophic level and each time some of the energy is lost. So the top consumer of a food chain receives the least energy. This loss of energy at each level limits typical food chains to only 4-6 links.

The provision of different amount of energy for different activities is called as energy budget.

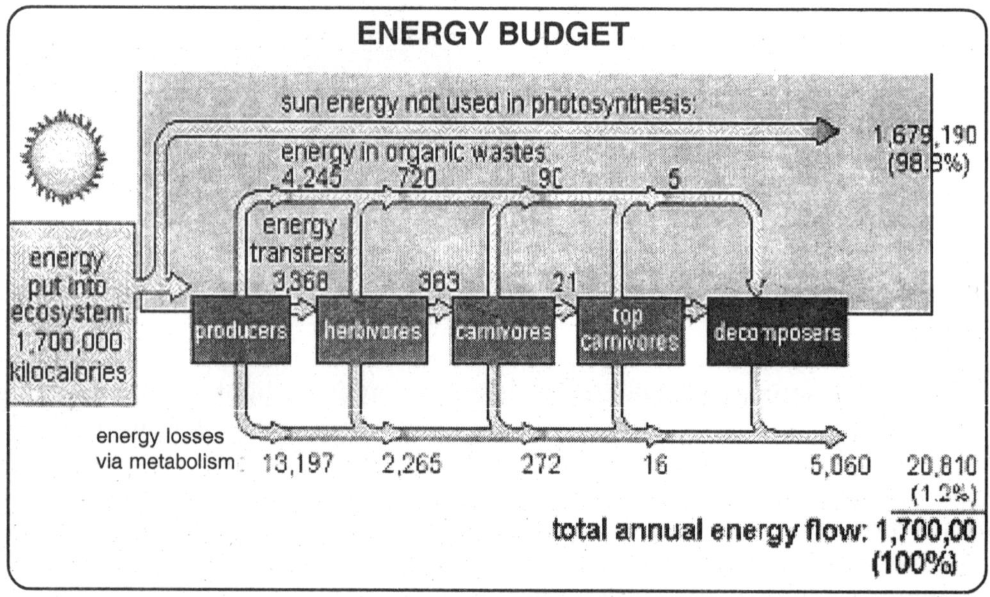

On an average, only 111 cal/cm^2/year of energy is trapped by the producers in producing organic food. According to Linderman only 0.2 per cent of the incident solar radiation is trapped by aquatic ecosystem and 1 per cent by terrestrial ecosystem. The modern crop plant can trap upto 5 per cent of the radiation falling on them. The maximum efficiency is recorded for sugarcane (10-12%).

IV. Nutrient / Biogeochemical Cycles

Biogeochemical cycle is a circuit or pathway by which a chemical element or molecule moves through both biotic ("bio-") and abiotic ("geo-") compartments of an ecosystem.

All chemical elements occurring in organisms are part of biogeochemical cycles. In addition to being a part of living organisms, these chemical elements also cycle through abiotic factors of ecosystems such as water (hydrosphere), land (lithosphere), and the air (atmosphere); the living factors of the planet can be referred to collectively as the biosphere. All the chemicals, nutrients, or elements—such as carbon, nitrogen, oxygen, phosphorous—used in ecosystems by living organisms operate on a *closed system*, which refers to the fact that these chemicals are recycled instead of being lost and replenished constantly such as in an open system. The energy of an ecosystem occurs on an *open system*; the sun constantly gives the planet energy in the form of light while it is eventually used and lost in the form of heat throughout the trophic levels of a food web.

(a) *Nitrogen Cycle*

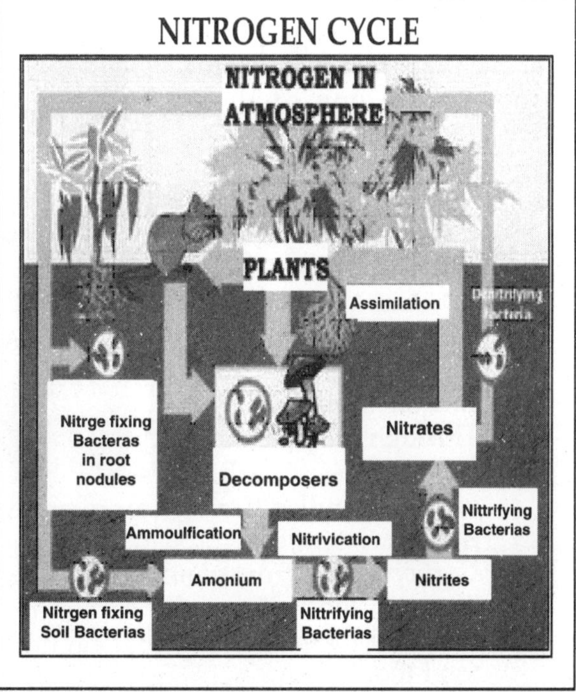

The nitrogen cycle is a much more complicated biogeochemical cycle but also cycles through living parts and non-living parts including the water, land, and air. Nitrogen is a very important molecule in that it is part of both proteins, present in the composition of the amino acids that make up proteins, as well as nucleic acids such as DNA and RNA, present in nitrogenous bases. The largest reservoir of nitrogen is the atmosphere, in which about 78 per cent of nitrogen is contained as nitrogen gas (N_2). Nitrogen gas is "fixed," in a process called nitrogen fixation. Nitrogen fixation combines nitrogen with oxygen to create nitrates (NO_3).

Nitrates can then be used by plants or animals (which eat plants or eat animals that have eaten plants). Nitrogen can be fixed either by lightning, industrial methods (such as for fertilizer), in free nitrogen-fixing bacteria in the soil, as well as in nitrogen-

nitrogen-fixing bacteria present in roots of legumes (such as rhizobium). Nitrogen-fixing bacteria use certain enzymes that are capable of fixing nitrogen gas into nitrates and include free bacteria in soil, symbiotic bacteria in legumes, and also cyanobacteria, or blue-green algae, in water.

After being used by plants and animals, nitrogen is then disposed of in decay and wastes. Detritivores and decomposers decompose the detritius from plants and animals, nitrogen is changed into ammonia, or nitrogen with 3 hydrogen atoms (NH_3). Ammonia is toxic and cannot be used by plants or animals, but nitrite bacteria present in the soil can take ammonia and turn it into nitrite, nitrogen with two oxygen atoms (NO_2). Although nitrite is also unusable by most plants and animals, nitrate bacteria changes nitrites back into nitrates, usable by plants and animals. Some nitrates are also converted back into nitrogen gas through the process of denitrification, which is the opposite of nitrogen-fixing, also called nitrification. Certain denitrifying bacteria are responsible for this.

(b) *The Carbon Cycle*

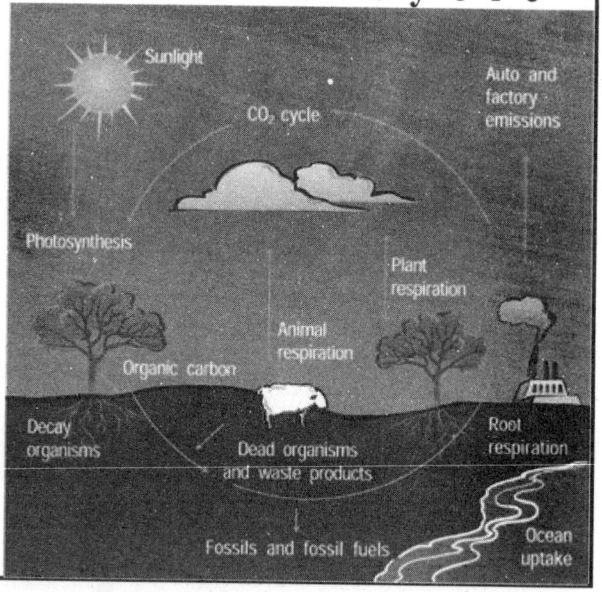

The *element* carbon is a part of *seawater*, the *atmosphere*, *rocks* such as *limestone* and coal, soils, as well as all *living things*. On our dynamic planet, carbon is able to move from one of these realms to another as a part of the *carbon cycle*.

Carbon cycle

- ***Carbon moves from the atmosphere to plants***
  In the *atmosphere*, carbon is attached to oxygen in a gas called carbon dioxide (CO_2). Through the process of *photosynthesis*, carbon dioxide is pulled from the air to produce food made from carbon for plant growth.
- ***Carbon moves from plants to animals***
  Through food chains, the carbon that is in *plants* moves to the *animals* those eat them. Animals that eat other animals get the carbon from their food too.
- ***Carbon moves from plants and animals to soils***
  When plants and animals die, their bodies wood and leaves decays bringing the carbon into the ground. Some is buried and will become fossil fuels in millions and millions of years.

- ***Carbon moves from living things to the atmosphere***
  Each time you exhale, you are releasing carbon dioxide gas (CO_2) into the atmosphere. Animals and plants need to get rid of carbon dioxide gas through a process called *respiration*.
- ***Carbon moves from fossil fuels to the atmosphere when fuels are burned***
  When humans burn fossil fuels to power factories, power plants, cars and trucks, most of the carbon quickly enters the atmosphere as carbon dioxide gas. Each year, five and a half billion tonnes of carbon is released by burning fossil fuels. Of this massive amount, 3.3 billion tonnes stays in the atmosphere. Most of the remainder becomes dissolved in *seawater.*
- ***Carbon moves from the atmosphere to the oceans***
  The oceans, and other bodies of water, absorb some carbon from the atmosphere. The carbon is dissolved into the water. *Marine animals* are able to use the carbon to build their skeletal material.

V. Balance in Ecosystem

An ecosystem develops over a long period. It reaches a State of delicate balance. All the species in the food webs get enough to eat. The food is just enough for them to multiply at the correct rate to keep the ecosystem going. Abiotic conditions like the climate, water availability, and sunlight are just right.

How do so many species live together in an ecosystem without fierce competition taking place? Organism do compete for food, but this does not lead generally to examination of species. The reason is that each species in an ecosystem has found its habitat.

The habitat of a species of plant or animal is the area where the species is particularly adapted to live. The environmental conditions of the area, such as the vegetation, climate, and the water availability, suit the species.

The habitats of different species in an ecosystem are generally different and this enables the species to live together in an ecosystem. For example, in a tropical rainforest, many species live on the same tree, but at different heights.

The balance in an ecosystem can be easily upset. Sometimes it is due to natural causes like fires or earthquackes. In recent times, however, human activities have been disturbing the balance of many ecosystems.

The interconnections in nature are so complex that we cannot predict all the consequences of degradation of ecosystems. Scientists agree, however, on effects like the following :

☞ Many species are becoming extinct, affecting many food webs.

☞ Global warming is taking place and naural disasters are increasing in frequency and severity.

☞ Natural resources like water are becoming scare.

VI. Ecological Succession / Adoption

Ecological succession, a fundamental concept in ecology, refers to more or less predictable and orderly changes in the composition or structure of an ecological community. Succession may be initiated either by formation of new, unoccupied habitat (*e.g.*, a lava flow or a severe landslide) or by some form of disturbance (*e.g.* fire, severe windthrow, waterlogging, etc.) of an existing community. The former case is often referred to as primary succession, the latter as secondary succession.

The idea of ecological succession goes back to the nineteenth century. In 1860 Henry David Thoreau read an address called "The Succession of Forest Trees" in which he described succession in an Oak-Pine forest. Henry Chandler Cowles, at the University of Chicago, developed a more formal concept of succession, following his studies of sand dunes on the shores of Lake Michigan (the Indiana Dunes). He recognized that vegetation on sand-dunes of different ages might be interpreted as different stages of a general trend of vegetation development on dunes, and used his observations to propose a particular sequence (sere) and process of primary succession.

Process of Succession

The process of succession takes place in a systamic order of sequential steps as follows :

1. *Nudation:* It is the development of the bare area without any life form.
2. *Invasion:* It is the successful establishment of one or more species on a bare area through dispersal or migration.
3. *Competition and coaction:* As the number of individuals grows there is competition, both inter-specific (between different species) and intra-specific (within the same species), for space, water and nutrition.They influence each other in a number of ways, known as coaction.
4. *Reaction:* The living organism grow, use water and nutrients from the substratum, in turn, they have a strong influence on the environment which is modified to a large extent and this is known as reaction.
5. *Stabilization:* The succession ultimately culminates in a more or less stable community called climax which is the equilibrium with the environment.

Ecological Adoption

All living organism adapt themselves against the unfavorable conditions of the atmosphere. Any such feature that the organism develops for coping up with the atmospheric condition is known as adoption. Plants being manufacturer of food are termed as food producers.

Plants have been divided into the following major ecological groups on the basis of their water relation.

- **Hydrophytes**—(hydro=water; Phyta=plants) Plants of water bodies.
- **Xerophytes** —(Xero=drying up; phytes=plants) Plants of Dry region.
- **Mesophytes**—(Meso=middle, Intermediate; phyton=plants) Plants of moderate atmospheric conditions.
- **Halophytes** —(Halo=salt; phytes=plants)—Plants of Salt region.
- **Epiphytes**—They grow on the plants but unlike parasites they manufacture their own food.

VII. Benefits of Ecosystem

The benefits that humans derive from ecosystems can be direct or indirect.

Direct benefits are harvested largely from the plants and animals in an ecosystem in the form of food and raw materials. These are the most familiar "products" an ecosystem yields as crops, livestock, fish, game, lumber, fuel wood, and fodder. Genetic resources that flow from the biodiversity of the world's ecosystems also provide direct benefits by contributing genes for improving the yield and disease resistance of crops, and for developing medicines and other products.

Indirect benefits arise from interactions and feedback among the organisms living in an ecosystem. Many of them take the form of services, like the erosion control and water purification and storage that plants and soil microorganisms provide in a watershed, or the pollination and seed dispersal that many insects, birds, and mammals provide. Other benefits are less tangible, but nonetheless highly valued: the scenic enjoyment of a sunset, for example, or the spiritual significance of a sacred mountain or forest grove. Every year, millions of people make pilgrimages to outdoor holy places, vacation in scenic regions, or simply pause in a park or their gardens to reflect or relax. As the manifestation of nature, ecosystems are the psychological and spiritual backdrop for our lives.

Some benefits are global in nature, such as biodiversity or the storage of atmospheric carbon in plants and soils. Others are regional; watershed protection that prevents flooding far downstream is an example. But many ecosystem benefits are local, and these are often the most important, affecting people directly in many aspects of their daily lives. Homes, industries, and farms usually get their water supplies from local sources, for instance. Jobs associated with agriculture and tourism are local benefits as well. Urban and suburban parks, scenic vistas, and the enjoyments of backyard trees and wildlife are all local products that define our sense of place.

Because so many ecosystem goods and services are enjoyed locally, it follows that local inhabitants often suffer most when these benefits are lost. By the same token, it is local inhabitants who usually have the greatest incentive to preserve the ecosystems they depend on. In fact, local people hold enormous potential both for managing ecosystems sustainably and for damaging them through careless use. But local communities rarely exert full control over the ecosystems they inhabit; with the market for ecosystem goods becoming increasingly global, outside economic forces and government policies can overwhelm the best local intentions.

VIII. Major Types of Ecosystem

Ecosystems can be categorized in different ways; some of them are as follows:

Ecosystem Types

- Natural
  - *(Acquatic)*
    1. Fresh Water
    2. Marine
  - *(Terrestrial)*
    1. Grassland
    2. Savanna
    3. Taiga
    4. Tundra
    5. Desert
    6. Forest
- Artificial (Man made)
  1. Agroecosystem etc.

The learned scientists of World Resource Institute, Washington DC, USA, under Pilot Analysis of Global Ecosystems (PAGE) studied the major ecosystem of the world which effects the human population of the world. The PAGE study assessed five of the world's major ecosystem types as follows.

- *Forest ecosystems* cover 22 per cent of the land surface (excluding Antarctica and Greenland) and contribute more than 2 per cent of global GDP through the production and manufacture of industrial wood products alone.
- *Grassland ecosystems* (including shrublands) cover 41 per cent of the land surface (excluding Antarctica and Greenland) and are critical producers of protein and fibre from livestock, particularly in developing countries.
- *Coastal ecosystems* (including marine fisheries) cover approximately 22 per cent of the total land area in a 100-km band along continental and island coastlines, as well as the ocean area above the continental shelf. The coastal zone is home to roughly 2.2 billion people or 39 per cent of the world's population and yields as much as 95 per cent of the marine fish catch.
- *Freshwater systems* cover less than 1 per cent of Earth's surface but they are the source of water for drinking, domestic use, agriculture, and industry;

freshwater fish and mollusks are also a major source of protein for humans and animals.

☞ *Agricultural ecosystems* or "agro ecosystems" cover 28 per cent of the land surface (excluding Antarctica and Greenland) and account for $ 1.3 trillion in output of food, feed, and fibre and for 99 per cent of the calories humans consume.

Together these five ecosystem types, which overlap in some places, cover the bulk of Earth's land area and a significant portion of the ocean area. They are also home to much of the world's population. Other ecosystems, such as polar zones, high mountains, ocean areas beyond the continental shelves, and even urban ecosystems account for the remainder of the area and are important in their own right. But the condition of the goods and services produced by these five major ecosystems will largely determine how well Earth's living systems meet human needs today and in the future.

Primary Goods and Services provided by Ecosystems

Ecosystem	*Goods*	*Services*
Forest Ecosystems	• Timber • Fuel wood • Drinking and irrigation water • Fodder • Non-timber products (vines, bamboos, leaves, etc.) • Food (honey, mushrooms, fruit, and other edible plants; game) • Genetic resources	• Remove air pollutants, emit oxygen • Cycle nutrients • Maintain array of watershed functions (infiltration, purification, flow control, soil stabilization) • Maintain biodiversity • Sequester atmospheric carbon • Moderate weather extremes and impacts • Generate soil • Provide employment • Provide human and wildlife habitat • Provide for aesthetic enjoyment and recreation
Grassland Ecosystems	• Livestock (food, game, hides, fibre) • Drinking and irrigation water • Genetic resources	• Maintain array of watershed functions (infiltration, purification, flow control, soil stabilization) • Cycle nutrients • Remove air pollutants, emit oxygen • Maintain biodiversity • Generate soil • Sequester atmospheric carbon • Provide human and wildlife habitat • Provide employment • Provide for aesthetic enjoyment and recreation

(Contd...)

Contd...

Ecosystem	*Goods*	*Services*
Coastal Ecosystems	• Fish and shellfish • Fishmeal (animal feed) • Seaweeds (for food and industrial use) • Salt • Genetic resources	• Moderate storm impacts (mangroves; barrier islands) • Provide wildlife (marine and terrestrial) habitat • Maintain biodiversity • Dilute and treat wastes • Provide harbours and transportation routes • Provide human habitat • Provide employment • Provide for aesthetic enjoyment and recreation
Freshwater Systems	• Drinking and irrigation water • Fish • Hydroelectricity • Genetic resources	• Buffer water flow (control timing and volume) • Dilute and carry away wastes • Cycle nutrients • Maintain biodiversity • Provide aquatic habitat • Provide transportation corridor • Provide employment • Provide for aesthetic enjoyment and recreation
Agro-ecosystems	• Food crops • Fibre crops • Crop genetic resources	• Maintain limited watershed functions (infiltration, flow control, partial soil protection) • Provide habitat for birds, pollinators, soil organisms important to agriculture • Build soil organic matter • Sequester atmospheric carbon • Provide employment

Sources : *Linking People and Ecosystems*, page no. 9, World Resources Institute, Washington, D.C. USA.

Major ecosystems of the world are as follows :

(a) *Forest Ecosystem*

These are the ecosystems having predominance of trees that are interspersed with a large number of species of herbs, shrubs, climbers, lichens, algae and a wide variety of wild animals and birds. Major sub-types of forest ecosystem are as follows :

1. The Tropical Rain Forest Ecosystem

Tropical rain forests are one of the most important areas on Earth. They are found in Congo basin of Africa, Amazon basin of South America, East Indies and India. These special ecosystems are homes to thousands of species animals and plants. Rain forests are not only densely packed plants, but are also full of tall trees that form a ceiling from the Sun above. This ceiling keeps smaller plants from growing. Areas where sunlight can reach the surface are full of interesting plants.

Tropical rain forests

Dark areas on the map show the locations

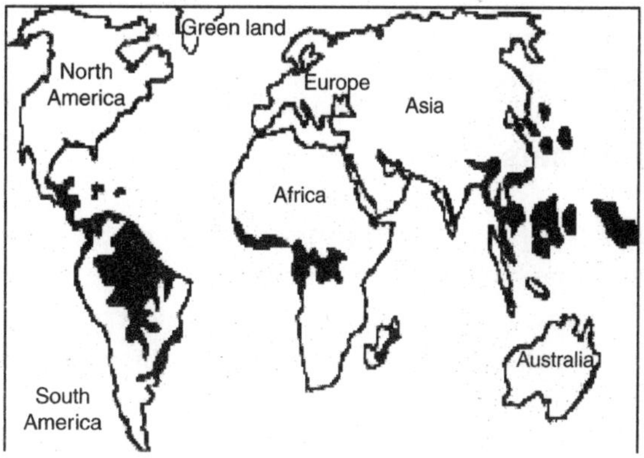

Rain forests get their name because they receive a lot of rain, on an average of 200 – 250 cm a year! The temperature does not change very much during the year. It is always warm and muggy.

Insects

The most feared spider in the world resides in the jungle. Tarantulas are one of the creepiest animals you will ever see. Most species of tarantula have poisonous fangs for killing prey and for protection. Although some are life-threatening to humans, others are harmless. Army ants are just one species of ant in the rain forest. They are called army ants because they march in a long, thick line through the jungle. Beautiful butterflies fill the forest.

Birds

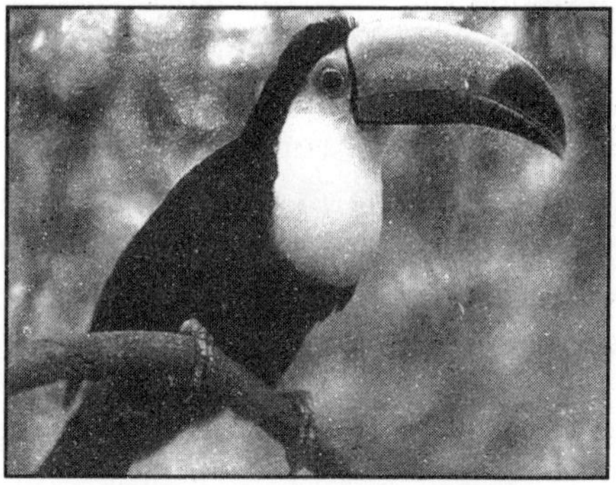

The birds of the rain forest are the most beautiful in the world. A wide range of colours can be seen flying through the trees. Many species of tropical birds are kept as pets because of their looks.

Hundreds of species of parrot live in the rain forest. The scarlet macaw is just one of these. It is also one of the longest, stretching to a length of 3 feet from its head to the tip of its tail. When these macaws eat a poisonous fruit, they eat a special type of clay that gets rid of the poison.

Toucans are also very colorful birds. They have large beaks that they use to reach fruit they can not get to. Scientists estimate that there are 33 species of toucan in the rain forest. Not every tropical bird was blessed with looks. The hoatzin looks more like a peacock without the pretty tail. Hoatzins are terrible flyers that crash land all the time ! The brown kiwi is a flightless bird that looks more like a rodent with a long beak and feathers. They have special claws used for running, digging and defence.

Mammals

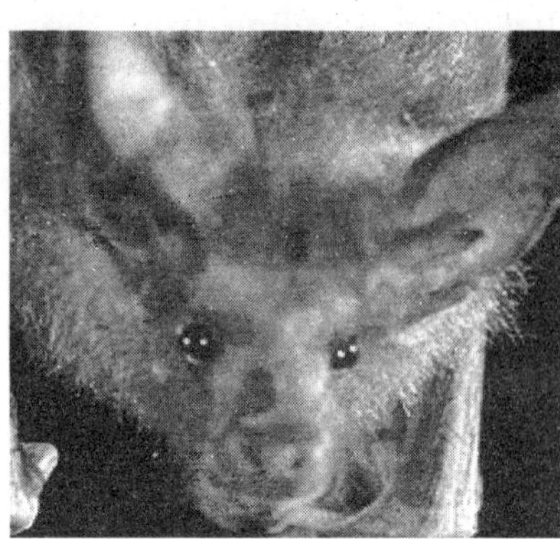

Several species of mammals live in the jungle. From the harmless fruit bat to the flying squirrel, the tropical rain forests are full of surprises.

The Indian flying fox is one of the largest bats in the world. Its wings can spread out to 5 feet in width ! Unlike bats in other parts of the world, these bats do not live in caves. They prefer to hang in trees during the day. Hundreds or even thousands of bats can be spotted in a single tree.

Vampire bats live in the Amazon jungle in South America. These bats do in fact drink the blood of their victims. They usually attack farm animals, but have also enjoyed the blood of humans.

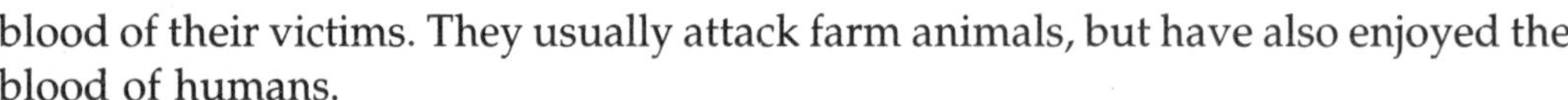

Reptiles

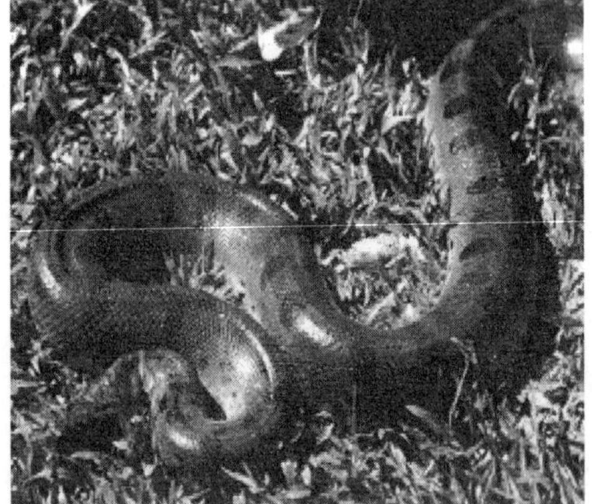

The tropical rain forests of the world are full of reptiles. Reptiles are cold blooded, which means their body temperature depends on their environment. So, it is important for them to stay in warm climates.

Snakes are reptiles, and there are plenty of them in the rain forests ! The mamba family is the most poisonous of all. They kill their prey by injecting poison with their sharp fangs.

Anacondas make up another snake family. They can reach 30 feet in length. Anacondas prefer to wrap themselves around their prey and squeeze, rather than inject poison. Anacondas swallow their prey whole and sleep while the food is digesting.

Chameleons are interesting lizards that can change colour. Geckos are very neat creatures. The flying gecko can glide from tree to tree to escape from predators.

Primates

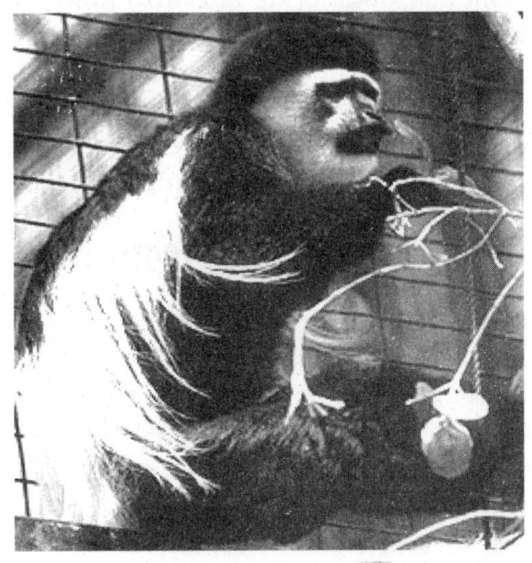

Monkeys and their cousins are all primates. Humans are also primates. There are many species of monkey in the tropical rain forests of the world. Monkeys can be divided into two groups: new world monkeys and old world monkeys.

New world monkeys live only in South and Central America. Spider monkeys live in the rain forests in the Andes Mountains. They look very strange with their long noses. Spider monkeys eat mostly fruit and nuts. They are joined by the howler monkeys. These primates are so named because they have a special sac that makes their sounds louder.

Old world monkeys live only in Africa and Asia. The colobus monkey is one such kind. These monkeys eat leaves. They live in small groups of 15, but other primates live in larger groups of up to 200.

There are too many species to discuss here, but we can name a few. Chimpanzees, orangutans and gorillas are all called pongids. Gorillas are too big to climb trees, so they are found on the forest floor.

2. Temperate Forest Ecosystem

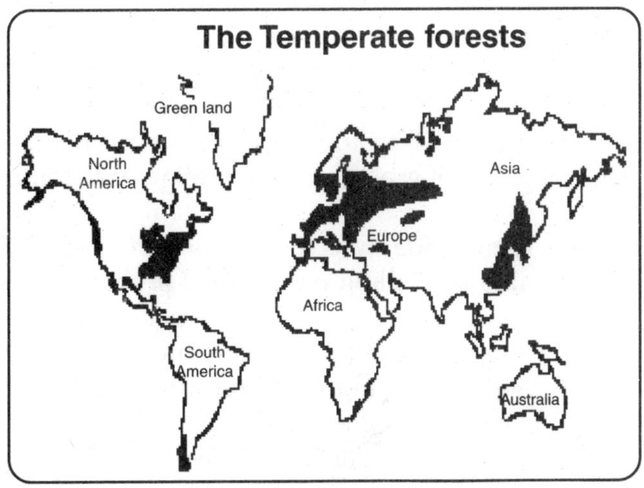

The temperate forest ecosystem is very important on Earth. Temperate forests are in regions where the climate changes a lot from summer to winter.

Temperate forests are made of two types of trees, deciduous and evergreen. Deciduous trees are trees that lose their leaves in the winter. Evergreens are trees that keep them all year long, like pine trees. Forests can either be one or the other, or a combination of both. A fourth kind of forest is a temperate rain forest. These are found in California, Oregon and Washington in the United States. These forests are made of redwoods and sequoias, the tallest trees in the world.

The amount of rainfall in an area determines if a forest is present. If there is enough rain to support trees, then a forest will usually develop. Otherwise, the region will become grassland.

(b) *Grassland Ecosystem*

Over one quarter of the Earth's surface is covered by grasslands. Grasslands are found on every continent except Antarctica, and they make up most of Africa and Asia. There are several types of grassland and each one has its own name such as Prairies in North America, Pampas in Argentina, Steppes in Eurasia, Puszter in Hungary, Veldts in South Africa, and Tussocks in New Zeland.

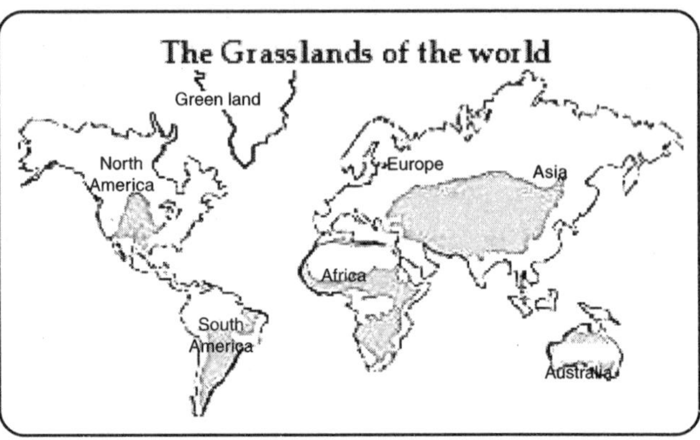

Grasslands develop where there is not enough rain for forests but too much rain for deserts. Grasslands are filled with grass.

There are many types of grass, though. Fields of wheat are considered grasslands, even though they are often cultivated by people. Grass is special because it grows underneath the ground. During cold periods the grass can stay dormant until it warms up.

World Resources Institute (WRI) report shows striking declines in world's grasslands. The world's grasslands have declined in their extent and condition, as well as their ability to support human, plant, and animal life. Some of the characteristics of grassland ecosystem are as follows :

- Grasslands, which cover 40 per cent of the earth's surface, are home to almost a billion people, half of them living in susceptible drylands.
- Agriculture and urbanization are transforming grasslands. For some North American prairies, conversion is already nearly 100 per cent. Road-building and human-induced fires also are changing the extent, composition, and structure of grasslands.
- All of the major foodgrains — corn, wheat, oats, rice, barley, millet, rye, and sorghum — originate in grasslands. Wild strains of grasses can provide

genetic material to improve food crops and to help keep cultivated varieties resistant to disease.

- Grasslands attract tourists willing to travel long distances and pay safari fees to hunt and view grassland fauna. Grasslands boast some of the world's greatest natural phenomena: major migratory treks of large herds of wildebeest in Africa, caribou in North America, and Tibetan antelope in Asia.

As habitat for biologically important flora and fauna, grasslands are found within 15 per cent of the Centres of Plant Diversity, 11 per cent of Endemic Bird Areas, and 29 per cent of ecoregions considered outstanding for biological distinctiveness.

(c) *Desert Ecosystem*

Desert occupy one-fifth of the earth's surface occurring in the region with an annual rainfall of less than 25 cms/year. There is at least one desert on every continent except Europe and Antarctica. In hot deserts the day temperature is 50^0 C or more and night temperature is low. Sand storms are very common in the desert ecosystem.

Deserts are more in southern hemisphere, some major are as Sahara desert in North Africa, Gobi desert in China, Arabian desert, Thar desert, Atakama and Patagonia in South America, Kalahari desert in South Africa.

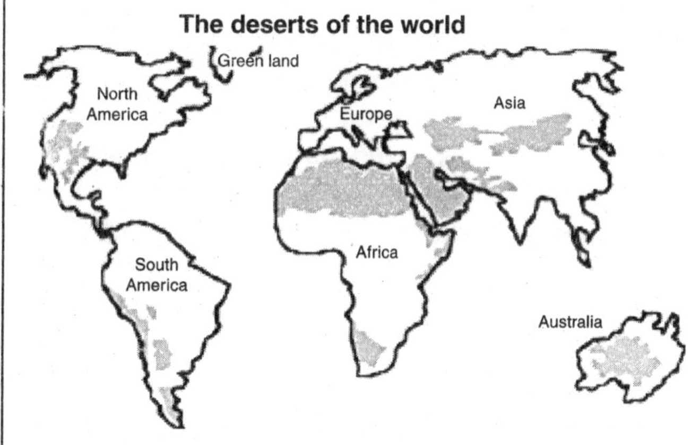

There are plenty of differences between the deserts of the world. Some deserts are made of very fine, red sand, others consists of sand mixed with pebbles and rocks. There are six types of desert as hot deserts, Warm semi desert scrub, Cold desert, Semi cold desert, Arctic alpine semi desert and Arctic or Alpine desert.

The desert sand started out as rock, but years of weathering by wind and water has created dunes in the deserts. These sands are mostly minerals, and sometimes oil can be found hidden deep within the rocks.

Desert Plants

The most famous desert plant is the cactus. There are many species of cacti. The saguaro cactus is the tall, pole shaped cactus you see on television. The saguaro can grow up to 40 feet tall. It can hold several tonnes of water inside its soft tissue. Like all cacti, the saguaro has a thick, waxy layer that protects it from the Sun.

Saguaro cactus

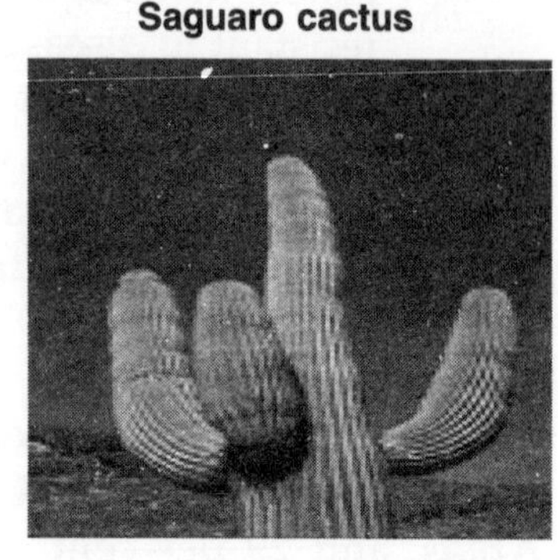

Other succulents include the desert rose and the living rock. This strange plant looks like a spiny rock. Its disguise protects it from predators. The welwitschia is a weird looking plant. It has two long leaves and a big root. This plant is actually a type of tree and it can live for thousands of years.

Desert Insects and Arachnids

One of the most common and destructive pests is the locust. A locust is a special type of grasshopper. They travel from place to place, eating all the plants they find. Locusts can destroy many crops in a single day.

Hairy Scorpion

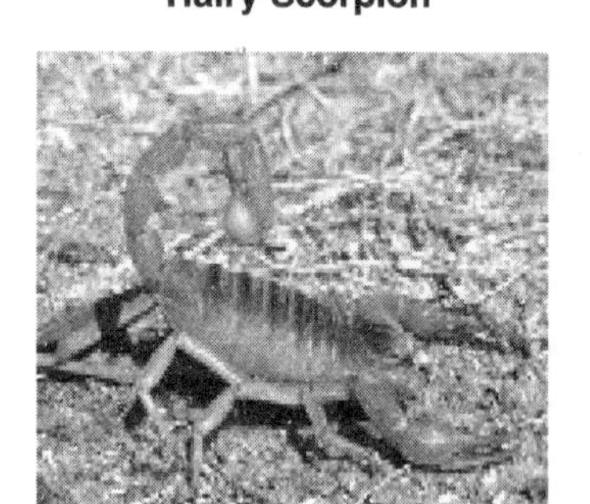

The darkling beetle has a hard, white, wing case that reflects the Sun's energy. This allows the bug to look for food during the day.

There are also several species of ants in the desert. The harvester ants gather seeds and store them for use during the dry season. There are also arachnids in the desert. Spiders are the most notable arachnids, but scorpions also belong in this group. Some species of scorpions have poison in their sharp tails. They sting their predators and their prey with the piercing tip.

Desert Birds

Like the other creatures of the desert birds come up with interesting ways to survive in the harsh climate. The sandgrouse has special feathers that soak up water. It can then carry the water to its young trapped in the nest.

Roadrunner

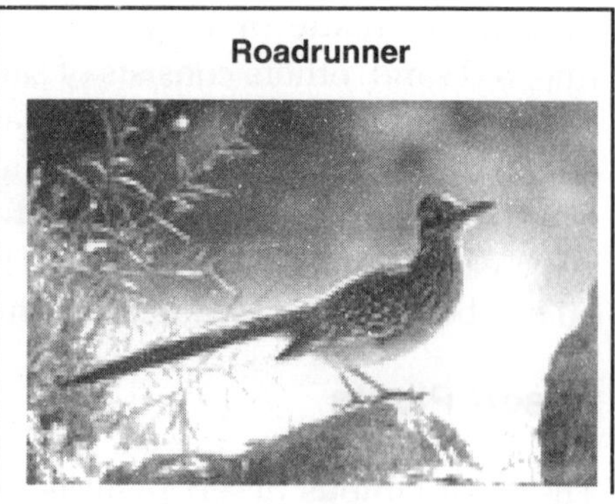

Other birds, like the gila woodpecker, depend on the giant saguaro as its home. This woodpecker hollows out a hole in the cactus for a nest. The cool, damp inside is safe for the babies.

The roadrunner is probably the most well known desert bird, thanks to the cartoon. Roadrunners are so named because they prefer to run rather than fly. Ostriches also prefer to use their feet. Even the young depend on walking to find food and water.

The galah is one of the prettiest desert birds. It is one of the few species that return to the same nest year after year. Galahs are interesting birds, in that the number of eggs they lay depends on the climate.

Desert Reptiles

Gila monster

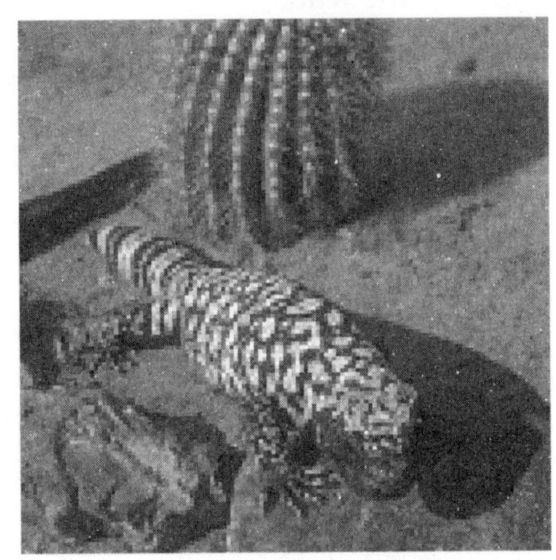

Reptiles are some of the most interesting creatures of the desert. Reptiles can withstand the extreme temperatures because they can control their body temperatures very easily. There are two main types of desert reptiles: snakes and lizards. Many species of rattlesnakes can be found in the desert. Other desert snakes include the cobra, kingsnake and the hognose. Lizards are probably the most bizarre looking animals in the desert. While some change colours and have sharp scales for defence, others change their appearance to look more threatening. One such creature is the frilled lizard.

Desert Mammals

Spiny anteater

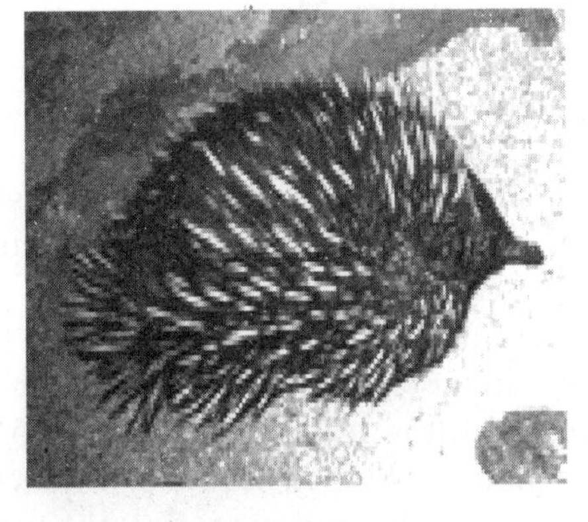

Many desert mammals dig holes in the ground and stay there during the hot days. They return to the surface at night to feed. Hamsters, rats and their relatives live in holes. The kangaroo and spiny anteater both live in the Australian desert region. Spiny anteaters are unusual mammals because they lay eggs.

The desert is also full of wild horses, foxes and jackals, which are part of the canine family. And we can not forget the cats. Lions are found all over the deserts of southern Africa.

Camels—The Cars of the Desert

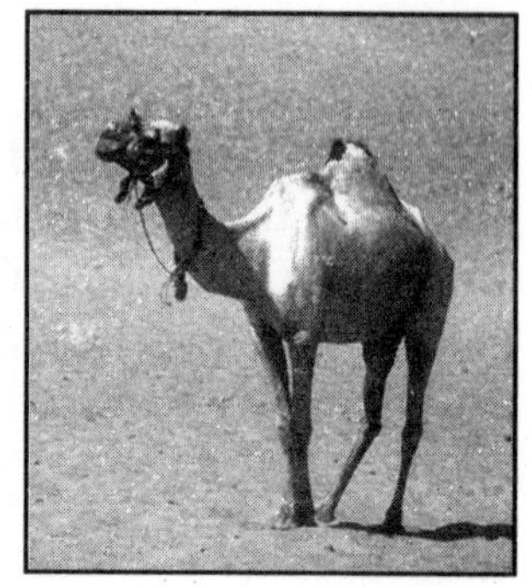

Camels could be included in the mammal section, but they are such an important part of the desert we devoted a whole page to them ! Camels are the cars of the desert. They are the main transportation for people that live in the desert.

There are two types of camels: bactrian and dromedary. The main difference between the two is the number of humps. Dromedaries have one hump, and bactrian have two. Both kinds are used by people, but only bactrians are found in the wild.

Camels are used because they need very little water. Camels can withstand very high temperatures without sweating. They also store fat in their humps for food. If a bactrian camel travels a long distance without eating, its hump will actually get smaller.

(d) *Tundra Ecosystem*

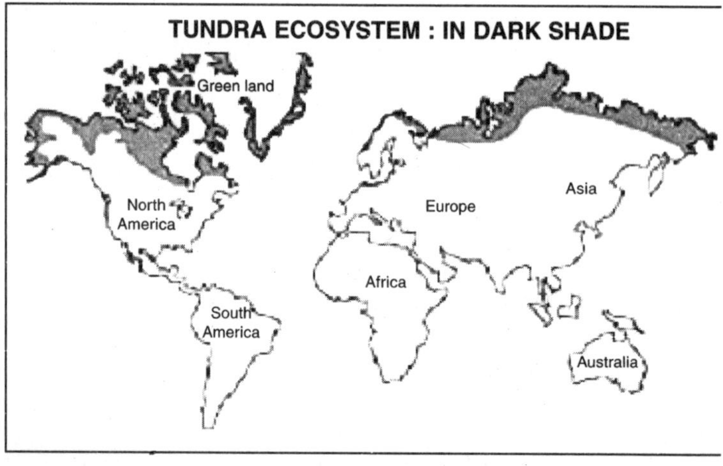

In the very cold places of the world, survival is not easy. The soil is frozen, its top surface thawing only during summer, and no trees can grow. Yet plants and animals that are adapted for the harsh conditions thrive. This ecosystem, or biome, is called tundra. Most of the world's tundra is found in the Arctic, as shown in the map. It is called Arctic tundra. There is a small amount of tundra on parts of Antarctica that are not covered with ice. Plus, tundra is found on mountains at high altitudes and is called alpine tundra.

Permafrost is the term given to frozen soil. During the winter months, permafrost reaches the surface of the tundra. It is very cold during the winter, with temperatures reaching negative 60 degrees F ! It is of course wondering how anything can live in such a cold place.

Well, in the summer time, the tundra changes. The Sun is out almost 24 hours a day, so the tundra starts to warm up. The permafrost melts at the surface, and plant life grows. However, the permafrost only disappears for a few inches below the surface. There is not enough soil for trees to grow, so only small plants are found in the tundra.

At the same time, a variety of animals come out to feast on the plants. Insects come to feed on the animals, and birds appear to enjoy the insects. What results is a very busy ecosystem !

(e) *Aquatic Ecosystem*

An *aquatic ecosystem* is an ecosystem located in a body of water. Abiotic environmental factors of aquatic ecosystems include temperature, salinity, and flow. The amount of dissolved oxygen in a water body is frequently the key substance in determining the extent and kinds of organic life in the water body. Fish need dissolved oxygen to survive. The salinity of the water body is also a determining factor in the kinds of species found in the water body. Organisms in marine ecosystems tolerate salinity, while many freshwater organisms are intolerant of salt.

The organisms (also called biota) found in aquatic ecosystems are either autotrophic or heterotrophic.

Autotrophic organisms are producers that generate organic compounds from inorganic material. Algae use solar energy to generate biomass from carbon dioxide and are the most important autotrophic organisms in aquatic environments. Chemosynthetic bacteria are found in benthic marine ecosystems. These organisms are able to feed on hydrogen sulphide in water that comes from volcanic vents. Great concentrations of animals that feed on this bacteria are found around volcanic vents.

Heterotrophic organisms consume autotrophic organisms and use the organic compounds in their bodies as energy sources and as raw materials to create their own biomass. Euryhaline organisms are salt tolerant and can survive in marine ecosystems, while stenohaline or salt intolerant species can only live in freshwater environments.

The two main types of aquatic ecosystems are marine ecosystems and freshwater ecosystems.

1. Marine Ecosystems

Marine ecosystems (ocean and seas) cover approximately 71 per cent of the Earth's surface and contain approximately 97 per cent of the planet's water. They generate 32 per cent of the world's net primary production. They are distinguished from freshwater ecosystems by the presence of dissolved compounds, especially salts, in the water. Approximately 85 per cent of the dissolved materials in seawater are sodium and chlorine. Seawater has an average salinity of 35 parts per thousand (ppt) of water. Actual salinity varies among different marine ecosystems.

Ocean water moves a lot, Tides, waves, surface currents, and deep water circulation are all types of ocean water movement. The oceans have a major effect on the weather, and they moderate the world's climate.

There are four major oceans. From biggest to smallest they are the Pacific, Atlantic, Indian and Arctic. The Pacific Ocean is so large it covers a third of the Earth's surface all by itself ! The largest sea is the South China Sea. People have used the oceans and seas for food and transportation for thousands of years.

Classes of organisms found in marine ecosystems include brown algae, dinoflagellates, corals, cephalopods, echinoderms, and sharks. Fish caught in marine ecosystems are the biggest source of commercial foods obtained from wild populations.

Environmental problems concerning marine ecosystems include unsustainable exploitation of marine resources (for example overfishing of certain species), water pollution, and building on coastal areas.

➢ Coastal Ecosystem

The continental margins, where coastal ecosystems reside, are regions of remarkable biological productivity and high accessibility. This has made them centres of human activity for millennia.

Coastal regions may define as "the intertidal and subtidal areas above the continental shelf (to a depth of 200 m) and adjacent land area up to 100 km inland from the coast."

Coastal ecosystems also includes marine fisheries because the bulk of the world's marine fish harvest as much as 95 per cent, by some estimates, is caught or reared in coastal waters.

Coral reefs, mangroves, tidal wetlands, sea grass beds, barrier islands, estuaries, peat swamps, and a variety of other habitats each provides its own distinct bundle of goods and services and faces somewhat different pressures.

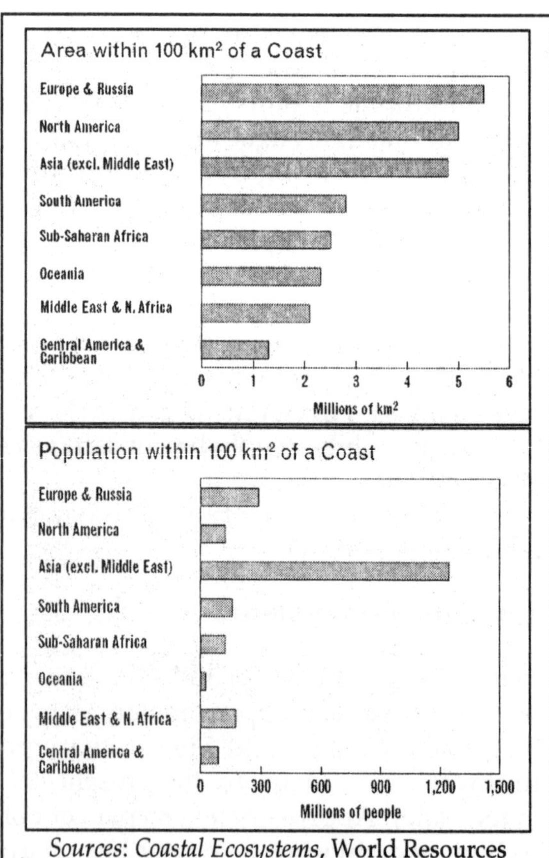

Sources: *Coastal Ecosystems*, World Resources Institute, Washington, D.C. USA

❖ Importance : Coastal Ecosystems

Coastal ecosystems provide a wide array of goods and services : they host the world's primary ports of commerce; they are the primary producers of fish, shellfish, and seaweed for both human and animal consumption; and they are also a considerable source of fertilizer, pharmaceuticals, cosmetics, household products, and construction materials.

➢ *Protection from Natural Calamities*

Healthy coastal ecosystems cannot completely protect communities from the impacts of storms and floods, but they do play an important role in stabilizing shorelines and buffering coastal development from the impact of storms, wind, and waves.

➢ *Food from Marine Fisheries*

Fish provided 16.5 per cent of the total animal protein consumed by humans in 1997. On an average this accounts for 6 per cent of all protein (plant and animal) that humans eat annually. Approximately 1 billion people rely on fish as their primary source of animal protein.

Global marine fish and shellfish production has increased six fold from 17 million tonnes in 1950 to 105 million metric tonnes in 1997.

The value of fishery exports in 1996 amounted to US$ 52.5 billion, 11 per cent of the value of agricultural exports that year.

➢ *Employment*

Fishing and aquaculture are major sources of employment as well, providing jobs for almost 29 million people worldwide in 1990. Some 95 per cent of these fish-related jobs were in developing countries.

➢ *Biodiversity*

Only 250,000 of the 1.75 million species catalogued to date in all ecosystems are found in marine environments, but experts believe that the majority of marine species have yet to be discovered and classified.

Life first evolved in the sea, and marine ecosystems still harbour an impressive variety of life forms.

➢ *Tourism*

In most countries, coastal tourism is the largest sector of this industry and in a number of countries; particularly Small Island developing states tourism contributes a significant and growing portion to GDP and foreign exchange. Travel and tourism in coastal zones can promote both conservation and economic development, if properly managed.

❖ Pressures on Coastal Ecosystems

A variety of factors are significantly altering coastal ecosystems. Chief among these are population growth, pollution, over harvesting, and the looming threat of climate change.

➢ *Population*

Globally, the number of people living within 100 km of the coast increased from roughly 2 billion in 1990 to 2.2 billion in 1995—39 per cent of the world's population.

However, the number of people whose activities affect coastal ecosystems is much larger than the actual coastal population because rivers deliver pollutants from inland watersheds and populations to estuaries and surrounding coastal waters.

Population Living Near a Coastline, 1995

Proximity to Coastline	*Population (in billion)*	*% of Total Population*
Within 25 km	1.143	20
Within 50 km	1.645	29
Within 100 km	2.212	39

➢ *Pollution*

A vast range of pollutants affects the world's coasts and oceans. These can be broadly classified into toxic chemicals (including organic chemicals, heavy metals, and radioactive waste), nutrients (including agricultural fertilizers and sewage), sediments, and solid waste. The occurrence of bacterial contamination is a special case, often associated with nutrient pollution. Oil pollution (from spills and seepage) includes toxic, nutrient, and sediment-based pollutants.

➢ *Over Harvesting*

Increasing fishing pressure have left many major fish stocks depleted or in decline. Yet over fishing is not a new phenomenon; it was recognized as an international problem as long ago as the early 1900s.

➢ *Climate Change*

Global climate change may compound other pressures on coastal ecosystems through the additional effects of warmer ocean temperatures, altered ocean circulation patterns, changing storm frequency, and rising sea levels. Changing concentrations of CO_2 in ocean waters may also affect marine productivity or even change the rate of coral calcification

❖ Modifications in Coastal Ecosystem

Overall, 19 per cent of all lands within 100 km of the coast is classified as highly altered, meaning they have been converted to agricultural or urban uses, 10 per cent semi altered (involving a mosaic of natural and altered vegetation), and 71 per cent are unaltered.

➢ *Mangroves and Coral Reefs*

Mangroves line approximately 8 per cent of the world's coastline. Some 112 countries and territories have mangroves within their borders. Although scientists cannot determine exactly how extensive mangroves were before people began to alter coastlines, based on historical records, anywhere from 5 to nearly 85 per cent of original mangrove area in various countries is believed to have been lost. Extensive losses have occurred in the last 50 years. For example, since 1975, much of the estimated 84 per cent of original mangroves were lost to Thailand. Overall, it is estimated that half of the world's mangroves forests have been destroyed

Coral reefs exist mostly in shallow tropical waters with minimal silt content. Shallow coral reefs occupy only 255,000 km^2 of the world's surface with more than 90 per cent in the Indo-Pacific region. Coral reefs are most extensive around the islands and coasts of the Western Pacific and Southeast Asia, which together encompass two-thirds of the world's coral ecosystems. These areas are also the richest in species diversity. Nonetheless, they support nearly 1 million species of plants and animals. Besides harbouring rich biodiversity, coral reefs provide an accessible area for small-scale fishing and help to protect coastlines from storm damage. Currently, on a global basis, coral reef degradation is a more serious problem.

➢ *Management Efforts to conserve Coastal Biodiversity*

Evidence of the declining condition of coastal biodiversity has stimulated a number of actions by local communities, NGOs, and national governments to slow the rate of loss of particular habitats and to protect the species that remain.

More than 3,600 marine protected areas have been designated throughout the world.

Sri Lanka spent US$ 30 million on revetments, groins, and breakwaters in response to severe coastal erosion that occurred in areas where coral reefs were heavily mined. Japan spent roughly 4.5 trillion yen (US$ 41 billion) on shoreline protection projects from 1970 to 1998 (Japanese Ministry of Commerce, 1998).

For many countries, protection of coastal ecosystems is likely to be one of the most cost-effective means of protecting coastal development from the impact of storms and floods.

Clearly, with the substantial loss in extent of various coastal ecosystems, the ability to provide this service of shoreline protection has significantly diminished in most nations.

2. Freshwater Ecosystems

Freshwater ecosystems cover 0.8 per cent of the Earth's surface and contain 0.009 per cent of its total water. They generate nearly 3 per cent of its net primary production. Freshwater ecosystems contain 41 per cent of the world's known fish species.

There are three basic types of freshwater ecosystems :

- *Lentic* : Slow-moving water, including pools, ponds, and lakes.
- *Lotic* : Rapidly-moving water, for example streams and rivers.
- *Wetlands* : Areas where the soil is saturated or inundated at least for some part of the time.

Lake Ecosystems

It can be divided into zones: pelagic (open offshore waters); profundal; littoral (nearshore shallow waters); and riparian (the area of land bordering a body of water). Two important subclasses of lakes are ponds, which typically are small lakes that integrade with wetlands, and water reservoirs. Many lakes, or bays within them, gradually become enriched by nutrients and fill in with organic sediments, a process called eutrophication. Eutrophication is accelerated by human activity within the water catchment area of the lake.

Pond Ecosystem

This is a specific type of freshwater ecosystem that is largely based on the autotroph algae which provide the base trophic level for all life in the area. The largest predator in a pond ecosystem will normally be a fish and in-between range smaller insects and microorganisms. It may have a scale of organisms from small bacteria to big creatures like water snakes, beetles, water bugs, and turtles.

River Ecosystems

The major zones in *river ecosystems* are determined by the river bed's gradient or by the velocity of the current. Faster moving turbulent water typically contains greater concentrations of dissolved oxygen, which supports greater biodiversity than the slow moving water of pools. These distinctions forms the basis for the division of rivers into upland and lowland rivers. The food base of streams within riparian forests is mostly derived from the trees, but wider streams and those that lack a canopy derive the majority of their food base from algae. Anadromous fish are also an important source of nutrients. Environmental threats to rivers include loss of water, dams, chemical pollution and introduced species.

Wetlands are dominated by vascular plants that have adapted to saturated soil. Wetlands are the most productive natural ecosystems because of the proximity of water and soil. Due to their productivity, wetlands are often converted into dry land with dikes and drains and used for agricultural purposes. Their closeness to lakes and rivers means that they are often developed for human settlement.

✶ Functions of Aquatic Ecosystem

Aquatic ecosystems perform many important environmental functions. For example, they recycle nutrients, purify water, attenuate floods, recharge ground water and provide habitats for wildlife. Aquatic ecosystems are also used for human recreation, and are very important to the tourism industry, especially in coastal regions. The health of an aquatic ecosystem is degraded when the ecosystem's ability to absorb a stress has been exceeded. *A stress* on an aquatic ecosystem can be a result of physical, chemical or biological alterations of the environment. Physical alterations include changes in water temperature, water flow and light availability. Chemical alterations include changes in the loading rates of biostimulatory nutrients, oxygen consuming materials, and toxins. Biological alterations include the introduction of exotic species. Human populations can impose excessive stresses on aquatic ecosystems.

IX. Polar Regions

An Emperor Penguin dives into the ocean through a hole in the ice

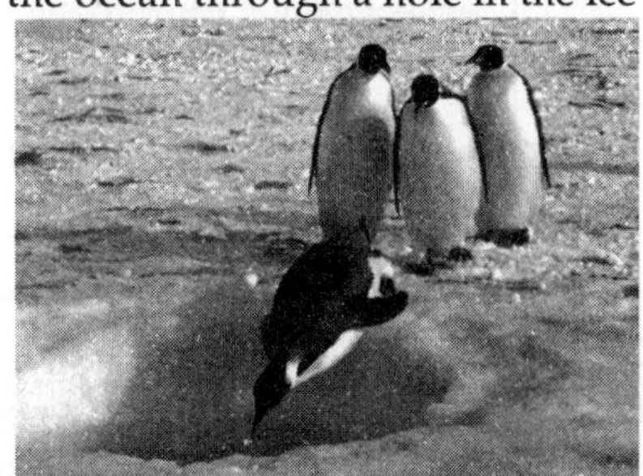

All sorts of living things call Earth's Polar Regions home – from tiny lichens encrusting the rocky landscapes of the Arctic tundra to huge blue whales swimming through the frigid waters of the Southern Ocean. Some animals are only part-time residents, migrating to warmer, lower latitudes during the winter months. Others live in polar

CASE STUDY

Kerala : Backwaters

The mangrove forests in particular have disappeared from the areas where retting predominate. Mangroves are the breeding grounds for fish fauna. The decimation of mangrove has led to precipitous decline in fish stocks. The solution to this problem is to evolve a technology which dispenses with the natural retting process. A recent development is the mechanical defibering process, which needs to be popularised.

The impact of developmental projects on the environment are a matter of serious concern. Kuttanad area is a typical example of such thoughtless developmental interventions. Kuttanad is a low-lying, shallow bay formed as a result of geological uplift. It has become an extensive brackish-water lagoon extending over 1100 km through the Vembanad Lake and Cochin estuary to the Arabian Sea. Five major rivers drain into it. It supports about 1.4 million people. The major economic activity is agriculture involving 40 per cent of the population. About 1.5 per cent of the people are engaged in aquaculture. However, human interventions, like salinity barrier at Thaneermukhom, extensive use of chemical fertilisers and pesticides, etc., have invited ecological disasters. The declining productivity has forced farmers and fisherfolk to change their traditional professions.

There are several reasons for shrinking of backwaters. The two major ones are natural and human interventions. Kerala has 41 rivers draining water from their catchment areas. Many of them drain into these backwaters. Increased deforestation in catchment areas has resulted in extensive soil erosion and silting of river mouths. A recent study found a very high annual sedimentation rate in one of the irrigation reservoirs. Apart from the silt from mountains, ocean currents also bring up sediment and deposit them in backwaters. Silting and sedimentation are the biggest problems in Cochin estuarine region. Cochin Port Trust spends enormous amount on dredging to keep the shipping channels open.

Population explosion and increased human activities are the most serious problems facing the country's ecosystems. The backwaters are no exception to it. The rate of urbanisation is unprecedented. The building boom due to defreezing of land and large inflow of money from Keralites living abroad will further strain the area's ecology, which is already under severe stress. A careful estimation of the ecosystem's carrying capacity and scientific development planning based on carrying capacity is essential to prevent an environmental catastrophe.

Dr. P. KUMARAN
National Environmental Engineering Research Institute
Regional Centre,
Kochi

locales year-round. Most have special adaptations that allow them to survive the extreme cold of the Earth's Polar Regions.

(a) Arctic

The windswept treeless plains of the Arctic tundra sometimes look barren, but they are inhabited by a multitude of plants and animals. A large amount of the land in the north polar region is part of Earth's tundra biome including the northern parts of Canada, Alaska (U.S.), Scandinavian countries, and Russia, as well as the northern fringes of Greenland that are not covered by ice. Travel south from the Arctic tundra, where temperatures are somewhat less frigid (although still really cold), and you are likely to find vast forests of conifer trees in the **taiga biome**. Travel north of the Arctic tundra you will find polar bears and the unique marine life in the Arctic Ocean.

(b) Antarctica

Antarctica is unique. It is the coldest, windiest, and driest continent on Earth. The land is barren and mostly covered with a thick sheet of ice. Antarctica is almost entirely south of the Antarctic Circle (66.5^0 S latitude). It is about one and a half times the size of the United States. Almost all of Antarctica is covered with a thick ice sheet. Ice shelves extend over the Ross and Weddell Seas. The little bits of land that are not covered by ice are very rocky. In several places under the ice sheet, there are freshwater lakes.

Antarctica

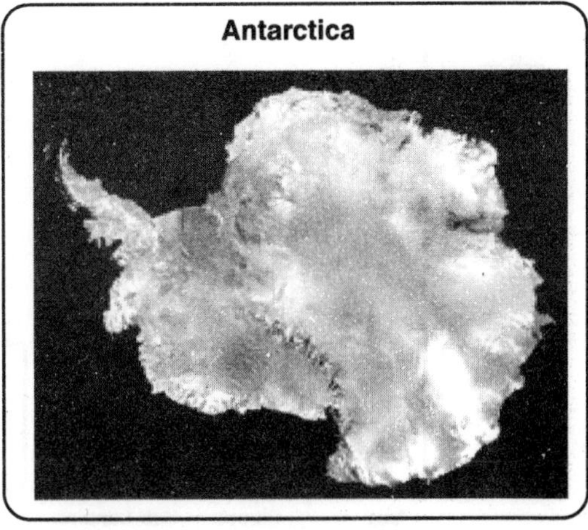

Temperatures can be very low. East Antarctica is colder than West Antarctica because it has a higher elevation. The Antarctic Peninsula has the warmest climate on the continent, however, high temperatures still average slightly below freezing point.

The tallest mountain of the continent of Antarctica is called Vinson Massif. It is 4,897 metres (16,050 feet) above sea level. This mountain formed as faults shifted, sending blocks of the Earth's crust up to higher elevations. Several of the other mountains in Antarctica are active volcanoes, including those on Deception Island and in remote parts of West Antarctica.

The Antarctic Treaty is an agreement between 45 countries that defines how Antarctica is to be shared as a place for scientific research. According to the treaty, no military from any country is allowed in Antarctica except to help with the scientific research. The treaty was first signed on December 1, 1959.

X. Conversion of Natural Ecosystems

Since the dawn of settled agriculture, humans have been altering the landscape to secure food, create settlements, and pursue commerce and industry. Croplands, pastures, urban and suburban areas, industrial zones, and the area taken up by roads, reservoirs, and other major infrastructure all represent conversion of natural ecosystems.

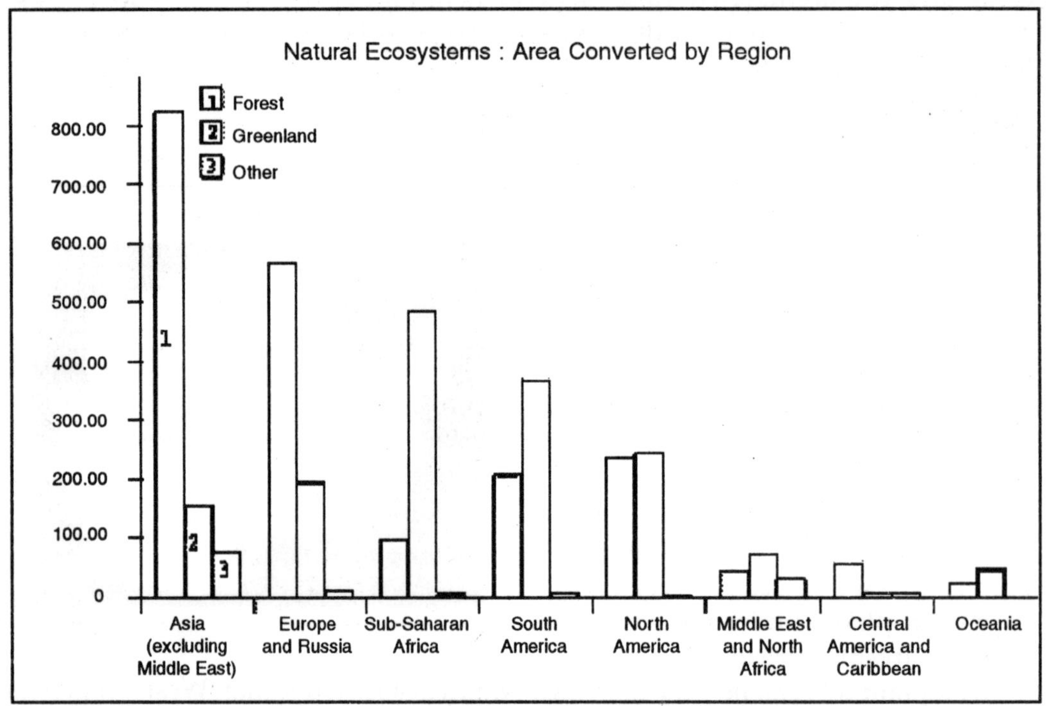

These transformations of the landscape are the defining mark of humans on Earth's ecosystems, yielding most of the food, energy, water, and wealth we enjoy, but they also represent a major source of ecosystem pressure.

Conversion alters the structure of natural ecosystems, and how they function, by modifying their basic physical properties— their hydrology, soil structure, and topography—and their predominant vegetation. This basic restructuring changes the complement of species that inhabits the ecosystem and disrupts the complex interactions that typified the original ecosystem. In many cases, the converted ecosystem is simpler in structure and less biologically diverse. In fact, habitat loss from conversion of natural ecosystems represents the primary driving force in the loss of biological diversity worldwide.

Historically, expansion of agriculture into forests, grasslands, and wetlands has been the greatest source of ecosystem conversion. Within the last century, however, expansion of urban areas with their associated roads, power grids, and other infrastructure, has also become a potent source of land transformation.

Worldwide, humans have converted approximately 29 percent of the land area almost 3.8 billion ha. to agriculture and urban or built-up.

Agricultural conversion to croplands and managed pastures has affected some 3.3 billion ha, roughly 26 per cent of the land area. All totalled, agriculture has displaced one-third of temperate and tropical forests and one-quarter of natural grasslands.

Agricultural conversion is still an important pressure on natural ecosystems in many developing nations, however, in some developed nations agricultural lands themselves are being converted to urban and industrial uses.

Natural Ecosystems : Area Converted by Region

Region	*Percentage of Land Converted*
Asia (excluding Middle East)	44
Central America & Caribbean	28
Europe & Russia	35
Middle East & North Africa	12
North America	27
Oceania	9
South America	33
Sub-Saharan Africa	25

Source: WRR calculations. World Resources Institute, Washington, D.C. USA, 2000.

Urban and built-up areas now occupy more than 471 million ha, about 4 per cent of land area. Almost half the world's population some 3 billion people live in cities. Urban populations increase by another 160,000 people daily, adding pressure to expand urban boundaries (UNEP 1999:47). Suburban sprawl magnifies the effect of urban population growth, particularly in North America and Europe. In the United States, the percentage of people living in urban areas increased from 65 per cent of the nation's population in 1950 to 75 per cent in 1990, but the area covered by cities roughly doubled in size during the same period.

Future trends in land conversion are difficult to predict, but projections based on the United Nations' intermediate range population growth model suggest that an additional one-third of the existing global land cover could be converted over the next 100 years.

Behind all the pressures impinging on ecosystems are two basic drivers : Human population growth and increasing consumption.

Primary Human-Induced Pressures on Ecosystems

Type of ecosystem	Direct Pressure	Indirect Pressure
Forest Ecosystems	• Conversion from agricultural or urban uses • Deforestation resulting in loss of biodiversity, release of stored carbon, air and water pollution • Acid rain from industrial pollution • Invasion of non-native species	• Population growth • Increasing demand for timber, pulp, and other fibre • Government subsidies for timber extraction and logging roads • Inadequate valuation of costs of industrial air pollution • Poverty and insecure tenure
Grassland Ecosystems	• Conversion due to agricultural or urban uses • grassland fires and loss of biodiversity, release of stored carbon, and air pollution • Soil degradation and water pollution from livestock herds	• Population growth • Increasing demand for agricultural products, especially meat • Inadequate information about ecosystem conditions • Poverty and insecure tenure • Accessibility and ease of conversion of grassland
Coastal Ecosystems	• Overexploitation of fisheries • Conversion of wetlands and coastal habitats • Water pollution from agricultural and industrial sources • Fragmentation or destruction of natural tidal barriers and reefs • Invasion of non-native species • Potential sea level rise	• Population growth • Increasing demand for food and coastal tourism • Urbanization and recreational development • Inadequate information about ecosystem conditions, especially for fisheries • Poverty and insecure tenure • Climate change
Freshwater Systems	• Over extraction of water for agricultural, urban, and industrial uses • Overexploitation of inland fisheries • Building dams for irrigation, hydropower, and flood control • Water pollution from agricultural, urban, and industrial uses • Invasion of non-native species	• Population growth • Widespread water scarcity and naturally uneven distribution of water resources • Government subsidies of water use • Inadequate valuation of costs of water pollution • Poverty and insecure tenure • Growing demand for hydropower
Agro-ecosystems	• Conversion of farmland to urban and industrial uses • Water pollution from nutrient runoff and siltation • Water scarcity from irrigation • Degradation of soil from erosion, shifting cultivation, or nutrient depletion • Changing weather patterns • Population growth	• Increasing demand for food and industrial goods • Urbanization • Government policies subsidizing • Agricultural inputs (water, research, transport) and irrigation, Poverty and insecure tenure • Climate change

Sources : World resources, Chapter-1, *Linking People and Ecosystems*, Page no. 19, World Resources Institute, Washington, D.C. USA.

Long answer type of questions

1. Define Ecology and Ecosystems.
2. What are the Biotic and Abiotic components of an Ecosystem?
3. Define Food Chain and Food Web? Give examples and discuss their significance.
4. Describe the flow of energy in an ecosystem.
5. What is an Ecological Pyramid? Write about its types.
6. What is Ecological Succession? Discuss in detail.
7. What are the Benefits of an Ecosystem?
8. What are the major types of Forest Ecosystem?
9. "Coastal Ecosystem is the regions of remarkable biological productivity and high accessibility" Explain in detail.
10. What are the primary human-induced pressures on ecosystems ?

Define the following terms

1. Food Chain
2. Food Web
3. Producers
4. Carnivores
5. Herbivores
6. Omnivores
7. Parasites
8. Detritivores
9. Trophic Levels

Fill in the blanks

1. The term Ecology was coined by................. in 1869.
2. Producers (autotrophs) utilize energy from the....................
3. In the ocean, ...is the primary producer.
4. Marine ecosystems cover approximately .... of the Earth's surface.
5. Food chain always starts with ....and culminates in top carnivorous.
6. Parasite is an organism that feeds on another living organism called.............
7. Tropical rain forests are found in Congo basin of ....

   Keys : 1. Earnst Haeckel; 2. sun; 3. Phytoplankton; 4. 71 per cent; 5. green plants; 6. Host; 7. Africa.

Tick the right answer

1. Forest ecosystems cover how much of the land surface (excluding Antarctica and Greenland)
   (a) 42 per cent
   (b) 32 per cent
   (c) 12 per cent
   (d) 22 per cent
2. Example of Herbivores is
   (a) deer
   (b) frogs
   (c) snakes
   (d) hawks
3. The modern crop plant can trap upto what per cent of the radiation falling on them?
   (a) 15%
   (b) 1%
   (c) 5%
   (d) 17%
4. The name of grassland found in North America is
   (a) Pampas
   (b) Steppes
   (c) Puszter
   (d) Prairies
5. The name of grassland found in Hungary is
   (a) Down
   (b) Steppes
   (c) Puszter
   (d) Zainu
6. The name of grassland found in South Africa is
   (a) Veldts
   (b) Steppes
   (c) Puszter
   (d) Hira
7. The name of grassland found in Eurasia is
   (a) Noreen
   (b) Steppes
   (c) Puszter
   (d) Prairies

   Keys : 1. d, 2. a, 3. c, 4. d, 5. c, 6. (a); 7. (b).

True / False types of questions.

1. **Herbivores** are those that eat only animals.
2. The amount of biomass produced for a given amount of solar energy is highest at the first level.
3. Interlinking of the food chains form a food web.
4. Food web helps in maintaining the stability in the ecosystem
5. On an average, only 52 Cal/cm^2/year of energy is trapped by the producers in producing organic food.
6. All chemical elements occurring in organisms are part of biogeochemical cycles.
7. The idea of ecological succession goes back to the nineteenth century

Keys : 1. false, 2. true, 3. true, 4. true, 5. false, 6. true, 7. true.

Unit - 4

Biodiversity and its Conservation

I. Introduction

Biodiversity or biological diversity is the diversity of life. There are a number of definitions and measures of biodiversity. The term *Biological Diversity* was coined by Thomas Lovejoy in 1980, while the word *Biodiversity* itself was coined by W.G. Rosen in 1985.

Biodiversity is the sum of all the different species of animals, plants, fungi, and microbial organisms living on Earth and the variety of habitats in which they live. Scientists estimate that upwards of 10 million—and some suggest more than 100 million—different species inhabit the Earth. Each species is adapted to its unique niche in the environment, from the peaks of mountains to the depths of deepsea hydrothermal vents, and from polar ice caps to tropical rain forests.

Biodiversity underlies everything from food production to medical research. Humans the world over use at least 40,000 species of plants and animals on a daily basis. Many people around the world still depend on wild species for some or all of their food, shelter, and clothing. All of our domesticated plants and animals came from wild-living ancestral species.

Healthy ecosystems are very important to biodiversity. They regulate many of the chemical and climatic systems that make available clean air and water and plentiful oxygen. Forests, for example, regulate the amount of carbon dioxide in the air, produce oxygen and control rainfall and soil erosion. Ecosystems, in turn, depend on the continued health and vitality of the individual organisms that compose them. Removing just one species from an ecosystem can prevent the ecosystem from operating optimally.

Scientists have discovered and named only 1.75 million species—less than 20 per cent of those estimated to exist. And of those identified, only a fraction has been examined for potential medicinal, agricultural, or industrial value. Much of the Earth's great biodiversity is rapidly disappearing, even before we know what is missing. Most biologists agree that life on Earth is now faced with the most severe extinction episode since the event that drove the dinosaurs to extinction 65 million years ago. Species of plants, animals, fungi, and microscopic organisms such as bacteria are being lost at alarming rates, in fact, that biologists estimate that three species go extinct every hour. Scientists around the world are cataloging and studying global biodiversity in hopes that they might better understand it, or at least slow the rate of loss.

(a) Levels of Biodiversity

Biodiversity can be studied at three different hierarchical levels. These levels of Biodiversity are interrelated but should be studied separately to understand the interconnections that support life on the earth.

There are three levels of biodiversity:

- Genetic Diversity.
- Species Diversity.
- Community and Ecosystem Diversity.

❖ Genetic Diversity

It is the basic source of biodiversity. Genes are the basic units of hereditary information transmitted from one generation to another. When the genes within the same species show different versions due to new combinations, it is called genetic variability. For example, all rice varieties belongs to the species *Oryza sativa*, but there are thousands of wild and cultivated varieties of rice which show variations at genetic level and differ in their colour, size, shape, aroma and nutrient content of the grain. This is the genetic diversity of the rice.

❖ Species Diversity

The richness of a species in an ecosystem is known as species diversity. This is the variability found within the population of a species or between different species of a community. It represents broadly the species richness and their abundance in a community.

❖ Community and Ecosystem Diversity

An ecosystem develops its own characteristics community of living organism (biotic community) which depends largely upon the amount of abiotic resources and conditions of the environment. Environment diversity has three following aspects:

- *Alpha Diversity* refers to diversity within a particular area, community or ecosystem, and is measured by counting the number of taxa within the ecosystem. It is a mixture of species richness and evenness, which is used to represent diversity within a community and habitat.

- *Beta Diversity* is species diversity between ecosystems; this involves comparing the number of taxa that are unique to each of the ecosystems. Greater the dissimilarity between communities,higher the beta diversity.
- *Gamma Diversity* is a measure of the overall diversity for different ecosystems within a region. It refers to the diversity of the habitats over the total land scape or geographical area.

(b) Value of Biodiversity

Biodiversity is the pillar upon which we build civilizations. Nature's products support such diverse industries as agriculture, cosmetics, pharmaceuticals, pulp and paper, horticulture, construction and waste treatment. There are three main reasons commonly cited in the literature for the benefits of biodiversity: Ecological role of biodiversity, Economic role of biodiversity, scientific role of biodiversity.

BENEFITS OF BIODIVERSITY

Linkages among Biodiversity, Ecosystem Services, and Human Well-being

Biodiversity represents the foundation of ecosystems that, through the services they provide, affect human well-being. These include provisioning services such as food, water, timber, and fiber; regulating services such as the regulation of climate, floods, disease, wastes, and water quality; cultural services such as recreation, aesthetic enjoyment, and spiritual fulfillment; and supporting services such as soil formation, photosynthesis, and nutrient cycling (CF2). The MA considers human well-being to consist of five main components: the basic material needs for a good life, health, good social relations, security, and freedom of choice and action. Human well-being is the result of many factors, many directly or indirectly linked to biodiversity and ecosystem services while others are independent of these.

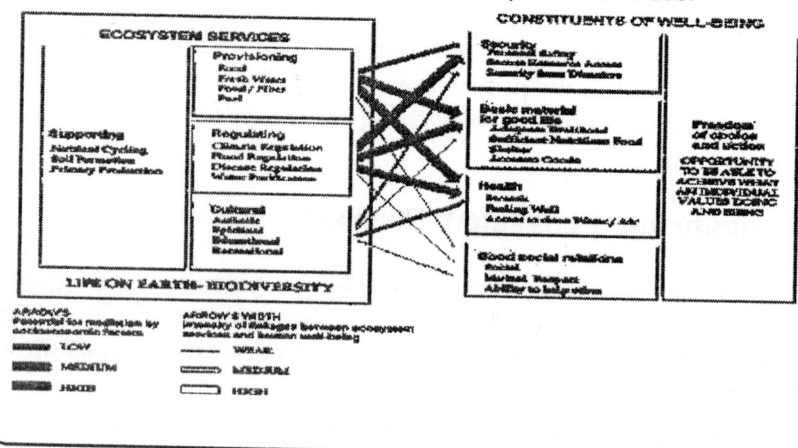

Medicinal Importance of Biodiversity

About 70 per cent of the medical drugs we use come from plants or are synthetics based upon plant drugs.

The oldest known medicinal plant is mahuang (*Ephedra sinica*), described in a pharmacopoeia by Chinese emperor Shen Nung in 2700 BC—it is a decongestant and modern decongestants contain drugs similar to those in mahuang.

Several drug companies are now doing screening tests on rainforest plants to detect medicinal activity—this is difficult because there are probably thousands of useful plants. Plants formerly used for arrow poisons or fish poisons often have medicinal activity.

Medicinal plants and their effect

Plant	*Drug*	*Effect*
Belladonna	Atropine	Inhibits parasympathetic nervous system, dilates eyes
Coffee	Caffeine	Stimulant
Opium poppy	Codeine, morphine	Pain killers
Madagascar periwinkle	Vinblastine	Anti-cancer
Chondrodendron species	Tubocurarine	Muscle relaxant
Pacific yew	Taxol	Anticancer
Foxglove	Digitoxin	Cardiac stimulant
Yellow cinchona	Quinine	Antimalarial
Wild yam	Diosgenin	Female contraceptive

Source: Biodiversity uses, China, 2005.

(c) Evolution of Biodiversity

Biodiversity found on Earth today is the result of 4 billion years of evolution. The origin of life is not well known to science, though limited evidence suggests that life may already have been well-established only a few 100 million years after the formation of the Earth. Until approximately 600 million years ago, all life consisted of bacteria and similar single-celled organisms.

The history of biodiversity during the Phanerozoic (the last 540 million years), starts with rapid growth during the Cambrian explosion—a period during which nearly every phylum of multicellular organisms first appeared. Over the next 400 million years or so, global diversity showed little overall trend, but was marked by periodic, massive losses of diversity classified as mass extinction events.

EVOLUTION OF BIODIVERSITIES / HABITAT

Date	*Event*
4600 *Ma	The planet Earth forms from the accretion disc revolving around the young Sun.
4100 Ma	The surface of the Earth cools enough for the crust to solidify. The atmosphere and the oceans form.
4000 Ma	The earliest life appears, possibly derived from self-reproducing RNA molecules. At this time, the atmosphere does not contain any free oxygen.
3500 Ma	Lifetime of the last universal ancestor; the split between the bacteria and the archaea occurs. Bacteria develop primitive forms of photosynthesis which at first do not produce oxygen.
3000 Ma	Photosynthesizing cyanobacteria evolve; they use water as a reducing agent, thereby producing oxygen as waste product. The moon is still very close to the earth and causes tides 1000 feet high. The earth is continually wracked by hurricane force winds. These extreme mixing influences are thought to stimulate evolutionary processes.
2500 Ma	Some bacteria evolve the ability to utilize oxygen to more efficiently use the energy from organic molecules such as glucose.
2100 Ma	More complex cells appear.
1200 Ma	Sexual reproduction evolves, leading to faster evolution.
1000 Ma	Multicellular organisms appear initially colonial algae, and later seaweeds, living in the oceans.
1000–750 Ma	The first known super continent, Rodinia, forms, and then breaks apart again.
950–780 Ma	Sturtian ice age, a time of multiple near-global glaciations, with periods oscillating between a Snowball Earth and a greenhouse Earth.
900 Ma	There are 481 18-hour days in a year. The rotation of the Earth has gradually slowed ever since.
750–580 Ma	According to the Snowball Earth hypothesis, the Precambrian Varangian ice age is so severe that the Earth's oceans freezed over completely; only in the tropics do oceans remain liquid.
600 Ma	Sponges (Porifera), the earliest multicellular animals, develop from cell colonies. Sponges are the simplest and most primitive animals, having partially-differentiated tissues but no muscles, nerves, internal organs, or capacity for locomotion. Cnidaria (jellyfish, etc.), Ctenophora, and other multicellular animals appear in the oceans
542–530 Ma	The first known footprints on land date to 530 Ma, indicating that early animal explorations may have predated the development of terrestrial plants.
475 Ma	The first primitive plants move onto land, having evolved from green algae living along the edges of lakes.
400 Ma	The first insects evolve, the wingless silverfish, springtails (no longer considered insects), and bristletails. First sharks appear.
450 Ma	Arthropods, with an exoskeleton that provides support and prevents water loss, are the first animals to move onto land. Among the first are Myriapoda (millipedes and centipedes), later followed by spiders and scorpions.
360 Ma	Plants evolve seeds, structures that protect plant embryos and enable plants to spread quickly on land.
365 Ma	The Late Devonian extinction is the period of mass extinction.
350-250 Ma	Karoo Ice Age, beginning with early Carboniferous and ending with late Permian. Two particular periods, in which much of Gondwanaland is glaciated from an early centre in Africa and South America, and a later centre in India and Australia, caused by polar wandering.

Note : Ma = Million years ago.

Date	*Event*
488 Ma	The first of the seven major extinction events over geological time occurs at the Cambrian-Ordovician transition. Soon after, the first of the jawed fishes, Placodermi, develop.
300 Ma	The super continent Pangea forms and will last for 120 million years; this is the last time all of the earth's continents fuse into one. Vast forests of clubmosses, horsetails, and tree ferns cover the land; when these decay they will eventually form coal and oil. Gymnosperms begin to diversify widely. Cycads, plants resembling palms, first appear.
250 Ma	The Permian-Triassic extinction event wipes out about 90% of all animal species; this fourth extinction event is the most severe mass extinction known.
220 Ma	The climate is very dry, and dry-adapted organisms are favoured
200 Ma	Fifth mass extinction event occurs at the Triassic-Jurassic transition.
180 Ma	The super continent Pangea begins to break up into several landmasses. The largest is Gondwana, made up of the landmasses, which are now Antarctica, Australia, South America, Africa, and India. Antarctica is still a land of forests. North America and Eurasia are still joined, forming the Northern supercontinent, Laurasia.
150 Ma	Giant dinosaurs are common and diverse
135 Ma	New dinosaurs *Iguanodon*, *Hylaeosaurus*, etc., appear after extinction of Jurassic forms. *Microraptor gui*, a 77 cm long dinosaur in Liaoning, Northeast China, has bird-like feathered wings on 4 limbs.
88 Ma	Breakup of Indo-Malagasy land mass.
80 Ma	India starts moving to Eurasia.
65 Ma	The Cretaceous-Tertiary extinction event (sixth extinction event) wipes out about half of all animal species including all non-avian dinosaurs, probably because of a cooling of the climate.
55 Ma	Australia breaks away from Antarctica.
50 Ma	The evolution of the horse starts.
43 Ma	Earliest elephant (Egypt): 1 m tall, size of a large pig, eats soft, juicy plants. It has a long nose, but no trunk nor tusks.
35 Ma	Grasses evolve from among the angiosperms.
22 Ma	India collides with Asia, causing the rise of Himalaya and the Tibetan plateau. Cut off from the humidity, Central Asia becomes a desert.
20 Ma	The African plate collides with Asia.
15 Ma	Apes from Africa migrate to Eurasia to become gibbons (lesser apes) and orangutans. Human ancestors speciate from the ancestors of the gibbon.
10 Ma	The climate begins to dry; savannas and grasslands take over the forests. Monkeys proliferate, and the apes go into decline. Human ancestors speciate from the ancestors of the gorillas.
7 Ma	Biggest primate *Gigantopithecus* is 2 m tall and lives in China (*Gigantopithecus blacki*), Vietnam, and northern India (*Gigantopithecus bilaspurensis*). Extinct by 300,000 years ago.
5.6 Ma	Drying up of the Mediterranean Sea.
5 Ma	Volcanoes erupt and create the small area of land that joins North and South America. Mammals from North America move South and cause extinction of mammals there. Human ancestors speciate from the ancestors of the chimpanzees. Chimpanzees and humans share 98 per cent of DNA: biochemical similarities are so great that their hemoglobin molecules differ by only one amino acid.
3 Ma	The bipedal australopithecines evolve in the savannas of Africa.
2 Ma	*Homo habilis* (handy man) uses primitive stone tools (choppers) in Tanzania.

Note : Ma = Million years ago.

Date	Event
500 ka	*Homo erectus* (Choukoutien, China) uses charcoal to control fire, though they may not know how to create or start it.
400 ka	Eastern gorillas diverge into the eastern lowland and mountain sub-species. Giant deer *Megaloceros giganteus*, Ireland; the antlers together span about 3.6 m or larger, extinct by 9.5 ka.
195 ka	Omo1, Omo2 (Ethiopia, Omo river) are the earliest known *Homo sapiens.*
160 ka	*Homo sapiens* (*Homo sapiens idaltu*) in Ethiopia, Awash River, Herto village, practice mortuary rituals and butcher hippos. Their dead bodies are later covered by volcanic rocks.
100 ka	The first anatomically modern humans (*Homo sapiens*) appear in Africa by this time or earlier. Modern humans enter Asia via two routes: one North through the Middle East, and another further South from Ethiopia, via the Red Sea and southern Arabia.
74 ka	Super volcanic eruption in Toba, Sumatra, Indonesia, causes *Homo sapiens* population to crash to 2,000. Six years without a summer are followed by a 1,000 year ice-age. Volcanic ash up to 5 m deep covers India and Pakistan.
70 ka	The most recent ice age, the Wisconsin glaciation, begins. Humans in the Blombos cave in South Africa make tools from bones, show symbolic thinking by creating ochre paintings. They also collect and pierce holes through sea shells to make necklaces.
60 ka	Y-chromosomal Adam lives in Africa. He is the last male human from whom all current human Y chromosomes are descended.
50 ka	Modern humans expand from Asia to Australia (to become today's Indigenous Australians) and Europe. Expansion along the coasts happens faster than expansion inland. Woolly rhino (*Coelodonta antiquus*) in Britain.
30 ka	Modern humans enter North America from Siberia. At least two of the first waves left few or no genetic descendants among Americans by the time Europeans arrive across the Atlantic Ocean. Humans reach Solomons. Humans move into Japan. Bow and arrows used in Sahara (grassland). Fired ceramic animal models made in Moravia (Czech Republic).
28 ka	Oldest known painting: in the Apollo 11 Rock Shelter, Namibia, and Africa. A 20 cm-long, 3 cm-wide object found in Hohle Fels Cave near Ulm in the Swabian Jura in Germany is the earliest sculpted stone penis.
27 ka	*Neanderthals* die out leaving *Homo sapiens* and *Homo floresiensis* as the only living species of the genus *Homo.* Czech invented textile and pressed weaving patterns into pieces of clay before firing them.
25 ka	Throwing sticks for hunting animals made from mammoth tusk (Poland).
23 ka	Venus of Willendorf, a small statuette of a female figure, discovered at a paleolithic site near Willendorf, Austria, dates from this era.
18 ka	*Homo floresiensis* existed in the Liang Bua limestone cave on Flores, remote Indonesian island.
15 ka	The last Ice Age ends. Sea levels across the globe rise, flooding many coastal areas, and separating former mainland areas into islands. Japan separates from Asia mainland. Siberia separates from Alaska. Tasmania separates from Australia. Java island forms. Sarawak, Malaysia and Indonesia separate. The cave paintings of Lascaux and Altamira were produced.
14 ka	Megafauna extinction starts (continuing to current day), where over 100 large mammal species disappear caused principally by the expanding human population.
11.5 ka	Extinction of the Sabertooth (*Smilodon*).
11 ka	Human population reaches 5 million. Domestication of dogs (first domesticated animal) from Gray Wolf subspecies (*Canis lupus pallipes*). All modern dogs today

Note : Ka = Thousands years ago.

Date	*Event*
	(5 main groups, about 400 breeds) belong to a single subspecies *Canis lupus familiaris.*
10 ka	Sahara is green with rivers, lakes, cattle, crocodiles and monsoons. Japan's hunter-gatherer Jomon culture creates world's earliest pottery. Humans reach Tierra del Fuego at the tip of South America, the last continental region to be inhabited by humans (excluding Antarctica).
8 ka	Common (Bread) wheat *Triticum aestivum* originates in southwest Asia due to hybridisation of emmer wheat with a goat-grass, *Aegilops tauschii.*
6.5 ka	Two rice species are domesticated: Asian rice *Oryza sativa* and African rice *Oryza glaberrima.*
3 ka	Humans start using iron tools.
AD 1	Human population 150 million.
AD 1835	Human population 1 billion.
AD 1969	Humans walk on the moon.
AD 2006	Human population approaching 6.5 billion. Holocene extinction event continues with the observed rate of extinction rising dramatically in the last 50 years. Most biologists believe that we are at this moment at the beginning of a tremendously accelerated anthropogenic mass extinction. Wilson estimates that at current rates of human destruction of the biosphere, one-half of all species of life will be extinct in 100 years.

*Ma — Million years ago *Source: Wikipedia Encyclopedia.*

II. Global Biodiversity

(a) Distribution on the Earth

Distribution of the global Biodiversity could be studied under the following two broad categories :

- Spatial Patterns of Biodiversity
- Temporal Patterns of Biodiversity

❖ Spatial Patterns of Biodiversity

Documenting spatial patterns in *biodiversity* is difficult because taxonomic, functional, trophic, genetic, and other dimensions of biodiversity have been relatively poorly quantified.

Estimates of the total number of species on Earth range from 5 million to 30 million. Irrespective of actual global species richness, however, it is clear that the 1.7–2 million species that have been

World: Approximate number of species which has been identified

Groups	*No. of species*
Higher plants	2,70,000
Algae	40,000
Fungi	72,000
Bacteria	4,000
Viruses	1,550
Mammals	4,650
Birds	9,700
Reptiles	7,150
Fish	26,959
Amphibians	4,780
Insects	10,25,000
Crustaceans	43,000
Molluscs	70,000
Nematodes and worms	25,000
Protozoa	40,000
Others	1,10,000

Source : Millennium Ecosystem Assessment, World-Resources Institute, Washington, D.C.

formally identified represent only a small portion of total species richness. More-complete biotic inventories are badly needed to correct for this deficiency.

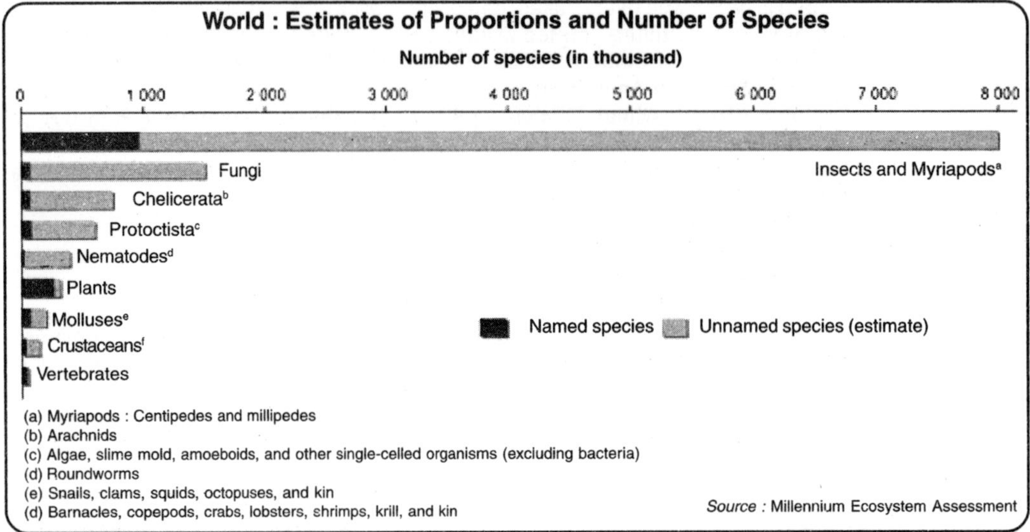

The 8 Biogeographical Realms and 14 Biomes

Biogeographic realms are large spatial regions within which ecosystems share a broadly similar biological evolutionary history. Eight terrestrial biogeographic realms are typically recognized, corresponding roughly to continents. Although similar ecosystems (such as tropical moist forests) share similar processes and major vegetation types wherever they are found, their species composition varies markedly depending on the biogeographic realm in which they are found. Assessing biodiversity at the level of biogeographic realms is important because the realms display substantial variation in the extent of change, they face different drivers of change, and there may be differences in the options for mitigating or managing the drivers. Terrestrial biogeographic realms reflect freshwater biodiversity patterns reasonably well, but marine biogeographic realms are poorly known and largely undefined.

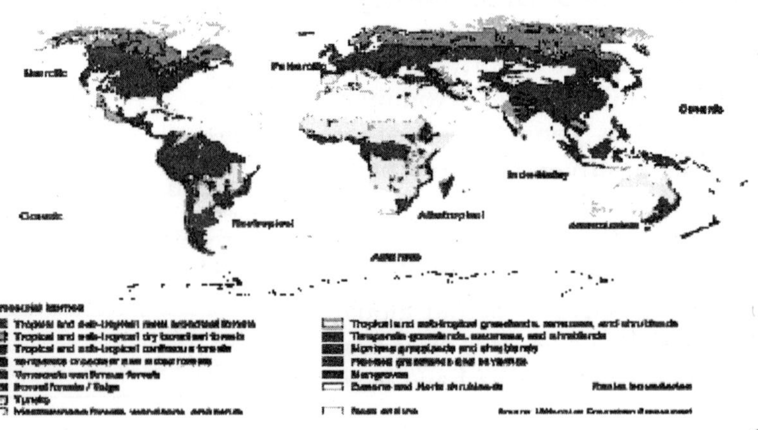

A large proportion of the world's terrestrial biodiversity at the species level is concentrated in a small part of the world, mostly in the tropics. Even among the larger and more mobile species, such as terrestrial vertebrates, more than one-third of all species have ranges of less than 1,000 square kilometres. In contrast, local and regional diversity of microorganisms tends to be more similar to large-scale and global diversity because of their large population size, greater dispersal, larger range sizes, and lower levels of regional species clustering.

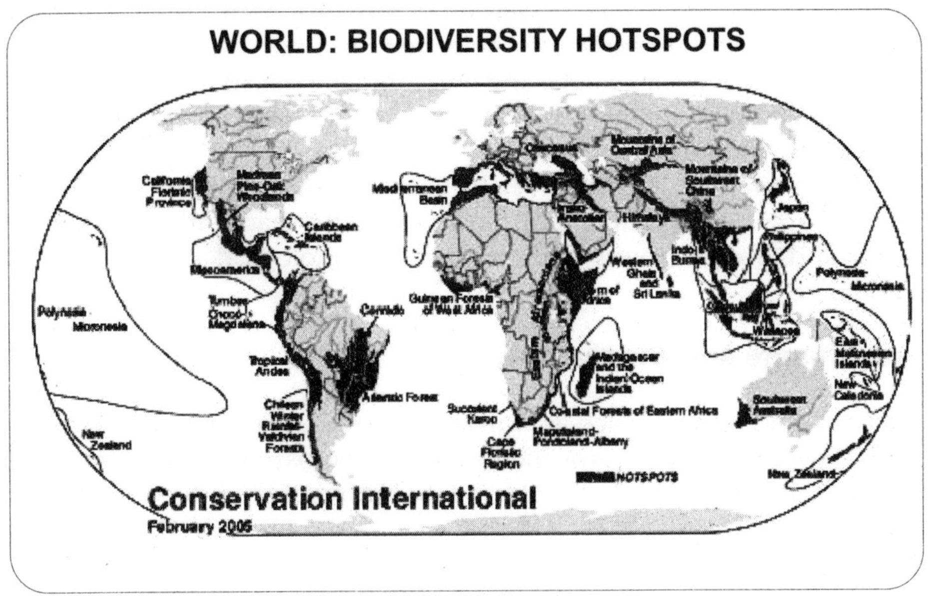

❖ Temporal Patterns of Biodiversity

Knowledge of patterns of biodiversity over time allow for only very approximate estimates of background rates of extinction or of how fast species have become extinct over geological time. Except for the last 1,000 years, global biodiversity has been relatively constant over most of human history, but the history of life is characterized by considerable change. The estimated magnitude of background rates of extinction is roughly 0.1–1.0 extinctions per million species per year. Most measurements of this rate have come from assessing the length of species' lifetimes through the fossil record: these ranges over 0.5–13 million years, and possibly 0.2–16 million years.

(b) Global Biodiversity Loss

➢ *Factors which lead to biodiversity loss*

Natural or human-induced factors that directly or indirectly cause a change in biodiversity are referred to as drivers.

- *Direct drivers* that explicitly influence ecosystem processes include land use change, climate change, invasive species, overexploitation, and pollution.
- *Indirect drivers,* such as changes in human population, incomes or lifestyle, operate more diffusely, by altering one or more direct drivers.

➢ *Direct Drivers*

Some direct drivers of change are easier to measure than others, for instance, fertilizer usage, water consumption, irrigation, and harvests. For other drivers, indicators are not as well developed and measurement data is less readily available. This is the case for non-native species, climate change, land cover conversion, and landscape fragmentation.

Changes in biodiversity are driven by combinations of drivers that work over time, on different scales, and that tend to amplify each other. For example, population and income growth combined with technological advances can lead to climate change.

Climate Change and Biodiversity

Recent changes in climate, such as warmer temperatures in certain regions, have already had significant impacts on biodiversity and ecosystems. They have affected species distributions, population sizes, and the timing of reproduction or migration events, as well as the frequency of pest and disease outbreaks. Projected changes in climate by 2050 could lead to the extinction of many species living in certain limited geographical regions. By the end of the century, climate change and its impacts may become the main direct driver of overall biodiversity loss.

While the growing season in Europe has lengthened over the last 30 years, in some regions of Africa the combination of regional climate changes and human pressures have led to decreased cereal crop production since 1970. Changes in fish populations have also been linked to large-scale climate variations such as "El Nio". As climate change will become more severe, the harmful impacts on ecosystem services will outweigh the benefits in most regions of the world. The Intergovernmental Panel on Climate Change (IPCC) project that the average surface temperature will raise by 2^0 to 6.4^0 C by 2100 compared to pre-industrial levels. This is expected to cause global negative impacts on biodiversity.

According to the projections :

- Climate change is likely to exacerbate the loss of biodiversity and increase the risk of extinctions.
- Water availability and quality will decrease in many arid and semiarid regions.

- The risk of floods and droughts will increase.
- The reliability of hydropower and biomass production in some regions will decrease.
- Diseases, such as malaria, dengue and cholera, are likely to become more frequent in many regions and so are other health problems linked to heat stress, malnutrition, and natural disasters.
- Agricultural productivity may decrease in the tropics and sub-tropics, and fisheries may be adversely affected as well.
- Changes in climate, in land use, and in the spread of invasive species will limit both the capability of species to migrate and the ability of species to survive in fragmented habitats.

❖ Direct Drivers are Critical in Different Ecosystems

Different direct drivers are critical in different ecosystems. Historically, habitat and land use change have had the biggest impact on biodiversity in all ecosystems, but climate change and pollution are projected to increasingly affect all aspects of biodiversity. Overexploitation and invasive species have been important as well and continue to be major drivers of changes in biodiversity.

Over the past 50 years, the most important direct drivers of change have been :

- *In terrestrial ecosystems:* Land cover change, mainly by conversion to cropland. Only areas unsuited to crop plants, such as deserts, boreal forests, and tundra, remain relatively intact. Deforestation and forest degradation are currently particularly extensive in the tropics. Nearly a quarter of the Earth's surface is currently covered by cultivated systems.

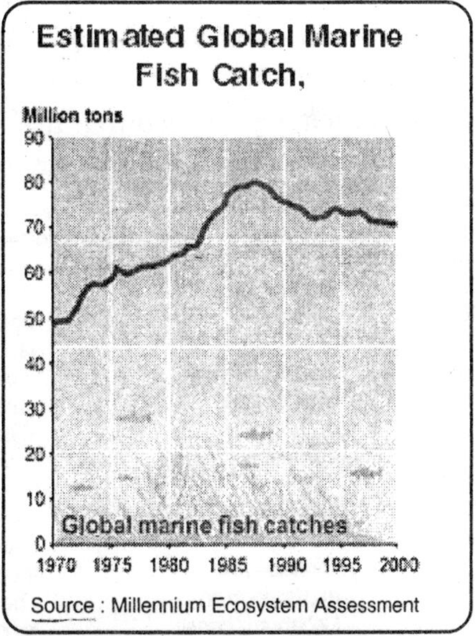

Source : Millennium Ecosystem Assessment

- *In marine ecosystems:* Fishing is the major direct human pressure affecting the structure, function, and biodiversity of the oceans. In all oceans, a number of fish stocks targeted in fisheries have collapsed because they have been overfished or fished above their maximum sustainable levels. After a peak in the late 1980s, the global amount fished has been declining.

➢ *In freshwater ecosystems:* Water regime changes, such as those following the construction of large dams; invasive species, which can lead to species extinction; and pollution, such as high levels of nutrients.

➢ *Indirect Drivers*

Five major indirect drivers that influence biodiversity are :

- *Change in Economic Activity* : Global economic activity is now nearly seven times what it was 50 years ago and it is expected to grow further. The many processes of globalization have been removing regional barriers, weakening national connections, and increasing the interdependence among people and between nations.
- *Population Change* : World population has doubled in the past forty years, reaching 6 billion in 2000. The fact that more and more people live in cities increases the demand for food and energy and thereby pressures on ecosystems.
- *Socio-Political Factors* : The trend toward democratic institutions over the past 50 years has enabled new forms of management of environmental resources.
- *Cultural and Religious Factors* : Culture conditions individuals' perceptions of the world, and their priority setting, for instance in terms of conservation.
- *Science and Technology* : The development and diffusion of scientific knowledge and technologies can on the one hand allow for increased efficiency in resource use and on the other hand provide the means to increase exploitation of natural resources.

Loss of Global Biodiversity in Civilizations

7000 BC–1800 BC	Mesopotamia/ Sumer *Salinization and waterlogging of Sumer's agroecosystem*	Around 7000 BC, people in this region (now, largely, Iraq) began to modify the natural environment. Lacking adequate rainfall, land had to be irrigated for Cultivation, and the demand for food increased as the population grew. The irrigated land became salinized and waterlogged. Records noting "the earth turned white" with salt date back to 2000 BC. By 1800 BC, the agricultural system—the foundation of Sumerian civilization—collapsed.
2600 BC–present	Lebanon *Overuse and exploitation of Lebanon's cedar forest*	At one time, Mount Lebanon was covered with a forest of cedars that were famous for their beauty and strength. In the third millennium BC, Byblos grew wealthy from its timber trade. The Egyptians used cedar timber for construction and used the resin for mummification. The exploitation continued through the centuries. Only four small groves remain today.

(Contd...)

(Contd...)

2500 BC–900	Mayan Empire *Soil erosion, loss of agroecosystem viability, and water siltation in Central America*	Mayans lived in what are now parts of Mexico, Guatemala, Belize, and Honduras.The agriculture techniques they used were creative and intensive—clearing hillsides of jungle, terracing fields to contain soil erosion. Soil erosion reduced crop yields, and higher levels of silt in rivers damaged the raised fields. Decreased food production and competition for the remaining resources may have led to that civilization's demise.
800 BC–200 BC	Greece *Conversion and deforestation in the Mediterranean*	In Homeric times, Greece was still largely covered with mixed evergreen and deciduous forests. Over time the trees were cleared to provide land for agriculture, fuel for cooking and heating, and construction materials. Overgrazing prevented regeneration. The olive tree, favoured for its economic value, began to flourish in ancient Greece because it grew well on the degraded land.
200 BC–present	China *Desertification along the Silk Road*	The fortification of the Great Wall during the Han dynasty gave rise to intensive cultivation of farmland in northern and western China and to the growth of a major travel and trade route that came to be known as the Silk Road. Deserts began irreversibly expanding in this area as a result of the demands of a growing population and gradual climate changes.
50 BC–450	Roman Empire *Desertification and loss of agroecosystem viability in North Africa*	The challenge of providing food for the population of Rome and its large standing armies plagued the empire. The North African provinces, once highly productive granaries, gradually became degraded as Roman demands for grain pushed cultivation onto marginal lands, prone to erosion. Scrub vegetation spread and some intensively cultivated areas became desertified
1400–1600	Canary Islands *Human and natural resource exploitation, degradation and extinctions in many regions*	Originally from North Africa, the Guanches were a people who inhabited the Canary Islands for more than 1,000 years before the Spanish arrived in the 1400s. The Spanish enslaved the Guanches, cleared the forests, and built sugar cane plantations. By 1600 the Guanches were dead, victims of Eurasian diseases and plantation conditions. As in the Canary Islands, regions in the Americas, Africa, and Asia where people were forced to grow and export cash crops such as sugar, tobacco, cotton, rubber, bananas, or palm oil, continue to suffer from deforestation, soil damage, biodiversity losses, and economic dependency instituted during colonization.
1800	Australia and New Zealand *Loss of biodiversity and proliferating invasive species in island ecosystems*	There were no hoofed animals in Australia and New Zealand before Europeans arrived at the end of the 18th century and began importing them. Within 100 years there were millions of sheep and cattle. The huge increase in grazing animals killed off many of the native grasses that were not well adapted to intensive grazing. Many island bird species, for example, were flightless and became easy prey for invaders. It is estimated that 90 percent of all bird extinctions occurred on islands.
1800	North America *Conversion, loss of habitat, and unrestrained killing of wildlife in North*	As land was cleared for settlement and cultivation around the world, animal habitats of almost every kind were reduced; animals were killed for food, hides, or recreation as commerce spread. In North America, herds of bison, totalling perhaps as many as 50 million, were hunted to near extinction by the end of the 19th century. Aquatic as well as terrestrial species became targets of exploitation and

(Contd...)

(Contd...)

	America	extinction. In the 19th century, whales were killed in large numbers to support industrializing economies in need of whale oil in great quantity, mainly for lighting and lubricants.
1800–1900	Germany and Japan *Industrial chemical poisoning of freshwater systems*	The industrial revolution had a profound impact on the waters of the world. Rivers that ran through industrial zones, like the Rhine in Germany, or rivers that ran through mining zones, like the Watarase in Japan, became heavily polluted in the 19th century.
1900	United States and Canada *Soil erosion and loss of biodiversity in the United States and Canada*	The Great Plains of the United States and Canada were ploughed in the late 19th and early 20th centuries and planted with new forms of drought-resistant wheat. Once the protective original grass cover was destroyed, drought in the 1930s enabled high, persistent wind storms to blow away much of the dry soil.
1928–present	Worldwide *Industrial chemicals deplete the world's protective ozone layer*	Chlorofluorocarbons (CFCs) are a family of volatile compounds invented in 1928. Thought to be the world's first nontoxic, nonflammable refrigerants, their use grew rapidly. They also were used as industrial solvents, foaming agents, and aerosol propellants. CFC production peaked in 1974, the same year researchers noted that CFC emissions could possibily damage human health and the ozone layer. In 1985, the discovery of an "ozone hole" over the Antarctic coincided with a first-ever coordinated international effort to phase out production of CFCs and other ozone-depleting substances. Worldwide phase out of CFC production is scheduled for 2010.

Sources : World resources, Chapter-1, Linking People and Ecosystems, Page no. 6 and 7, World Resources Institute, Washington, D.C. USA.

Current Trends in Biodiversity

For all aspects of biodiversity, current pace of change and loss is hundreds of times faster than previously in recorded history and the pace shows no indication of slowing down.

Virtually all of Earth's ecosystems have been dramatically transformed through human actions, for example, 35 per cent of mangrove and 20 per cent of coral reef areas have been lost.

Land areas where the changes have been particularly quick over the past two decades include :

- The Amazon basin and Southeast Asia (deforestation and expansion of croplands);
- Asia (land degradation in drylands); and
- Bangladesh, Indus Valley, parts of Middle East and Central Asia, and the Great Lakes region of Eastern Africa.

Conversion has been slower in areas, such as Mediterranean forests, where most suitable land for agriculture had already been converted by 1950 and where the majority of native habitats had already been lost.

Species extinction is a natural part of Earth's history. However, over the past 100 years humans have increased the extinction rate by at least 100 times compared to the natural rate. The current extinction rate is much greater than the rate at which new species arise, resulting in a net loss of biodiversity.

Within well-studied groups (conifers, cycads, amphibians, birds, and mammals), between 12 per cent and 52 per cent of species are threatened with extinction, according to the IUCN Red List. In general the most threatened species are those that are higher up the food chain, have a low population density, live long, reproduce slowly, and live within a limited geographical area. Within many species groups, such as amphibians, African mammals, and birds in agricultural lands, the majority

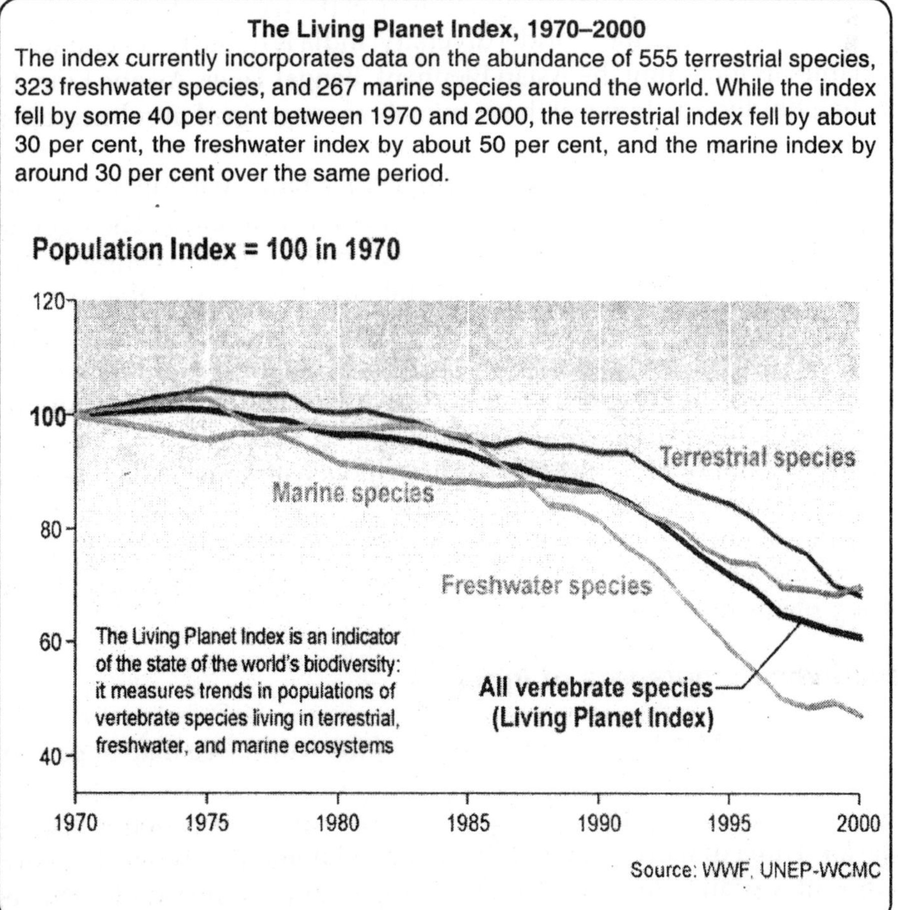

The Living Planet Index, 1970–2000

The index currently incorporates data on the abundance of 555 terrestrial species, 323 freshwater species, and 267 marine species around the world. While the index fell by some 40 per cent between 1970 and 2000, the terrestrial index fell by about 30 per cent, the freshwater index by about 50 per cent, and the marine index by around 30 per cent over the same period.

of species have faced a decline in the size of their population, in their geographical spread, or both. The Living Planet Index compiled by the WWF is an indicator of trends in the overall abundance of wild species. Between 1970 and 2000, it indicates declines in all environments.

Since 1960, intensification of agricultural systems coupled with specialization by plant breeders and the harmonizing effects of globalization have led to a substantial reduction in the genetic diversity of domesticated plants and animals. Today a third of the 6,500 breeds of domestic species are threatened with extinction.

III. BIODIVERSITY IN INDIA

(a) India as a mega-diversity nation

India is one of the 12-mega diversity countries of the world, which together possess more than 60 per cent of the world's diversity. India is home to several well known large mammals including the Asian Elephant, Bengal Tiger, Asiatic Lion, Leopard and Indian Rhinoceros. Some of these animals are engrained in culture, often being associated with deities.

These large mammals are important for wildlife tourism in India. The popularity of animals have helped greatly in conservation efforts in India. The tiger has been particularly important and Project Tiger was a major effort to conserve the tigers.

There are about 2,546 species of fishes (about 11 per cent of the world species) found in Indian waters. About 197 species of amphibians (4.4 per cent of the world total) and more than 408 reptile species (6 per cent of the world total) are found in India. Among these groups the highest levels of endemism are found in the amphibians.

There are about 1,250 species of birds from India with some variations depending on taxonomic treatments accounting for about 12 per cent of the world species.

There are about 410 species of mammals known from India which is about 8.86 per cent of the world species. WCMC gives an estimate of about 15,000 species of flowering plants in India.

(b) Biodiversity hotspots of India

India is one of the high biodiversity regions of the world (see map at page no. 159) with three biodiversity hotspots — the Western Ghats, the Eastern Himalayas and the Indo-Burma regions. These hotspots have a number of endemic species.

The land area of more than 3 million square kilometres shows diversity in the habitats with variation in rainfall, altitude, topography and latitude. The region is also under the influence of the monsoons which are a major seasonal factor.

INDIA: MAJOR BIOGEOGRAPHIC REGIONS

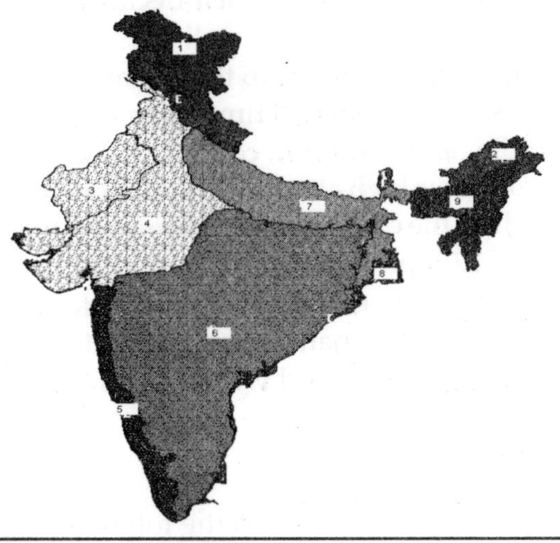

No.	*Biogeographic Region*	*Biotic Province*	*Total Area* (km^2)	*Percent (%)*
1.	Trans-Himalayan	Upper Region	186200	5.5
2.	Himalayan	NW Himalayas	6900	6.4
		West Himalayas	720000	
		Central Himalayas	123000	
		East Himalayas	83000	
3.	Desert	Kutch	45000	5.6
		Thar	180000	
		Ladakh	NA	
4.	Semi Arid	Central India	107600	16.6
		Gujarat- Rajwara	400400	
5.	Western Ghat	Malabar Coast	59700	4.0
		Western Ghat Mt.	99300	
6.	Deccan Peninsula	Deccan Plateau South	378000	42.0
		Central Plateau	341000	
		Eastern Plateau	198000	
		Chhota Nagpur	217000	
		Central Highland	287000	
7.	Gangetic Plain	Upper Gangatic Plain	206400	10.8
		Lower Gangatic Plain	153000	
8.	Coasts	West Coast	6500	2.5
		East Coast	6500	5.2
9.	North East India	Brahmaputra Valley	65200	
		North- Eastern Hill	106200	
10.	Islands	Andaman Island	6397	0.3
		Nicobar Island	1930	
		Lakshadweep Island	180	

Source : Zoological Survey of India

The Western Ghats : It is a chain of hills that run along the western edge of peninsular India. Their proximity to the ocean and through orographic effect, they receive high rainfall. These regions have moist deciduous forest and rain forest. The region shows high species diversity as well as high levels of endemism. The region shows bio geographically affinities to the Malayan region, and the Satpura.

The Eastern Himalayas : The Eastern Himalayas is the region encompassing Bhutan, northeastern India, and southern, central, and eastern Nepal. The region is geologically young and shows high altitudinal variation. It has nearly 163 globally threatened species including the One-horned Rhinoceros, the Water Buffalo and in all 45 mammals, 50 birds, 17 reptiles, 12 amphibians, 3 invertebrate and 36 plant species. The Relict Dragonfly is an endangered species found here, the only other species in the genus being found in Japan. The region is also home to the Himalayan Newt, the only salamander species found within Indian limits.

(c) Eco-Regions in India

The main land of India could be divided into the following 10 major eco-regions:

A. Tropical and subtropical moist broadleaf forests

1. Meghalaya subtropical forests
2. Brahmaputra Valley semi-evergreen forests
3. Eastern Highlands moist deciduous forests
4. Sundarbans freshwater swamp forests
5. Orissa semi-evergreen forests
6. Lower Gangetic plains moist deciduous forests
7. Upper Gangetic Plains moist deciduous forests
8. Malabar Coast moist forests
9. North Western Ghats moist deciduous forests
10. North Western Ghats montane rain forests
11. South Western Ghats moist deciduous forests
12. South Western Ghats montane rain forests

B Tropical and subtropical dry broadleaf forests

1. Chota Nagpur dry deciduous forests
2. East Deccan dry evergreen forests
3. Kathiarbar-Gir dry deciduous forests
4. Narmada Valley dry deciduous forests
5. Northern dry deciduous forests
6. South Deccan Plateau dry deciduous forests

C. Tropical and subtropical coniferous forests

1. Himalayan subtropical pine forests
2. Northeast India-Myanmar pine forests

D. Temperate broadleaf and mixed forests

E. Temperate coniferous forests
F. Tropical and subtropical grasslands, savannas, and shrublands
G. Montane grasslands and shrublands
H. Flooded grasslands and savannas
I. Deserts and xeric shrublands
J. Mangrove

A. Tropical and Subtropical Moist Broadleaf Forests

Tropical and subtropical moist broadleaf forests, also known as tropical wet forests, are a tropical and subtropical forest biome. The biome includes several types of forests, including lowland tropical rain forests, which receive high rainfall year-round; moist deciduous and semi-evergreen forests, with high overall rainfall marked by strong seasonal variations; montane rain forests found in cooler-climate mountainous areas; and freshwater swamp forests and peat swamp forests.

Tropical and subtropical moist broadleaf forests are found in a belt around the equator and in the humid subtropics, and are characterized by warm, humid climates with high year-round rainfall. Tropical and subtropical forest regions with lower rainfall are home to Tropical and subtropical dry broadleaf forests and Tropical and subtropical coniferous forests. Temperate rain forests also occur in certain humid temperate coastal regions.

Rainforests are characterized by high rainfall, with definitions setting minimum normal annual rainfall between 200 cm and 170 cm . The soil can be poor because high rainfall tends to leach out soluble nutrients.

The undergrowth in a rainforest is restricted in many areas by the lack of sunlight at ground level. This makes it possible for people and other animals to walk through the forest. If the leaf canopy is destroyed or thinned for any reason, the ground beneath is soon colonised by a dense tangled growth of vines, shrubs and small trees called *jungle.*

1. Meghalaya Subtropical Forests

The Meghalaya subtropical forests is a montane subtropical moist broadleaf forest ecoregion of eastern India. The ecoregion covers an area of 41,700 square kilometres, encompassing the Khasi Hills, Garo Hills, and Jaintia Hills of India's Meghalaya State, and adjacent portions of Assam State.

The ecoregion is one of the wettest in the world, with some places, notably Mawsynram and Cherrapunji, receiving up to eleven meters of rain in a year.

The ecoregion is considered one of the most species-rich in India, with a rich diversity of birds, mammals, and plants.

Over 320 species of orchids are native to Meghalaya. The endemic pitcher plant *(Nepenthes khasiana)* is now endangered in the wild.

The ecoregion is home to 110 species of mammals, none of which are endemic. Species include the Tiger, Clouded Leopard, Asian Elephant, Dhole or Asiatic Wild Dog, Sun Bear, Sloth Bear, Smooth-coated Otter, Indian Civet, Chinese Pangolin, Indian Pangolin, Assamese Macaque, Bear Macaque, Capped Leaf Monkey, and Hoolock Gibbon.

2. Brahmaputra Valley semi-evergreen forests

The Brahmaputra Valley semi-evergreen forests is a tropical moist broadleaf forest ecoregion of eastern India. The ecoregion covers 56,700 square kilometres , which encompasses the alluvial plain of the Brahmaputra River in India's Assam State.

3. Eastern Highlands moist deciduous forests

The Eastern Highlands moist deciduous forests is a tropical moist broadleaf forest ecoregion of east-central India. The ecoregion covers an area of 341,100 square kilometres, extending across portions of Andhra Pradesh, Chhattisgarh, Jharkhand, Madhya Pradesh, Maharashtra, and Orissa States.

The Eastern Highlands moist deciduous forests extend from the Bay of Bengal coast in northern Andhra Pradesh and southern Orissa, across the northern portion of the Eastern Ghats range and the northeastern Deccan Plateau, to the eastern Satpura Range and the upper Narmada River valley.

The forests of the ecoregion are sustained by the moisture-bearing monsoon winds from the Bay of Bengal, which lies to the southeast

The ecoregion's forests are dominated by Sal. The flora of the ecoregion shares many affinities with the moist forests of the Western Ghats and the eastern Himalayas.

The ecoregion is considered globally outstanding by the World Wildlife Fund for its assemblage of large mammals, including tiger, wolf, gaur, and sloth bear. The Asian Elephant has been extirpated from the ecoregion.

4. Sundarbans freshwater swamp forests

The Sundarbans freshwater swamp forests are a tropical moist broadleaf forest ecoregion of India and Bangladesh. The ecoregion covers an area of 14,600 square kilometres of the vast Ganges-Brahmaputra Delta, extending from India's West Bengal State into eastern Bangladesh. The Sundarbans freshwater swamp forests lie between the upland Lower Gangetic plains moist deciduous forests and the brackish-water Sundarbans mangroves bordering the Bay of Bengal.

The fertile soils of the delta have been subject to intensive human use for centuries, and the ecoregion has been mostly converted to intensive agriculture, with few enclaves of forest remaining. The remaining forests, together with the Sundarbans mangroves, are important habitat for the endangered tiger.

5. Orissa semi-evergreen forests

The Orissa semi-evergreen forests are a tropical moist broadleaf forest ecoregion of eastern India. The ecoregion covers an area of 22,300 square kilometres on the coastal plain of Orissa State.

6. Lower Gangetic plains moist deciduous forests

The Lower Gangetic plains moist deciduous forests is a tropical moist broadleaf forest ecoregion eastern India. The ecoregion covers an area of 254,100 square kilometres, covering most of States of West Bengal, Bihar, and Tripura, and extending into adjacent portions of Assam, Uttar Pradesh, and Orissa States.

The Lower Gangetic plains moist deciduous forests extends across the alluvial plain of the lower Ganges and Brahmaputra rivers, which form the world's largest river delta. The ecoregion is currently one of the most densely-populated regions on earth, and the forests have largely been replaced with intensive agriculture. To the north, the ecoregion extends to the base of the Himalayas.

7. Upper Gangetic plains moist deciduous forests

The Upper Gangetic plains moist deciduous forests is a tropical moist broadleaf forest ecoregion of northern India. It lies on the alluvial plain of the Ganges and Yamuna rivers, with an area of 263,100 square kilometres (101,600 square miles), covering most of the State of Uttar Pradesh and adjacent portions of Uttarakhand, Haryana, Madhya Pradesh and Bihar.

The ecoregion has a tropical climate. Rainfall is highly seasonal, falling mainly during the June to September southwest monsoon.

In ancient times the region was mostly forested, with sal the predominant tree. Many trees lose their leaves during the winter dry season. The ecoregion is currently densely populated, and the fertile plains have largely been converted to intensive agriculture, with only a few enclaves of forest remaining.

8. Malabar Coast moist forests

The Malabar Coast moist forests is a tropical moist broadleaf forest ecoregion of southwestern India. It lies along India's Konkan and Malabar coasts, in a narrow strip between the Arabian Sea and the Western Ghats range, which runs parallel to the coast. It has an area of 35,500 square kilometres, and extends from northern Maharashtra through Goa, Karnataka and Kerala to Kanyakumari in southernmost Tamil Nadu.

The ecoregion extends from sea level to the 250 metres contour of the Western Ghats. Very little of the natural vegetation of the ecoregion remains; it has largely been cleared for agriculture, grazing, and teak plantations.

9. North Western Ghats moist deciduous forests

The North Western Ghats moist deciduous forests is a tropical moist broadleaf forest ecoregion of southwestern India. It lies between 250 and 1000 metres elevation in the northern portion of the Western Ghats range, from their northern end in Maharashtra State, through Karnataka to the transitional forests of Wayanad in Kerala.

10. North Western Ghats montane rain forests

The North Western Ghats montane rain forests is a tropical moist broadleaf forest ecoregion of southwestern India. It covers an area of 30,900 square kilometres, extending down the spine of the Western Ghats range, from Maharashtra State in the north through Karnataka to Kerala State in the south. The montane rain forests are found above 1000 metres elevation, and are surrounded at lower elevations by the North Western Ghats moist deciduous forests.

Unlike the lowland forests, which are composed largely of drought-deciduous trees, the montane rain forests are predominantly evergreen laurel forest.

11. South Western Ghats moist deciduous forests

The South Western Ghats moist deciduous forests is a tropical moist broadleaf forest ecoregion of southern India. It covers the southern portion of the Western Ghats range and the Nilgiri Hills between 250 and 1000 metres elevation in Kerala, Karnataka and Tamil Nadu States.

The ecoregion has an area of 23,800 square kilometres. It includes the southern ranges of the Western Ghats, including the Agastyamalai and Anamalai, and the eastward spurs of the Nilgiri Hills and Palni Hills.

12. South Western Ghats montane rain forests

The South Western Ghats montane rain forests are an ecoregion of southern India, covering the southern portion of the Western Ghats range in Kerala and Tamil Nadu, at elevations over 1000 metres. They are cooler and wetter than the lower elevation South Western Ghats moist deciduous forests, which surround the montane rain forests.

The ecoregion is the most species-rich in peninsular India, and is home to numerous endemic species. It covers an area of 22,600 square kilometres. It is estimated that two-thirds of the original forests have been cleared, and only 3,200 square kilometres, or 15 per cent of the intact area, is protected.

The southern portion of the Western Ghats contains the highest peaks in the range, notably Anai Mudi in Kerala, at 2,695 metres elevation. The Ghats intercept the moisture-laden monsoon winds off the Arabian Sea, and the average annual precipitation exceeds 2,800 mm. The northeast monsoon from October to November supplements the June to September southwest monsoon. The South Western Ghats are the wettest portion of peninsular India, and are surrounded by drier ecoregions to the east and north.

The montane evergreen forests support a great diversity of species. The trees generally form a canopy at 15 to 20 m, and the forests are multistoried and rich in epiphytes, especially orchids.

The ecoregion also supports a rich fauna, which is also high in endemism: of 78 mammal species, 10 are endemic, along with 42 per cent of the fishes, 48 per cent of the reptiles, and 75 per cent of the amphibians. Of 309 bird species, 13 are endemic.

The ecoregion supports India's largest elephant population, along with populations of threatened tiger, leopard, sloth bear, gaur, and wild dog. The rare and endemic Nilgiri tahr is limited to a 400 km band of *shola*-grassland mosaic, from the Nilgiri Hills in the north to the Ashambu Hills in the south. The lion-tailed macaque and Nilgiri macaque are endangered endemic primate species.

B. Tropical and Subtropical Dry Broadleaf Forests

The tropical and subtropical dry broadleaf forest biome, also known as tropical dry forest, is located at tropical and subtropical latitudes. Though these forests occur in climates that are warm year-round, and may receive several hundred centimetres of rain per year, they deal with long dry seasons which last several months and vary with geographic location. These seasonal droughts have great impact on all living things in the forest. Deciduous trees predominate in most of these forests, and during the drought a leafless period occurs, which varies with species type. Because trees lose moisture though their leaves, the shedding of leaves allows trees such as teak and mountain ebony to conserve water during dry periods.

Though less biologically diverse than rainforests, tropical dry forests are home to a wide variety of wildlife including monkeys, large cats, parrots, various rodents, and ground dwelling birds. Mammalian biomass tends to be higher in dry forests than in rain forests, especially in Asian and African dry forests. Many of these species display extraordinary adaptations to the difficult climate.

This biome is alternately known as the tropical and subtropical dry forest biome or the tropical and subtropical deciduous forest biome. Locally some of these forests are also called monsoon forests, and they tend to merge into savannas.

1. Chota Nagpur dry deciduous forests

The Chota Nagpur dry deciduous forest is a tropical dry broadleaf forest ecoregion in eastern India. It is located in the Chota Nagpur Plateau in the States of Jharkhand, Orissa and Chhattisgarh.

Forests range from dry to wet. It is also swampy in some places. In some regions it is made up of grasslands of bamboo and bushes. Tigers, Asian elephants and bears are some of the animals found here.

2. East Deccan dry evergreen forests

The East Deccan dry evergreen forests are an ecoregion of southeastern India. The ecoregion includes the coastal region behind the Coromandel Coast on the Bay of Bengal, between the Eastern Ghats and the sea. It covers eastern Tamil Nadu State and southeastern Andhra Pradesh State.

The East Deccan dry evergreen forests cover lie in the rain shadow of the Western Ghats and Eastern Ghats, which block the rain-bearing summer southwest monsoon. Rainfall averages 800 mm/year, and mostly falls during the highly variable northeast monsoon between October and December.

The ecoregion covers an area of 25,500 square kilometres, extending from Ramanathapuram District of Tamil Nadu to Nellore District of Andhra Pradesh.

The ecoregion is home to two important wetlands, Kaliveli Lake north of Pondicherry in Viluppuram District of Tamil Nadu, and Pulicat Lake north of Chennai. Kaliveli lake is the one of the largest wetlands in peninsular India, and is deemed a wetland of national and international importance by the IUCN. Predominant species are ebony, strychnine tree, etc. A few small enclaves of deciduous Sal forest exist, but are under intensive human pressure.

Only five per cent of the ecoregion remains in forest, which is found in isolated pockets. Less than one per cent of the ecoregion lies in reserves or protected areas.

3. Kathiarbar-Gir dry deciduous forests

The Kathiawar-Gir dry deciduous forests are a tropical dry broadleaf forest ecoregion of western India.The Kathiawar-Gir forests have a disjunct distribution. The main part of the ecoregion comprises the Aravalli Range and the eastern half of Rajasthan State, extending into eastern Gujarat and the Malwa region of Madhya Pradesh. A small enclave of the ecoregion covers the peak of Girnar on the Kathiawar peninsula of western Gujarat.

The ecoregion has tropical monsoon climate, with most of the rainfall during the southwest monsoon (June-September), and arid for the remaining months of the year. Rainfall averages 550 to 700 mm/year. Temperatures often exceed 40° C.

Higher elevations of the Aravallis stay cooler, and the windward slopes (generally southeast-facing) receive higher rainfall.

The composition of the ecoregion's forests varies with moisture and soils. The highest elevations of Mount Abu are covered with conifer forests.

Top predators include the Asiatic Lion, Bengal Tiger Leopard, and Indian Wolf. Other mammal fauna include the Hyena, Chousingha, Blackbuck, , and Chinkara. Bird species include the endangered Indian Bustard, and Lesser Florican, and the near-endemic White-naped tit.

4. Narmada Valley dry deciduous forests

The Narmada Valley dry deciduous forests are a tropical dry forest ecoregion of central India. The ecoregion lies mostly in Madhya Pradesh State, but extends into portions of Chhattisgarh, Maharashtra, and Uttar Pradesh States.

The Narmada Valley dry deciduous forests cover an area of 169,900 km^2 (65,600 square miles) of the lower Narmada River Valley and the surrounding uplands. The Narmada Valley is an east-west flat-bottomed valley, or graben.

Rainfall in the ecoregion is highly seasonal.

The natural vegetation of the region is a three-tiered forest. The forests typically have an upper canopy at 15-25 metres, a 10-15 meter understory of smaller trees and large shrubs, and a 3-4 metre undergrowth. Teak is the dominant canopy tree, in association with Coromandel Ebony, Dhaora, etc.

The ecoregion is home to 76 species of mammals, none of which are endemic, although several of which, including tiger, gaur, dhole or asiatic wild dog, sloth bear, chousingha, and blackbuck, are threatened.

The ecoregion is home to 276 bird species, none of which are endemic. Large threatened birds include the Lesser Florican and Indian Bustard.

5. Northern dry deciduous forests

The Northern dry deciduous forests is a tropical dry broadleaf forest ecoregion of east-central India. It covers an area of 58,300 square kilometres, extending across portions of Andhra Pradesh, Chhatisgarh, Orissa, and Jharkhand States. The region extends north and south in the dry western rain shadow of the Eastern Ghats range, which block the moisture-laden monsoon winds from the Bay of Bengal to the east. It is completely surrounded by the more humid Eastern Highlands moist deciduous forests ecoregion.

6. South Deccan Plateau dry deciduous forests

The South Deccan Plateau dry deciduous forests is an ecoregion of southern India. The ecoregion lies in the eastern foothills of the Western Ghats; the dry forests lie in the Ghats' rain shadow, and receive considerably less rainfall than the North

Western Ghats moist deciduous forests and South Western Ghats moist deciduous forests that lie to the west. The ecoregion covers the southern portion of Karnataka's Malnad region, extending south into the Kongu Nadu region of eastern Tamil Nadu.

The ecoregion includes the cities of Bangalore and Mysore in Karnataka, and Coimbatore, Karur, and Salem in Tamil Nadu.

C. Tropical and Subtropical Coniferous Forests

Tropical and subtropical coniferous forests are a forest biome. They are located in regions of semi-humid climate at tropical and subtropical latitudes.

1. Himalayan subtropical pine forests

The ecoregion extends across the lower elevations of the great Himalaya range, States of Jammu and Kashmir, Himachal Pradesh, and Uttarakhand, Nepal, the Indian State of Sikkim, to Bhutan in the east.

The predominant tree in the ecoregion is the drought-resistant Chir Pine.

2. Northeast India-Myanmar pine forests

The Northeast India-Myanmar pine forests is a subtropical coniferous forest ecoregion of northeastern India and adjacent portions of Myanmar.

The ecoregion covers an area of 9700 km^2 of the Naga Hills, part of the belt of folded mountains that make up the India-Myanmar border region. The pine forests are found between 1500 and 2500 metres elevation, and occur in three enclaves; the largest straddles the boundary between India's Nagaland State and Myanmar, with two smaller enclaves in the southern portion of India's Mizoram State, near Myanmar border. The pine forests are surrounded at lower elevations by the predominantly broadleaf Mizoram-Manipur-Kachin rain forests.

Flora Pines are the predominant trees, associated with conifers, including hemlocks and firs, and broadleaf trees, including oaks and maples *(Acer)*. *Rhododendron*, *Ilex*, *Prunus*, and bamboo are understory shrubs.

D. Temperate Broadleaf and Mixed Forests

Temperate broadleaf and mixed forests are a temperate and humid biome.Typically, they occur in warm and rainy climates, sometimes with a distinct dry season. A dry season occurs in the winter in East Asia and in summer on the wet fringe of the Mediterranean climate zones. Other areas have a fairly even distribution of rainfall, and annual rainfall is typically over 600 millimetres (24 inches) and often over 1500 millimetres (60 inches). Temperatures are typically moderate except in parts of Asia such as Ussuriland where temperate forests can occur despite extremely harsh winters due to the heavy summer monsoon rains. Elsewhere winter temperatures typically range from maximum of 10-15°C (50-59°F) to minimum of 0-8°C (32-4 6°F). Except for old palaeosols in southern Australia, most soils in this region are fertile and usually influenced by glaciation or mountain building. In southern Australia, extremely infertile, nutrient deficient soils give a very different biome with evergreen eucalypt trees whose small, hard leaves are adapted to stay on the tree for a long period as replacement more often is far too costly as there is almost no available phosphorus. On the much more fertile soils of other continents, deciduous trees with star-shaped leaves that are shed every autumn predominate.

E. Temperate Coniferous Forests

Temperate coniferous forests are found with warm summers and cool winters and adequate rainfall to sustain a forest. In most temperate coniferous forests, evergreen conifers predominate, while some are a mix of conifers and broadleaf evergreen trees and/or broadleaf deciduous trees. Temperate evergreen forests are common in the coastal areas of regions that have mild winters and heavy rainfall, or inland in drier climates or mountain areas. Many species of trees inhabit these forests including cedar, cypress, douglas-fir, fir, juniper, kauri, pine, podocarpus, spruce, redwood and yew. The understory also contains a wide variety of herbaceous and shrub species.

This region does not support deciduous trees or flowering plants, since the climate does not support insects. Coniferous forests also have limited rainfall, requiring deciduous trees to shed their leaves soon after producing them.

Structurally, these forests are rather simple, generally consisting of two layers: an overstory and understory. Some forests may support an intermediate layer of shrubs.

Coniferous forests are currently the largest terrestrial biome on earth, although they will be surpassed by desert in the near future. This is due to extensive logging and desertification.

F. Tropical and Subtropical Grasslands, Savannas, and Shrublands

Tropical and subtropical grasslands, savannas, and shrublands are a grassland biome located in semi-arid to semi-humid climate regions of subtropical and trcpical latitudes. Grasslands are dominated by grass and other herbaceous plants. Savannas are grasslands with scattered trees. Shrublands are dominated by woody or herbaceous shrubs.

Rainfall in tropical and subtropical grasslands, savannas, and shrublands is between 50 and 150 centimetres a year, and can be highly seasonal, with the entire year's rainfall sometimes occurring within a couple of weeks. Much of the plant life on savannas is adapted to seasonal aridity.

Tropical and subtropical grasslands, savannas, and shrublands ecoregions Terai

The Tarai ("moist land") is a belt of marshy grasslands, savannas, and forests at the base of the Himalaya range from the Yamuna River in the west to the Brahmaputra River in the east. The Terai zone is inundated yearly by the monsoon-swollen rivers of the Himalaya. Below the Terai lies the great alluvial plain of the Yamuna, Ganges, Brahmaputra, and their tributaries.

Terai-Duar savanna and grasslands

The Terai-Duar savanna and grasslands is an ecoregion that stretches across the middle of the Terai belt, from Uttarakhand State through southern Nepal to northern West Bengal. The Terai-Duar savanna and wetlands are a mosaic of tall grasslands, savannas and evergreen and deciduous forests. The grasslands are among the tallest in the world, and are maintained by silt deposited by the yearly monsoon floods. Important grasses include Kans grass and Baruwa grass. The ecoregion is home to the endangered Indian Rhinoceros, as well as elephants, tigers, bears, leopards and other wild animals. Much of the ecoregion has been converted to farmland.

G. Montane Grasslands and Shrublands

Montane grasslands and shrublands is biome defined by the World Wildlife Fund. The biome includes at high altitude (montane, subalpine, and alpine) grasslands and shrublands around the world.

Montane grasslands and shrublands, particularly in subtropical and tropical regions, often evolved as virtual islands, separated from other montane regions by warmer, lower elevation regions, and are frequently home to many distinctive and endemic plants.

Montane grasslands and shrublands located above the treeline are commonly known as alpine tundra, which occurs in mountain regions around the world. Below the treeline are subalpine and montane grasslands and shrublands. Stunted subalpine forests are known as krummholz, and occur just below the treeline, where harsh, windy conditions and poor soils create dwarfed and twisted forests of slow-growing trees.

H. Flooded Grasslands and Savannas Rann of Kutch

The Rann of Kutch is a seasonally marshy region located in the Thar Desert biogeographic province in Gujarat State of northwestern India . The name "Rann" comes from the Hindi word *ran* meaning "salt marsh". Kutch is the name of the district wherein it is situated. The Rann of Kutch comprises some 10,000 square miles between the Gulf of Kutch and the mouth of the Indus River in southern Pakistan.

The Rann is famous for the Indian Wild Ass sanctuary, the Little Rann of Kutch, where the last of three species of Asiatic Wild Ass (*Equus hemionus khur* or *khar*), the only ones in Asia, still exists along with wolves, foxes, jackals, *chinkara* gazelles, nilgai antelope and blackbucks. The Rann of Kutch is also the only place in India which plays host to migrating flamingoes. There are 13 species of lark in the Rann of Kutch.

I. Deserts and Xeric Shrublands

Deserts and xeric shrublands is a biome characterized by a dry climate. Deserts and xeric shrublands occur in tropical, subtropical, and temperate climate regions.

It is characterized by :

- ☞ Rainfall : almost none
- ☞ Temperature : hot or cold
- ☞ Soil : very limited
- ☞ Plants : very sparse (succulents)
- ☞ Animal : very sparse (insect, reptiles, arachnids, nocturnal birds).

Due to the diversified habitat, the vegetation and animal life in this arid region is very rich. About 23 species of lizard and 25 species of snakes are found here and several of them are endemic to the region.

Some wildlife species, which are fast vanishing in other parts of India, are found in the desert in large numbers such as the Great Indian Bustard the Blackbuck, the Indian Gazelle and the Indian Wild Ass in the Rann of Kutch.

The Desert National Park, Jaisalmer, spread over an area of 3,162 km^2, is an excellent example of the ecosystem of the Thar Desert, and its diverse fauna. Great Indian bustard, blackbuck, chinkara, desert fox, Bengal fox, wolf, desert cat etc. can be easily seen here. Tal Chhapar Sanctuary is a very small sanctuary in Churu District, 210 km from Jaipur, in the Shekhawati region. This sanctuary is home to a large population of graceful blackbuck. Desert fox and desert cat can also be spotted along with typical avifauna such as partridge and sand grouse.

J. Mangroves Plants

Mangroves plants are that which survive high salinity, tidal extremes, strong wind velocity, high temperature and muddy anaerobic soil— a combination of conditions hostile for other plants. Mangroves not only protect the coastal communities from the fury of cyclones and coastal storms, but also promote sustainable fisheries and prevent sea erosion. In addition, they provide medicine and fuelwood. They also serve as the home of a wide range of flora and fauna.

State-wise list of Mangroves areas in India

State / UT	*Mangrove Area*
West Bengal	1. Sunderbans
Orissa	2. Bhaitarkanika, 3. Mahanadi, 4. Subernarekha, 5. Devi, 6. Dhamra, 7. MGRC, 8. Chilka
Andhra Pradesh	9. Coringa, 10. East Godavari, 11. Krishna
Tamil Nadu	12. Pichavram, 13. Muthupet, 14. Ramnad, 15. Pulicat, 16. Kazhuveli
A & N. Islands	17. North Andamans, 18. Nicobar
Kerala	19. Vembanad
Karnataka	20. Coondapur, 21. Dakshin Kannada / Honnavar
Goa	22. Karwar
Maharashtra	23. Achra-Ratnagiri, 24. Devgarh-Vijay Dur, 25. Veldur, 26. Kundalika-Ravdana, 27. Mumbra-Diva, 28.Vikroli, 29. Shreevardhan, 30. Vaitarna, 31. Vasasi-Manori, 32. Malvan
Gujarat	33. Gulf of Kutchh, 34. Gulf of Khambat

The *Sundarbans* delta is the largest mangrove forest in the world. It lies at the mouth of the Ganges and is spread across areas of Bangladesh and West Bengal in India. It is listed in the UNESCO world heritage list. There are now 400 Bengal tigers and about 30,000 spotted deer in the area

(d) Wildlife in India

India possesses an enormous wealth of animal life spread all over the subcontinent. It is estimated that nearly 40,000 species of insects, 2,000 of birds, and 500 of mammals exist in the country today. A brief description of each is given as following.

Some Important Endangered Animals of India

1 Lion tailed macaw
2. Nilgiri langoor
3. Hoolock gibbon
4. Snow leopard
5. Great one horned rhinoceros
6. Musk deer
7. Great Indian Bustard
8. Common Indian monitor varanus
9. Reticulated python
10. Peacock

Insects

Among the animals species occurring in astronomical numbers are the insects. As many as 39,150 species have been listed so far and research is still in progress, describing at least one additional species each day. They occur in all habitat types and include beautiful butterflies and moths in the part of the country and massive locusts in the western desert.

Reptiles

India is known for its variety of snakes. About 428 species are found in India. Only 50 species of snake have poisonous fangs. Notable among them are cobras including the king cobra, kraits, vipers etc .There are 150 species of lizards and 30 species of turtles and tortoises.

Birds

There are over 2,000 species of birds in India. Over 1,700 species are residents of India and breed here. About 300 species, mostly water birds such as ducks, geese, teals, cranes, and waders and a few land birds like the Imperial sand grouse, houbara, rosy paster, starling come from the Palaearctic Region of the Himalayas, Central and Northern Asia and Eastern and Northern Europe.

Large congregations of water fowl are also seen in Bihar, Chilka Lake of Orissa, Point Calimere in Tamil Nadu and Nalsarovarin Gujarat. Among the five nesting sites of the flamingos, the Great and the Little Rann of Kutch are on the world map where both the greater flamingos heronaries are Keoladeo, Sajonakholi, Ranganathittu, and Vedanthangal where thousands of storks, egrets and herons nest during the rain.

Partridges, quails and chukor are prized upland game birds. The list below gives some of the beautiful and colour designed game birds :

- ★ Black partridge
- ★ Painted gouse
- ★ Tragopans
- ★ Gray jungle fowl
- ★ Painted spurfawl
- ★ Monal pheasants

The other colourful birds include bee-eaters, parakeets, rollers and wood peckers, kingfishers, barbets minvets and sunbirds .They are rich in metallic colours. The Indian roller combine both metallic and pastel colours of the blue sky and the emerald green of the shades. Green pigeon, golden orioes, bulbuls, laughing thrush, Malabar whistling thrush, shamas, babblers, Robins and larks are our song birds which delight by the melodious soothing notes.

The favourite talking birds are the hill myna, large Alexander parakeet and blossom headed parakeets. The cuckoo are the noisy one, rightly called brain fever bird due to their harsh call. The koel has a comparatively milder melody.

The peacock is a legendary bird of Indian mythology and now a national bird. It has no parallel in the design of its colorful tail feathers called train, consisting of moon and crescents and metallic blue neck. It is too common in western India due to religious protection given to these birds. The Great Indian Bustard, a grassland bird, is a miniature Ostrich. The tallest flight bird of India is the Saras crane, conspicuously seen breeding in the north Indian plains during the monsoons. The rare black neck crane nest in Laddakh. Common crane, Demoiselle crane and Siberian cranes migrate to India in winter. The first two arrive in hundred and thousands in the western India and the third only in a small number at Bharatpur in Rajasthan. The black neck stork is the most colourful among the six stocks of India.

Birds of prey are represented by hawks, eagles, vultures, and falcons. The largest raptor is the tawny eagle with a wing spread over to two metres. Hawk eagle, Bonelli's eagle, crested serpent eagle, lagger falcon, marsh harrier, shikra and shahin are considered as the tiger of the desert sky. Owl include collared scopes owl, forest eagle owl and forest spotted owlet. Those who enjoy scoring flights are vultures, particularly Indian white backed vulture.

Mammals

India has a unique distinction of having as many as 372 species of mammals distributed a wide variety of habitat types, varying from luxurious tropical rain forest to the hot Thar desert of Rajasthan and Arctic cold desert of Laddakh. They represent all the major mammals of the world, including prime predators. Of these tigers and common leopard, are well distributed in the country while snow leopards are confined to the higher Himalayas. Another variety—the clouded leopard is actually not a member of the Panthera genus. It is found only in the northeastern India where it leads an arboreal life as a nocturnal predator. The lion is highly localized in the Gir forest of northwestern India. The hunting cheetah is also said to have existed in India though there is no record of this prior to the Mughal rule. Presently it is extinct in India. There are eight species of cats; all of them are endangered species. These include as Lynx, Caracal, Desert cat, Jungle cat, Fishing cat, Leopard cat, Pella's cat, Marbled cat.

There also exist civets such as Bear cat binturang, Marbled polecat, Chinese fervet badger and Burmese ferrat bodgeer.

Three species of mangoose are also common in India. These are the common mangoose, small Indian mongoose, and stripped necked mongoose. The stiped variety is the only species of hyena found in India. The wolf, wild dog, jackal and a variety of foxes of the vulpus genera are also effective predators. Four species of bears must be added to the list. The brown bear is confined to the northwestern Himalayas and the smaller Malayan sun bear to the eastern Himalayas. The Himalayan black bear is found throughout the mountain range. But the widest distribution from the foothills of the Himalayas is that of the sloth bear ranging through the country excluding the Himalayas and the deserts. The red panda, is also called cat bear, does not belong to the bear family but to the sub-family of raccoons. There are ten species of the weasel's family like the ratel and otter, four species of mastins and weasels and three species of badgers. The insectivores include shrews, hedgehogs and moles. The bats are flying mammals and are represented by eleven extent species in India. The order of the primates consist of fourteen species sadly, eleven of them, including the golden langur, and the lion tailed macaque, are endangered. India has only one ape—the hoolock. The commonest of the primates are the common langur and the rhesus macaw. The slow loris and slender loris are clownish primates forms found in the northeast and in the Western Ghats.

The principal prey species for the predators are the antelopes and the deer. The four species of antilopes seen in India includes the Tibetan gazelle or chiru, black buck chinkara. Four horned antelope and the nilgai. Of the seven species of deer, hangul in the northwest, and thamin in the northeast are endangered. Other like sambar, chital, barking dear are common all over India. Musk dear is confined to higher reaches of the Himalayas and hog dear and swamp dear in the gangetic tarai and Assam valley and a small population in central India. Mouse dear is found in deciduous forest of the peninsula.

The wild boar is the common but its miniature version, the pygmy hog, is endangered and is confined to a few northeastern grasslands. For smeller killers a hundred odd species of rodents provide the food base. The curious among them is the flying squirrel. There are no rabbits in India. Among hares, hispid hare, once thought to be extinct, is a miniature hare.

Wild cattle include the massive gaur in woodlands, the wild buffaloes, in the tall grassland of Assam, the banteng and the yack in the trans-Himalayas.

The Indian Elephant, a different species to the African one, and the great Indian one horned rhinoceros still exist in safer numbers of 22,000 and 1,300 respectively. The Asiatic wild ass and its Tibetan race, the kiang, dominate the hot and the cold desert respectively. They have no predators except man.

Aquatic Animals

The blue whale and sperm whale, common dolphin, gangetic dolphin and the dugong are mammals which live an aquatic life. They seem to have returned to a specialised way of life in water after they work evolved as terrestrial mammals.

(e) Conservation of Biodiversity in India

The sustainable use of biodiversity is fundamental to sustainable development.

However, during the past few decades, industrialization has put a strain on the ecosystem, altering and even destroying it. The loss of biodiversity stems from destruction of the habitat, extension of agriculture, filling up of wetlands, conversion of rich biodiversity sites for human settlement and industrial development, destruction of coastal areas and commercial exploitation.

The following major steps have been taken to conserve biodiversity :

- Establishment of protected area network of 88 national parks and 490 wild life sanctuaries.
- A programme of eco-development involving local communities is being implemented.
- Another programme of biosphere reserve is under implementation.
- A specific programme for the conservation of wetlands, mangroves and coral reefs is also being implemented.
- Six internationally significant wetlands of India have been declared as Ramsar sites under the Ramsar Convention.
- A centrally sponsored programme of National Lake Conservation was launched in 1993.
- The Wild Life Protection Act (1972) is being revised.
- Under the World Heritage Convention, five natural sites have been declared as World Heritage Sites.
- Project Tiger, initiated in 1973, has created 27 tiger reserve that led to the doubling of the tiger population.
- Project Elephant, initiated in 1991-92, assists States in ensuring the long-term survival of elephants in their natural habitats.
- The Government of India has put a ban on performance of lion, tiger, panther, bear and monkeys by circuses.
- The National Committee on the Conservation and Management of Mangroves and Coral Reefs, set up in September 1998, has recommended the establishment of an Indian coral reef monitoring network. Financial assistance from UNDP and Global Environment Facility (GEF) has been availed for strengthening the Gulf of Mannar Biosphere Reserves and a project relating to the Andamans Coral Reefs.

❖ *Biosphere Reserves in India*

Biosphere Reserves are areas of terrestrial and coastal ecosystems which are internationally recognized within the framework of UNESCO's Man and Biosphere (MAB) Programme. These reserves are required to meet a minimal set of criteria and adhere to a minimal set of conditions before being admitted to the World

Network of Biosphere Reserve designated by UNESCO for inclusion in the World Network of Biosphere Reserves.

List of Operational Biosphere Reserves in India

S. No.	*Biosphere Reserve*	*States*
1.	Nilgiri	Karnataka, Tamil Nadu and Kerala
2.	Nanda Devi	Uttrakhand
3.	Nokrek	Meghalaya
4.	Great Nicobar	Andaman and Nicobar Islands
5.	Gulf of Mannar	Tamil Nadu
6.	Manas	Assam
7.	Sunderbans	West Bengal
8.	Similipal	Orissa
9.	Dibru-Saikhowa	Assam
10.	Dehang Debang	Arunachal Pradesh
11.	Pachmarhi	Madhya Pradesh
12.	Kanchanjunga	Sikkim
13.	Agasthyamalai	Tamil Nadu and Kerala

These reserves are rich in biological and cultural diversity and encompass unique features of exceptionally pristine nature. The goal is to facilitate conservation of representative landscapes and their immense biological diversity and cultural heritage, foster economic and human development which is culturally and ecologically sustainable and to provide support for research, monitoring, education and information exchange.

The thirteen Biosphere Reserves set up in the country so far not only aim to protect representative ecosystem, but also serve as laboratories for evolving alternative models of development. A list of Biosphere Reserves set up so far along with their area and location is given in the Table.

On the basis of the proposal submitted by this Ministry to the International Coordinating Council (ICC) of Man and Biosphere Reserve (MAB) Programme of UNESCO, three Biosphere Reserves; Sunderban (West Bengal), Mannar (Tamil Nadu) and Nilgiri (Tamil Nadu) have been included in the International Network of Biosphere Reserves. Efforts are on for getting other Biosphere Reserves included in the World Network of Biosphere Reserves. This facilitates international recognition and attracts additional funding in these sites.

❖ National Parks in India

A national park is an area which is strictly reserved for the batterment of the wild life and where activities like forestry, grazing and cultivation are not permitted.

India's first National Park was *Hailey National Park*, now Jim Corbett National Park, established in 1935. By 1970, India had only 5 National Parks; while today she has 92 (as on May 2004). Currently, 38,000 km^2 of surface area are covered by National Parks, a mere 1.2 per cent of India's total surface area.

A total number of 166 National Parks have been authorized, and plans are underway to complete the remaining scheduled parks, like the *Kambalakonda National Park* in Andhra Pradesh and the *Anamudi Shola* and *Pampadum Shola* in Kerala.

Animals have been kept in captivity as pets since very early times, as is evident from the *Vedas*, the *Upanishads*, the *Puranas*, and the *epics*, the *Ramayana* and the *Mahabharata*.

❖ Zoo in India

The modern zoo was introduced in India in Madras (now Chennai) by the British in 1855. This was followed by several others, in the Princely States as well as the British-administered regions: Trivandrum (1857), Junagadh and Mumbai (1863), Hyderabad (1872), Jaipur and Kolkata (1875), Mysore (1892), Lucknow (1921), and Trichur, Udaipur, and Bikaner (1935). At present there are over 200 zoo-like facilities in the country.

Earlier, the role of zoos in India was mainly to provide recreation and add to the prestige of rulers. From the 1950s onwards, the focus changed to conservation, education, research (cultural and ecological), and lastly to tourism and recreation. Now, the emphasis is shifting to thematic and specialized displays. The centre of attention at the Junagadh zoo, for instance, are the Indian lion and the Indian wild ass; Thiruvananthapuram focuses on lion-tailed macaws; hoolock gibbons at Guwahati; and the wolf at Hyderabad.

The display of animals may take several forms. Zoogeographic displays exhibit animals according to the continent of origin (for instance, Asia, Africa, and South America), habitat (the tundra, temperate, sub-tropical, equatorial regions), or geographical regions (Indo-Malaysian, Himalayan, Palaeoarctic, and Australian). This approach began in the 1960s and is used in the renovation of older zoos.

A combination of several displays is adopted according to the suitability of the site. The availability of space in existing zoos is the prime reason they adopt such an approach, while the zoo-cum-botanical garden concept is gaining popularity where plants and animals are closely interrelated and dependent on one another. This concept has been adopted where forest areas were taken up for zoos as in Tirupati and Visakhapatnam (Andhra Pradesh), Bhopal (M.P.), Bannerghata (Karnataka), and Vandalur (Tamil Nadu), using the indigenous vegetation.

Wildlife Sanctuaries

Wildlife sanctuaries are also the protected areas where killing, hunting, shooting, or capturing of wild life is prohibited except under the control of highest authority. However, private ownership rights are permissible and forestry operations are also permitted to an extent that they do not affect the wildlife adversely.

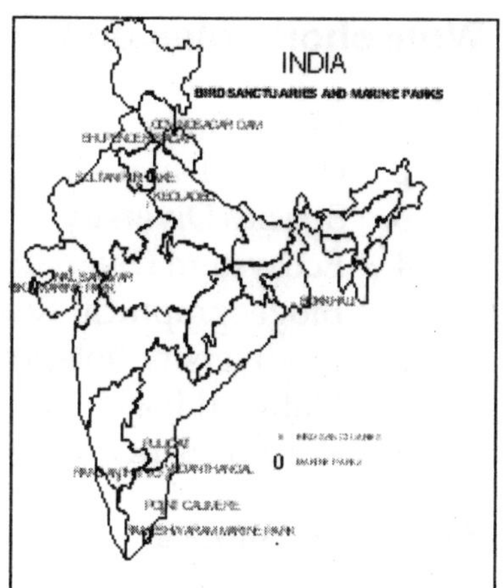

INDIA : IMPORTANT WILDLIFE SANCTUARIES		
Name of Sanctuary	State	Major Wild Life
Ghana Bird Sanctuary	Rajasthan	300 species of birds
Hazaribagh Bird Sanctuary	Bihar	Tiger, Leopard
Sultanpur Bird Sanctuary	Haryana	Migratory birds
Nal Sarovar Bird Sanctuary	Gujarat	Water birds
Abohar Bird Sanctuary	Punjab	Black buck
Mudamalai Bird Sanctuary	Tamil Nadu	Tiger, elephant, Leopard
Veanthangal Bird Sanctuary	Tamil Nadu	Water birds
Jalapara Bird Sanctuary	West Bengal	Rhinoceros, Elephant, Tiger
Wild Ass Sanctuary	Gujarat	Wild Ass, Wolf, Chinkara

Questions

Long answer type of questions

1. Define Biodiversity. How can you classify bio-diversity? Discuss the importance of biodiversity.
2. Write down about the evolution of biodiversity.
3. Explain the factors which are responsible for biodiversity loss.
4. Give an account of biodiversity in India.
5. Describe the eco-regions of India.
6. What are the steps, which have been taken to conserve bio-diversity in India?

Write short notes on the following:

1. Biodiversity
2. Genetic Diversity.
3. Species Diversity.
4. Ecosystem Diversity.
5. Biogeographical Realms.
6. Biodiversity hotspots.
7. National Park.
8. Wildlife Sanctuaries.

Fill in the blanks

1. Scientists have discovered and named only .... million species.
2. World population has ....in the past forty years.
3. The tallest flight bird of India is the ....
4. The modern zoo was introduced in India in ....by the British in 1855.
5. The ....is a legendary bird of Indian mythology and now a national bird.
6. There are over........... species of birds in India.
7. India's first National Park was...................., established in 1935.

Keys : 1. 1.75; 2. Doubled; 3. Saras crane; 4. Chennai; 5. Peacock; 6. 2000; 7. Jim Corbett.

Tick the right answer

1. The estimated population of Tigers in the country is :
   (a) 1500
   (b) 1000
   (c) 500
   (d) Over 3,500
2. The estimated population of Elephants in the country is :
   (a) Over 27,000
   (b) Over 15,000
   (c) Over 37,000
   (d) Over 47,000
3. The estimated population of Asiatic Lion in the country is :
   (a) Over 600
   (b) Over 200
   (c) Over 300

(d) Over 150

4. The estimated population of Rhinoceros in the country is :
   (a) Over 2, 700
   (b) Over 3, 700
   (c) Over 4, 700
   (d) Over 1, 700
5. Project Elephant, initiated in
   (a) 1975-76
   (b) 1980-81
   (c) 1991-92
   (d) 1995-96
6. As of May 2004, India has
   (a) 92 National Park
   (b) 65 National Park
   (c) 75 National Park
   (d) 115 National Park
7. National Lake Conservation was launched in
   (a) 1974
   (b) 1993
   (c) 1983
   (d) 1964

Keys : 1. (d); 2. (a); 3. (c); 4. (d); 5. (c); 6. (a); 7. (b).

True/False types of questions

1. India is not one of the 12-mega diversity countries of the world.
2. Humans the world over use at least 40,000 species of plants and animals on a daily basis.
3. India is known for its variety of snakes. About 428 species are found in India.
4. The Wild Life Protection Act (1972) is being revised.
5. Biodiversity is not the pillar upon which we build civilizations.
6. Beta diversity is species diversity between ecosystems.
7. Alpha diversity refers to diversity within a particular area

Keys : 1. false; 2. true; 3. true; 4. true; 5. false; 6. true; 7. true.

Unit - 5

Environmental Pollution

I. Definition

The word Pollution is derived from Latin word *"pollutionem"* means to defile or make dirty. Pollution may be defined as the contamination of Earth's environment with materials that interfere with human health, the quality of life, or the natural functioning of ecosystems (living organisms and their physical surroundings). Although some environmental pollution is a result of natural causes such as volcanic eruptions, most is caused by human activities.

II. Pollutants

There are two main categories of polluting materials, or pollutants.

1. Biodegradable
2. Non-degradable pollutants.

EXAMPLES OF MAJOR POLLUTANTS

1.	Solid wastes	Garbage, rubbish, ashes, dead animals, demolition wastes, mining waste, crop residues etc.
2.	Liquid wastes	Sewage, Kitchen waste, soil washing.
3.	Gaseous wastes	Smog gases (carbon monoxide, SO_2, NO_2), Ozone, Hydrogen sulphide.
4.	Deposited matter	Soot, smoke, tar, grit, dust etc.
5.	Radioactive waste	Argon-41, Cobalt- 60, Krypton-85, Strontium-90, Plutonium–235
6.	Gases	Oxides of Nitrogen and Sulphur, Halogens, carbon monoxides, ozone, ammonia.
7.	Acids	Nitric Acid, Sulphuric Acid, and other acids.(e.g. acid rain)
8.	Metal Mercury	Cadmium, chromium, iron, zinc, lead, tin, nickel.
9.	Agrochemicals	Insecticides, pesticides, herbicides, rodenticides, fungicides, weedicides, and fertilizers, e.g. – DDT, BHC.
10.	Organic Substances	Benzene, aldehydes, detergents, ether, phosgenes, acetic acid, etc.

Biodegradable pollutants are materials, such as sewage, that rapidly decompose by natural processes. These pollutants become a problem when added to the environment faster than they can decompose. Nondegradable pollutants are materials that either do not decompose or decompose slowly in the natural environment. Once contamination occurs, it is difficult or impossible to remove these pollutants from the environment.

Nondegradable compounds such as dichlorodiphenyltrichloroethane (DDT), dioxins, polychlorinated biphenyls (PCBs), and radioactive materials can reach dangerous levels of accumulation as they are passed up the food chain into the bodies of progressively larger animals. For example, molecules of toxic compounds may collect on the surface of aquatic plants without doing much damage to the plants. A small fish that grazes on these plants accumulates a high concentration of the toxin. Larger fish or other carnivores that eat the small fish will accumulate even greater, and possibly life-threatening, concentrations of the compound. This process is known as bioaccumulation.

Pollution exists in many forms and affects many different aspects of Earth's environment. *Point-source* pollution comes from specific, localized, and identifiable sources, such as sewage pipelines or industrial smokestacks. *Nonpoint-source* pollution comes from dispersed or uncontained sources, such as contaminated water runoff from urban areas or automobile emissions.

The effects of these pollutants may be immediate or delayed. Primary effects of pollution occur immediately after contamination occurs, such as the death of marine plants and wildlife after an oil spill at sea. Secondary effects may be delayed or may persist in the environment into the future, perhaps going unnoticed for many years. DDT, a nondegradable compound, seldom poisons birds immediately, but gradually accumulates in their bodies. Birds with high concentrations of this pesticide lay thin-shelled eggs that fail to hatch or produce deformed offspring. These secondary effects, publicized by Rachel Carson in her 1962 book, *Silent Spring*, threatened the survival of species such as the bald eagle and peregrine falcon, and aroused public concern over the hidden effects of nondegradable chemical compounds.

III. Types of Pollution

- *Air pollution*, the release of chemicals and particulates into the atmosphere. Common examples include carbon monoxide, sulfur dioxide, chlorofluorocarbons (CFCs), and nitrogen oxides produced by industry and motor vehicles. Ozone and smog are created as nitrogen oxides and hydrocarbons react to sunlight.
- *Water pollution* affects oceans and inland bodies of water. Examples include organic and inorganic chemicals, heavy metals, petrochemicals, chloroform, and bacteria. Water pollution may also occur in the form of thermal pollution and the depletion of dissolved oxygen.
- *Soil contamination* often occurs when chemicals are released by spill or

underground storage tank leakage. Contaminants include hydrocarbons, heavy metals, MTBE, herbicides, pesticides and chlorinated hydrocarbons. Often leads to water pollution via surface runoff and leaching to groundwater.

- *Radioactive contamination*, added in the wake of twentieth century discoveries in atomic physics.
- *Noise pollution*, which encompasses roadway noise, aircraft noise, industrial noise as well as high-intensity sonar.
- *Light pollution*, includes light trespass, over-illumination and astronomical interference.
- *Visual pollution*, which can refer to the presence of overhead power lines, highway billboards, scarred landforms (as from strip mining), open storage of junk or municipal solid waste.

(a) Air Pollution

Air pollution is a broad term applied to any chemical, physical (e.g. particulate matter), or biological agent that modifies the natural characteristics of the atmosphere. The atmosphere is a complex, dynamic natural system that is essential to support life on planet earth. Stratospheric ozone depletion due to air pollution has long been recognized as a threat to human health as well as to the earth's ecosystems.

The World Health Organization (WHO)-estimates that 4.6 million people die each year from causes of directly attributable to air pollution. Many of these mortalities are attributable to indoor air pollution. Worldwide more deaths per year are linked to air pollution than to automobile accidents. Research published in 2005 suggests that 310,000 Europeans die from air pollution annually. *Direct causes of air pollution related deaths include aggravated asthma, bronchitis, emphysema, lung and heart diseases, and respiratory allergies.*

Urban air pollution is commonly known as smog. The dark London smog is generally a smoky mixture of carbon monoxide and organic compounds from incomplete combustion (burning) of fossil fuels such as coal, and sulfur dioxide from impurities in the fuels. As the smog ages and reacts with oxygen, organic and sulfuric acids condense as droplets, increasing the haze. Smog developed into a major health hazard by the twentieth century. In 1952, about 4,000 Londoners died of its effects.

A second type of smog, photochemical smog, began reducing air quality over large cities like Los Angeles in the 1930s. This smog is caused by combustion in car, truck, and airplane engines, which produce nitrogen oxides and release hydrocarbons from unburned fuels. Sunlight causes the nitrogen oxides and hydrocarbons to combine and turn oxygen into *ozone, a chemical agent that attacks rubber, injures plants, and irritates lungs.* The hydrocarbons are oxidized into materials that condense and form a visible, pungent haze.

Eventually most pollutants are washed out of the air by rain, snow, fog, or mist, but only after travelling large distances, sometimes across continents. As pollutants build up in the atmosphere, sulfur and nitrogen oxides are converted into acids that mix with rain. This acid rain falls in lakes and on forests, where it can lead to the death of fish and plants, and damage entire ecosystems. Eventually the contaminated lakes and forests may become lifeless. Regions that are downwind of heavily industrialized areas, such as Europe and the eastern United States and Canada, are the hardest hit by acid rain. Acid rain can also affect human health and man-made objects; it is slowly dissolving historic stone statues and building facades in London, Athens, and Rome.

The worst short-term civilian pollution crisis in India was the 1984 Bhopal Disaster. Leaked industrial vapours killed more than 2,000 people outright and injured anywhere from 150,000 to 600,000 others, some 6,000 of whom would later die from their injuries. The United Kingdom suffered its worst air pollution event when the December 4th Great Smog of 1952 formed over London. In six days more than 4,000 died, and 8,000 more died within the following months. An accidental leak of anthrax spores from a biological warfare laboratory in the former USSR in 1979 near Sverdlovsk is believed to have been the cause of hundreds of civilian deaths.

There are many available air pollution control technologies and urban planning strategies available to reduce air pollution, however, worldwide costs of addressing the issue are high. The most immediate method of improving air quality would be the use of bioethanol fuel, biodiesel, solar energy, and hybrid vehicle technologies.

➢ Sources of Air Pollution

Air pollutants are classified as either directly released or formed by subsequent chemical reactions. A direct release air pollutant is one that is emitted directly from a given source, such as the carbon monoxide or sulfur dioxide, all of which are byproducts of combustion; whereas, a subsequent air pollutant is formed in the atmosphere through chemical reactions involving direct release pollutants. The formation of ozone in photochemical smog is the most important example of a subsequent air pollutant.

◆ Anthropogenic Sources

Anthropogenic sources (human activity) related to burning different kinds of fuel as follows :

- Combustion-fired power plants.
- Controlled burn practices used in agriculture and forestry management.
- Motor vehicles generating air pollution emissions.
- Marine vessels, such as container ships or cruise ships, and related port air emissions.

- Wood, coal, fuel oil or natural gas burning fireplaces, stoves, furnaces and incinerators.
- Oil refining, power plant operation and industrial activity in general.
- Chemicals, dust and crop waste burning in farming.
- Fumes from paint, varnish, aerosol sprays and other solvents.
- Waste deposition in landfills, which generate methane.
- Military uses, as nuclear weapons, toxic gases, germ warfare and rocketry.

◆ Natural Sources

- Dust from natural sources, usually large areas of land with little or no vegetation.
- Methane, emitted by the digestion of food by animals, for example cattle.
- Pine trees, which emit volatile organic compounds (VOCs).
- Radon gas from radioactive decay within the Earth's crust.
- Smoke and carbon monoxide from wild fires.
- Volcanic activity, which produce sulfur, chlorine, and ash particulates.

❖ Unit and Methods of Measurement of Air Pollution

➢ **Units of measurement :** There are two main units to measure the concentration of air pollution :

- Part per million (ppm) – It is based on volume measurement and indicates the volume of pollutant contained in one million volume of air (at standard temperature of 25^0 C and pressure of 760 mm)
- Micrograms per cubic metre ($\mu g/m^3$)—Concentration of air pollutants can also be expressed by relating the mass of the pollutant to the volume of the air containing it. The unit of microgrammes per cubic metre ($\mu g/m^3$), where one microgram is equal to 10^{-6} gms. In densely polluted air the concentration can also be expressed in milligrams per cubic metre.

➢ **Methods of measurement :** The Methods of measurement of air pollution followed by the Central Pollution Control Board, Delhi are as follows :

A. Sulphur Dioxide (SO_2)

The SO_2 is absorbed from air in a solution of potassium tetrachloromercurate (TCM). The resultant complex is made to react with pararosaniline and formaldehyde to form the coloured pararosaniline methylsulphuric acid, the absorbance of this solution is measured by means of a suitable spectrophotometer at 560 µm.

B. Nitrogen Dioxide (NO_2)

The NO_2 in ambient air is collected by bubbling it through a solution of sodium hydroxide and sodium arsenate. The resultant nitrite ion concentration is calorimetrically determined by reacting it with sulfanilamide and N- (1-napthyl) - ethylene diamine dihydrochloride, the absorbance is then measured at 540 μm.

C. Suspended Particulate Matter (SPM)

SPM is measured gravimetrically high volume sampling with whatman filter paper is used at average flow rate being not less than 1.1 cubic metre per minute.

National Ambient (Surrounding) Air Quality Standards

Pollutants	*Time-weighted average*	*Concentration in ambient air*			*Method of measurement*
		Industrial Areas	*Residential, Rural & other Areas*	*Sensitive Areas*	
Sulphur Dioxide (SO_2)	Annual Average*	80 μg/m³	60 μg/m³	15 μg/m³	Improved West and Geake Method Ultraviolet-Fluorescence
	24 hours**	120 μg/m³	80 μg/m³	30 μg/m³	
Oxides of Nitrogen as (NO_2)	Annual Average*	80 μg/m³	60 μg/m³	15 μg/m³	Jacob & Hochheiser (Na-Arsenite) Method Gas Phase Chemiluminescence
	24 hours**	120 μg/m³	80 μg/m³	30 μg/m³	
Suspended Particulate Matter (SPM)	Annual Average*	360 μg/m³	140 μg/m³	70 μg/m³	High Volume Sampling, (at flow rate not less than 1.1 m³/minute).
	24 hours**	500 μg/m³	200 μg/m³	100 μg/m³	
Respirable Particulate Matter (RPM) (size less than 10 microns)	Annual Average*	120 μg/m³	60 μg/m³	50 μg/m³	Respirable particulate matter sampler
	24 hours**	150 μg/m³	100 μg/m³	75 μg/m³	
Lead (Pb)	Annual Average*	1.0 μg/m³	0.75 μg/m³	0.50 μg/m³	ASS Method after sampling using EPM 2000 or Filter paper
	24 hours**	1.5 μg/m³	1.00 μg/m³	0.75 μg/m³	
Ammonia	Annual Average*-	0.1 mg/ m³	0.1 mg/ m³	0.1 mg/m³	—
	24 hours**	0.4 mg/ m³	0.4 mg/m³	0.4 mg/m³	
Carbon Monoxide (CO)	8 hours**	5.0 mg/m³	2.0 mg/m³	1.0 mg/ m³	Non Dispersive Infra Red (NDIR)
	1 hour	10.0 mg/m³	4.0 mg/m³	2.0 mg/m³	

* Annual Arithmetic mean of minimum 104 measurements in a year taken twice a week 24 hourly at uniform interval.

** 24 hourly/8 hourly values should be met 98 per cent of the time in a year. However, 2 per cent of the time, it may exceed but not on two consecutive days.

Source: Central Pollution Control Board, New Delhi.

Effects of Air Pollutants on Human Health

Pollutants	*Source*	*Pathological effect on man*
Sulphur Dioxide	Coal and Oil burning	Chest constriction, headache, vomiting, and death from respiratory ailments.
Nitrogen dioxides	Soft coal, Automobile	Dust penetrate far into the lungs
Hydrogen sulphide	Refineries, and chemical industries	Causes nausea, irritate eyes and throat.
Carbon Monoxide	Oil burning, gasoline, and motor exhaust	Reduces oxygen carrying capacity.
Ammonia	Explosives, dye making, fertilizers	Inflame upper respiratory tracks.
Suspended Particles (Ash, soot, smoke)	Incinerators and all manu-facturing process	Cause eraphysema, eye irritation and cancer
Arsenics	Metal or acid containing arsenic soldering	Damage red cells in the blood, kidneys and cause jaundice.

❖ Air Pollution in India

Industrialization and urbanization have resulted in a profound deterioration of India's air quality. India has more than 20 cities with populations of at least 1 million, and some of them, including New Delhi, Mumbai, Chennai, and Kolkata are among the world's most polluted. Urban air quality ranks among the world's worst. Of the 3 million premature deaths in the world that occur each year due to outdoor and indoor air pollution, the highest number are assessed to occur in India. Sources of air pollution, India's most severe environmental problem, come in several forms, including vehicular emissions and untreated industrial smoke. Continued urbanization has exacerbated the problem of rapid industrialization, as more and more people are adversely affected and cities are unable to implement adequate pollution control mechanisms.

One of the most affected cities in New Delhi, where airborne particulate matter (PM) has been registered at levels more than 10 times India's legal limit. Vehicles are the major source of this pollution, with more than three million cars, trucks, buses, taxis, and rickshaws already on the roads. With vehicle ownership rising along with population and income, India's efforts to improve urban air quality have focused in this area. In New Delhi, emissions limits for gasoline—and diesel-powered vehicles came into effect in 1991 and 1992, respectively, and the city has prohibited the use of vehicle more than 15 years old. Emissions standards for passenger cars and commercial vehicles were tightened in 2000 at levels equivalent to the Euro-1 standards of the European Union, while the even-more-stringent Euro-2 standards have been in place for the metropolitan areas of Delhi, Mumbai, Chennai, and Kolkata since 2001. Furthermore, the sulfur content of motor fuels sold in the four cities has been restricted to 500 parts per million (PPM) since 2001 in order to be compatible with tighter vehicle emissions standards. Motor fuel sulfur content in all other regions of India has been limited to 2,500 PPM since January 2000.

India's high concentration of pollution is not due to the absence of a sound environmental legal regime, however, but to a lack of environmental enforcement at the local level. In 1998, India's Supreme Court issued a ruling requiring all the city's buses to be run on compressed natural gas (CNG) by March 31, 2001.

In addition, India's reliance on coal-fired power plants for its electricity generation has undermined some of the vehicular-oriented air quality improvement initiatives. Despite the fact that India is a large coal consumer, its Central Pollution Control Board has been slow to set sulfur dioxide (SO_2) emissions limits for coal-fired power plants, mainly because most of the coal mined in India is low in sulfur content. Coal-fired power plants do not face any nitrogen oxide (NO_x) emissions limits either, although thermal plants fuelled by other fossil fuels are subject to particulate matter emission standards. Again, however, the government's support for air quality standards has been undermined by the lack of enforcement of these standards.

India : Seven Locations having highest concentration of SPM during the year 2002

Industrial			*Residential*		
Location	*State*	*Annual Mean Conc. (μg/m³)*	*Location*	*State*	*Annual Mean Conc. (μg/m³)*
Basni Ind. Area, Jodhpur	Raj	528*	Town Hall, Delhi	Delhi	534*
M/s A.C. Pvt. Ltd., Fazalganj, Kanpur	U.P.	507*	Sojati Gate, Jodhpur	Rajasthan	526*
Shahzada Bagh, Delhi	Delhi	468*	Gandhi Test Centre, Patna	Bihar	509*
Shivalic Ind., Faridabad	Haryana	465*	Nal Stop, Pune	Maharashtra	507*
Shahdara, Delhi	Delhi	415*	Off. - HSPCB, Faridabad	Haryana	474*
Lajpat Nagar, Kanpur	U.P.	414*	Deputy ka Parao, Kanpur	U.P.	459*
Raunaq Auto Ltd., Gajraula	U.P.	408*	Janakpuri, Delhi	Delhi	442*

Source : Pollution Control Board, India, 2002.

* Locations where annual mean concentration of SPM exceeded the respective standards of 360 μg/m³ for Industrial and 140 μg/m³ for Residential areas.

❖ Government Policies on Air Pollution in India

The air quality has been, therefore, an issue of social concern in the backdrop of various developmental activities. The norms for ambient air quality and industry specific emissions have been notified. For control of air pollution, with a view to initiate policy measures and to prepare ambient air quality management plans, 326 Air Quality Monitoring Stations have been installed covering 32 States and Union Territories. Out of these, on-line data display is available in respect of 215 stations. Presently, only the criteria pollutants namely, sulphur dioxide, oxides of nitrogen and respirable suspended particulate matter are monitored by Pollution Control Boards, Universities and Research Institutes. Besides this, additional parameters for other toxic trace matters and polycyclic aromatic hydrocarbons are also being monitored in selected cities of the country. For continuous air quality monitoring, Automatic Air Quality Monitoring Stations have been set up in four cities namely, Jodhpur, Patna, Pune and Sholapur. In addition such stations are also being provided in the cities of Kanpur, Varanasi, Jharia and Kolkata.

Keeping in view the monitored data available on air quality, the Hon'ble Supreme Court in its various judgements have identified sixteen cities namely, Hyderabad, Patna, Ahmedabad, Faridabad, Jharia, Bangalore, Pune, Mumbai, Sholapur, Jodhpur, Chennai, Agra, Kanpur, Lucknow, Varanasi and Kolkata as equal to or more polluted than Delhi for which Action Plans for improvement of air quality have been drawn. The CPCB has evolved a format for preparation of action plans, which has been circulated to all State Pollution Control Boards/ Committees. The Action Plans emphasize identification of sources of air pollution, assessment of pollution load and adoption of abatement measures for identified sources. Setting up interdepartmental task force for implementation of city specific action plan has also been suggested. A Review Meeting for ascertaining implementation of these plans was held in the Ministry and the respective Boards have been advised to undertake bench marking of pollution levels and sources for evolving necessary plans.

In order to control vehicular pollution, a road map has been adopted as per the schedule proposed in Auto Fuel Policy, which includes use of cleaner fuels, automobile technologies and enforcement measures for in use vehicles through improved Pollution Under Control (PUC) certification system. As per the Auto Fuel Policy, Bharat Stage-II norms for new vehicles have been introduced throughout the country from 1st April, 2005. However, EURO-III equivalent emission norms for all new vehicles, except 2-3 wheelers, have been introduced in 11 major cities from 1st April, 2005. To meet Bharat Stage-II, EURO-III and EUROIV emission norms, matching quality of petrol and diesel is being made available. Due to multiplicity and complexity of air polluting sources, apportionment of contribution to ambient air pollution from these sources is important for planning cost effective pollution control strategies. In view of this, a study on "Air Quality Assessment, Emission inventory/Source Apportionment Studies for Indian Cities" has been initiated for major Indian cities. In the first phase, the study would cover six cities viz; Delhi, Bangalore, Pune, Kanpur, Mumbai and Chennai with focus on apportionment of fine particulate matter (RSPM). A Steering Committee under the chairmanship of Secretary (E&F) for overall supervision and a Technical Committee under the chairmanship of Chairmanship, CPCB to look into and to guide on the technical aspects of the projects have been set up. A common methodology for conducting the study has been finalized with identification of technical institutions for completing the study.

❖ Measures to Control Air Pollution

There is an immediate need to improve and upgrade the existing monitoring network. Following measures would greatly enhance the quality and reliability of data and monitoring activities as such :

- Old air quality monitoring equipment needs replacement.
- Adequate infrastructure may be provided and manpower may be trained for proper sampling, preservation and analysis, data reporting, etc.
- Monitoring of additional parameters such as Carbon Monoxide, Lead, PAHs, Benzene, 1.3 butadine, Ozone, etc. may be carried out.
- Existing network of 295 stations may be expanded and continuous monitoring of air pollutants may be carried out, wherever appropriate.
- Epidemiological studies may be carried out in various cities where levels of air pollutants are exceeding the standards.
- More sensitive areas may be identified and notified.
- Background stations may be included in the network to assess the anthropogenic impact.
- Calibration of air quality monitoring instruments may be carried out regularly.
- By planting trees and growing vegetation.
- Maximum use of alternative source of energy.
- Use of pollution control equipments.

(b) Noise Pollution

Noise pollution is unwanted human-created sound that disrupts the environment. In other words noise pollution, means human-created noise harmful to health or welfare.

❖ Causes of Noise Pollution

The dominant cause of noise pollution is from transportation sources,vehicles are the worst offenders, with aircraft, railroad stock, trucks, buses, automobiles, and motorcycles all producing excessive noise. Besides transportation noise, other prominent sources are office equipment, factory machinery, appliances, power tools, festivals, lighting hum and audio entertainment systems. With the popularity of digital audio player devices, individuals in a noisy area might increase the volume in order to drown out ambient sounds. Construction equipment also produces noise pollution.The word *noise* comes from the Latin word *nausea* meaning seasickness.

Sources of noise pollution

Transportation	Aircrafts, trains, trucks, tractors, three-wheelers, etc.
Industries/Construction machinery	Factory equipment, generators, pile drivers, road rollers, etc.
Events	Loudspeakers, Religious and Political meeting, etc.

Noise intensity is measured in decibel units. The decibel scale is logarithmic; each 10-decibel increase represents a tenfold increase in noise intensity. Human perception of loudness also conforms to a logarithmic scale; a 10-decibel increase is perceived as roughly a doubling of loudness. Thus, 30 decibels is 10 times more intense than 20 decibels and sounds twice as loud; 40 decibels is 100 times more intense than 20 and sounds 4 times as loud; 80 decibels is 1 million times more intense than 20 and sounds 64 times as loud. Distance diminishes the effective decibel level reaching the ear. Thus, moderate auto traffic at a distance of 100 ft (30 m) rates about 50 decibels. To a driver with a car window open or a pedestrian on the sidewalk, the same traffic rates about 70 decibels; that is, it sounds 4 times louder. At a distance of 2,000 ft (600 m), the noise of a jet takeoff reaches about 110 decibels—approximately the same as an automobile horn only 3 ft (1 m) away.

Typical average decibel level (dbA) of some common sounds

Source	*dbA*
Threshold of hearing	0
Quiet whisper (1m)	30
Normal conversation	60
Loud singing (1m)	75
Motorcycle (10m)	88
Diesel truck (10m)	100
Pneumatic drill (1m)	115
Amplified pop music (2m)	120
Jet plane (30m)	130
Threshold of Pain	
Rocket Engine	180

Subjected to 45 decibels of noise, the average person cannot sleep. At 120 decibels the ear registers pain, but hearing damage begins at a much lower level, about 85 decibels. The duration of the exposure is also important. There is evidence that among youngsters hearing sensitivity is decreasing year by year because of exposure to noise, including excessively amplified music. Apart from hearing loss, such noise can cause lack of sleep, irritability, heartburn, indigestion, ulcers, high blood pressure, and possibly heart disease. One burst of noise, as from a passing truck, is known to alter endocrine, neurological, and cardiovascular functions in many individuals; prolonged or frequent exposure to such noise tends to make the physiological disturbances chronic. In addition, noise-induced stress creates severe tension in daily living and contributes to mental illness.

The Central Pollution Control Board (CPCB) of India has recommended permissible noise level for the different locations as following:

Area Category	*Noise level in dBA leq*	
	Day	*Night*
Industrial	75	70
Commercial	65	55
Residential	55	45
Silence Zone	50	40

❖ Effects of Noise pollution on human health

Principal noise health effects are both health and behavioural in nature. The mechanism for chronic exposure to noise leading to hearing loss is well established. The elevated sound levels cause trauma to the cochlear structure in the inner ear, which gives rise to irreversible hearing loss. The pinna (visible portion of the human ear) combined with the middle ear amplifies sound levels by a factor of 20 when sound reaches the inner ear. The findings proved that ageing is an almost insignificant cause of hearing loss, which instead is associated with chronic exposure to moderately high levels of environmental noise.

High noise levels can contribute to cardiovascular effects and exposure to moderately high (e.g. above 70 dBA) during a single eight hours period causes a statistical rise in blood pressure of five to ten mm of mercury; a clear and measurable increase in stress; and vasoconstriction leading to the increased blood pressure noted above as well as to increased incidence of coronary artery disease.

Noise pollution constitutes a significant factor of annoyance and distraction in modern artificial environments such as :

- ☞ The meaning listeners attribute to the sound influences annoyance, so that, if listeners dislike the noise content, they are annoyed.
- ☞ If the sound causes activity interference, noise is more likely to annoy (for example, sleep disturbance).
- ☞ If listeners feel they can control the noise source, the less likely the noise will be annoying.
- ☞ If listeners believe that the noise is subject to third party control, including police, but control has failed, they are more annoyed.

- The inherent unpleasantness of the sound causes annoyance. What is music to one is noise to another.
- *Contextual sound.* If the sound is appropriate for the activity it is in context. If one is at a race track the noise is in context and the psychological effects are absent. If one is at an outdoor picnic the race track noise will produce adverse psychological and physical effects.

Noise pollution can also be harmful to animals. High noise levels may interfere with the natural cycles of animals, including feeding behaviour, breeding rituals and migration paths. The most significant impact of noise to animal life is the systematic reduction of usable habitat, which in the case of endangered species may be an important part of the path to extinction. Perhaps, the most sensational damage caused by noise pollution is the death of certain species of beaked whales, brought on by the extremely loud (up to 200 decibels) sound of military SONAR.

❖ Noise Pollution and Government Policies in India

Noise levels have been a matter of concern due to various activities, religious functions, festivals and related celebrations. The main sources of noise pollution include industrial activities, use of public address system, construction activities, use of generator sets, pressure horns and fire crackers, etc. Keeping in view the increasing trend in noise levels, Ministry has issued various regulations from time to time to control noise pollution in ambient air, at source and at manufacturing stage. To control community noise, Noise Pollution (Regulation and Control) Rules, 2000 were issued in February 2000, which makes it mandatory for local authorities to control noise levels in their respective areas.

- In Civil Writ Petition No. 72 of 1998 regarding noise pollution – implementation of laws for restricting use of loudspeakers and high volume producing sound system, the Hon'ble Supreme Court in its judgment of July 2005 has given detailed directions regarding implementation of laws for controlling noise. Subsequently, referring to the amendment of October 2002 issued by the Ministry in respect of notification of February 2000 permitting the use of loudspeaker or public address system during the night hours between 10.00 p.m. to 06:00 a.m. on or during any cultural or religious festive occasions of a limited duration not exceeding 15 days in all during a calendar year, Hon'ble Supreme Court had further observed that a limited power of exemption from operations of noise rules granted by the Central Government in exercise of its statutory power cannot be held unreasonable.
- In pursuance of these judgments and to collect benchmark data, all the

CASE STUDY

Delhi during Deepawali Festival

During Deepawali days, noise level increases due to the bursting of crackers. In order of assess the air pollution and noise caused due to bursting of crackers, ambient air quality was measured at selected locations in Delhi during 2003. The observations are as follows:

Location	*Noise Levels in dB(A)*		
	Normal Day	*Deepawali Day*	*Standard Limit*
AIIMS Crossing	60	76	55
Lajpat Nagar	66	89	55
Friends Colony	56	90	55
Arjun Nagar	63	81	55
Connaught Place	70	74	65
India Gate	63	69	50
Mayur Vihar II	59	81	55
Patel Nagar	71	73	55
Kamla Nagar	68	78	55
Kidwai Nagar	62	76	55
Dilshad Garden	67	80	55
Pusa R. Crossing	79	77	55
ITO Crossing	—	77	55

Source: Pollution Control Board, India, 2002.

regulatory agencies of the State Government/Union Territories have been advised to comply with stipulated norms and to draw an Action Plan for ensuring the compliance of the directions. The concerned agencies have also been advised to strengthen/establish environmental cells at the State and district levels to check noise pollution and also to undertake surveys in major cities especially before and after the festivals to ensure compliance. Intensive campaigns were also launched in print and electronic media about deleterious effects of noise pollution. For creating awareness, most of the State governments have sent their monitoring reports of survey undertaken before and on Diwali day and the reports reveal that there has been a reasonable success in arresting menace of noise pollution.

- The noise limits for Diesel Generator (DG) set up to 1000 KVA were notified in May 2002. After review of the preparedness by the manufacturers to comply with the standards, the time for implementation was extended up to 1st January, 2005. While the emission norms for DG sets above 19 KW and up to 800 KW have been made operational since November 2004, these norms for DG sets up to 19 KW have come into effect from 1st July 2005.

Measures to Control Noise Pollution

- Roadways noise is the most widespread environmental component of noise pollution worldwide. There are a variety of effective strategies for mitigating adverse sound levels including: use of noise barriers, limitation of vehicle speeds, alteration of roadway surface texture, limitation of heavy duty vehicles, use of traffic controls that smooth vehicle flow to reduce braking and acceleration, innovative tire design and other methods.

- Using ear protective devices e.g., ear plugs, headphones, etc.
- Public awareness and Implementation of legislation against noise pollution.
- Plantation because plants absorb noise.
- Use of sound absorption silencers.

(c) Water Pollution

When toxic substances enter lakes, streams, rivers, oceans, and other water bodies, they get dissolved or lie suspended in water or get deposited on the bed. This results in the pollution of water whereby the quality of the water deteriorates, affecting aquatic ecosystems. Pollutants can also seep down and affect the groundwater deposits.

❖ Causes of Water Pollution

1. Domestic sewage

Water pollution has many sources. The most polluting of them are the city sewage and industrial waste discharged into the rivers. The facilities to treat waste-water are not adequate in any city in India. Presently, only about 10 per cent of the waste-water generated is treated; the rest is discharged as it is into our water bodies. Due to this, pollutants enter groundwater, rivers, and other water bodies. Such water, which ultimately ends up in our households, is often highly contaminated and carries disease-causing microbes. Agricultural run-off, or the water from the fields that drains into rivers, is another major water pollutant as it contains fertilizers and pesticides.

Sources and types of major water pollution

Source	*Types of Pollutants*
Agriculture	Fertilizers (principally nitrogen and phosphorous), animal wastes, sediments
Industry	Synthetic organic chemicals, including (PCBs) and dioxin, toxic inorganic chemicals, including heavy metals, radioactive materials, heat discharge
Mining	Acids, chlorides, heavy metals
Municipalities and residences	Nutrients, organic materials, heavy metals, toxic chemicals, chlorides, sewage

The amount of organic material that can rot in the sewage is measured by the biochemical oxygen demand (BOD). BOD is the amount of oxygen required by micro-organisms to decompose the organic substances in sewage. Therefore, the more organic material there is in the sewage, the higher the BOD. It is among the most important parameters for the design and operation of sewage treatment plants. BOD levels of industrial sewage may be many times that of domestic sewage.

Dissolved Oxygen (DO) is the amount of oxygen dissolved in a given quantity of water at a particular temperature and atmospheric pressure. The saturation value of DO varies from 8-15 mg/litre. For active fish species 5-8 mg/litre is required whereas less desirable species can survive at 3.0 mg./litre. Dissolved oxygen is an important factor that determines the quality of water in lakes and rivers. The higher the concentration of dissolved oxygen, the better the water quality.

When sewage enters a lake or stream, micro-organisms begin to decompose the organic materials. Oxygen is consumed as micro-organisms use it in their metabolism. This can quickly deplete the available oxygen in the water. When the dissolved oxygen levels drop too low, many aquatic species perish. In fact, if the oxygen level drops to zero, the water will become septic. When organic compounds decompose without oxygen, it gives rise to the undesirable odours usually associated with septic or putrid conditions.

Sewage generated from the urban areas in India has multiplied manifold since 1947. Today, many people dump their garbage into streams, lakes, rivers, and seas, thus making water bodies the final resting place of cans, bottles, plastics, and other household products. The various substances that we use for keeping our houses clean add to water pollution as they contain harmful chemicals. In the past, people mostly used soaps made from animal and vegetable fat for all types of washing. But most of today's cleaning products are synthetic detergents and come from the petrochemical industry. Most detergents and washing powders contain phosphates, which are used to soften the water among other things. These and other chemicals contained in washing powders affect the health of all forms of life in the water.

2. Eutrophication

When fresh water is artificially supplemented with nutrients, it results in an abnormal increase in the growth of water plants. This is known as eutrophication. The discharge of waste from industries, agriculture, and urban communities into water bodies generally stretches the biological capacities of aquatic systems. Chemical run-off from fields also adds nutrients to water. Excess nutrients cause the water body to become choked with organic substances and organisms. When organic matter exceeds the capacity of the micro-organisms in water that break down and recycle the organic matter, it encourages rapid growth, or blooms, of algae. When they die, the remains of the algae add to the organic wastes already in the water; eventually, the water becomes deficient in oxygen. Anaerobic organisms (those that do not require oxygen to live) then attack the organic wastes, releasing gases such as methane and hydrogen sulphide, which are harmful to the oxygen-requiring (aerobic) forms of life. The result is a foul-smelling, waste-filled body of water. This has already occurred in such places as Lake Erie and the Baltic Sea, and is a growing problem in freshwater lakes all over India. Eutrophication can produce problems such as bad tastes and odours as well as green scum algae. Also the growth of rooted plants increases, which decreases the amount of oxygen in the deepest waters of the lake. It also leads to the death of all forms of life in the water bodies.

3. Agricultural Run-Off

The use of land for agriculture and the practices followed in cultivation greatly affect the quality of groundwater. Intensive cultivation of crops causes chemicals from fertilizers (e.g. nitrate) and pesticides to seep into the groundwater, a process commonly known as leaching. Routine applications of fertilizers and pesticides for agriculture and indiscriminate disposal of industrial and domestic wastes are increasingly being recognized as significant sources of water pollution.

The high nitrate content in groundwater is mainly from irrigation run-off from agricultural fields where chemical fertilizers have been used indiscriminately.

4. Industrial Effluents

Industrial waste-water usually contains specific and readily identifiable chemical compounds. Water pollution is concentrated within a few sub-sectors of industries, mainly in the form of toxic wastes and organic pollutants. Out of this a large portion can be traced to the processing of industrial chemicals and to the food products industry. In fact, a number of large and medium sized industries in the region covered by the Ganga Action Plan do not have adequate effluent treatment facilities. Most of these defaulting industries are sugar mills, distilleries, leather processing industries, and thermal power stations. Most major industries have treatment facilities for industrial effluents. But this is not the case with small scale industries, which cannot afford enormous investments in pollution control equipment, as their profit margin is very slender.

❖ Treatment of Waste Water

The sewage and factory waste have to be cleaned to some extent before they flow into waste water. There are two ways:

(i) Primary treatment; and
(ii) Secondary treatment.

Primary treatment employs physical processes such as screening, shredding, sedimentation and floatation. It results in the settlement and most suspended particulates as well as of some oxygen demanding wastes.

Secondary treatment makes use of microbial activity to oxidized waste material. There are two common methods:

Intickling Filters : Waste water is passed through a thick bed of gravel stones where bacteria consume most of the organic matter. The resulting water, which is now much less polluted trickles out through the bottom of the bed and is transported elsewhere through pipes for further treatment.

Activated Sludge Process : The sewage is pumped after primary treatment, into an aeration tank where it mixes with air and sludge containing some algae and bacteria. These bacteria break down up to 80-90 per cent of the organic matter and the algae generate oxygen for bacterial growth and multiplication. The water is then chlorinated to kill the disease producing germs.

❖ Effects of Water Pollution

The five main kinds of physical and chemical effects of pollutants are as addition of poisonous substances, addition of suspended solids, addition of non-toxic salts, water deoxygenation and heating of water.

Polluted water can spread many epidemic diseases as cholera, typhoid, dysentery etc. The effects of water pollution are not only devastating to people but also to animals, fish, and birds. Polluted water is unsuitable for drinking, recreation, agriculture, and industry. It diminishes the aesthetic quality of lakes and rivers. More seriously, contaminated water destroys aquatic life and reduces its reproductive ability. Eventually, it is a hazard to human health. Nobody can escape the effects of water pollution.

Human health is one of the most important factors in economic development.A healthy workforce is essential for the development of an economy. A healthy work force requires a healthy environment, which is clean air, water, recreation and wilderness. Pearce and Warford (1993) have argued that the most important and immediate consequence of environmental degradation in the developing world take the form damage to human health. Further, the argued that diarrhoea is common occurrence in many developing countries with three million to five million cases recorded every year, Each case is estimated to involve a loss of 3-5 working days, amounting to nine billion working days lost in a single year.

It has been found that developing countries are facing serious water-borne diseases due to lack of safe drinking water. Walsh and Warren have estimated mortality and morbidity from water-borne disease in Africa an Asia. According to them water-borne diseases due to water pollution have a definite impact on the morbidity and mortality and morbidity from water-borne diseases in Africa. According to them water-borne diseases due to water pollution have a definite impact on morbidity and mortality. And ultimately it has serious negative impact on economic activities in the form of loss of working days, death of trained workers, expenditure on hospitalisation and so on. Besides, a number of attempts have been made to estimate the economic cost of health damage due to water pollution ,in developed countries. Pearce *et al.* (1978) have reviewed some of the studies conducted in the US to estimate national health costs of polluted water. Outbreaks of the disease were monetarised on the basis of 10 days lost income and resources cost of five days stay in hospital. It was estimated that the unit social cost per case was $100 and that there were approximately one million cases of gastroenteritis each year in the US. Two million working days are lost in the US each year due to acute gastroenteritis and diarrhoea at an average wage loss of $30 a day. It is estimated that the value of the 1,000 death due to hepatitis infection per year is around $100,000 per life.

Another attempt was made by Phan Tumvanit in the Thailand to compare the damage cost due to water pollution and the abatement cost in order to compare it with the abatement cost of a pollution control programme. He adopted the direct questioning method (CVM) along with the available scientific finding. The relationship between the damage cost and the water quality were examined. It was concluded that treatment level had to be kept above 75 per cent in order to maintain the river quality above 4mg/litre dissolved oxygen, above which no damage costs are assumed. At the macro level, countries like Poland, the Netherlands and Germany seem to have high environmental degradation costs. For instance in the Netherlands the estimated cost of pollution damage was 0.5-0.8 per cent of GNP in 1986. Ethiopia has estimated the cost of deforestation as $300 million in 1983, or 6 per cent of GNP.

❖ Water Pollution in India

The major rivers of the country suffer from reduction in flow while entering the plains and passing through cities (because of water being drawn for irrigation and drinking water supply in cities). At the same time, they receive polluted discharge, the main pollutants being untreated municipal sewage, fertilizers /insecticides and industrial effluents.

Central Pollution Control Board (CPCB) in collaboration with concerned SPCBs/ PCCs established a nationwide network of water quality monitoring comprising 1019 stations in 27 States and 6 Union Territories. The monitoring is done on monthly or quarterly basis in surface waters and on half yearly basis in case of ground water. The monitoring network covers 200 Rivers, 60 Lakes, 5 Tanks, 3 Ponds, 3 Creeks, 13 Canals, 17 Drains and 321 Wells. Among the 1019 stations, 592 are on rivers, 65 on lakes, 17 on drains, 13 on canals, 5 on tanks, 3 on creeks, 3 on ponds and 321 are groundwater stations.

The water quality monitoring results obtained during 1995 to 2006 indicate that the organic and bacterial contamination are continued to be critical in water bodies. This is mainly due to discharge of domestic waste water mostly in untreated form from the urban centres of the country. The municipal corporations at large are not able to treat increasing the load of municipal sewage flowing into water bodies without treatment. Secondly, the receiving water bodies also do not have adequate water for dilution. Therefore, the oxygen demand and bacterial pollution is increasing day by day. This is mainly responsible for water borne diseases.

The water quality monitoring results were analyzed with respect to indicator of oxygen consuming substances (Bio-chemical demand) and indicator of pathogenic bacteria (total colliform and faecal colliform). The result of such analysis shows that there is gradual degradation in water quality. The number of observations having BOD and coliform density has increased during 1995 to 2006.

The major initiatives taken by government to control water pollution are as follows :

National River Conservation Plan (1995)

Under this scheme, polluted stretches of major rivers have been identified for sewage collection and treatment. At present, 153 towns have been considered under the National River Conservation Plan (NRCP), out of which 74 towns are located on Ganga, 21 on Yamuna, 12 on the Damodar, six on the Godavari, nine on the Cauvery, four each on the Tungabhadra and Sutlej, three each on the Subarnarekha, Betwa, Wainganga, Brahmini, Chambal and Gomti, two on the Krishna and one each on the Sabarmati, Khan, Kshipra, Narmada and Mahanadi. This project was started with 100 per cent funding by the Centre. However, given resource constraints, States have to share 30 per cent of the cost during the Tenth Plan.

The scheme plans to tackle river pollution by setting up additional sewage treatment plants where there is a shortage, diverting raw sewage flowing in open drains to these plants, construction of low cost sanitation facilities to prevent open defecation on river banks, setting up improved crematoria, etc.

The works under NRCP, including that of Ganga Phase-I, are expected to cost Rs. 3,780 crore. Till January 2002, Rs. 1,295 crore has been spent on the scheme. About 45 per cent of the cleaning of the Ganga has been completed. However, overall progress is poor because of delays in land acquisition and slow pace of work by municipal corporations.

National Lake Conservation Plan (1994)

The National Lake Conservation Plan was initiated in 1994 for cleaning important urban lakes with high levels of silting and pollution. Initially, ten lakes were identified for coverage – Ooty, Kodaikanal, Powai, Dal, Sukhna, Sagar, Nainital, Udaipur, Rabindra Sagar and Hussain Sagar. However, work has started on only one lake and project reports for three lakes namely Ooty, Powai and Kodaikanal have been prepared and approved till date. The progress regarding other lakes is extremely slow because of delays in the finalisation of detailed project (DPRs), tender procedures and award of contract. The progress of work on Dal Lake has been hampered by the delay in approval of the DPR by the State Government.

CASE STUDY

The Ganga Basin

The Ganga rises on the southern slopes of the Himalayan ranges from the Gangotri glacier at 4,000 m above mean sea level. After entering the plains at Haridwar, it winds its way to the Bay of Bengal, covering 2,500 km through the provinces of Uttar Pradesh, Bihar and West Bengal. In the plains it is joined by Ramganga, Yamuna, Sai, Gomti, Ghaghara, Sone, Gandak, Kosi and Damodar along with many other smaller rivers. The Ganga receives over 60 per cent of its discharge from its tributaries.

The Ganga River carries the highest silt load of any river in the world and the deposition of this material in the delta region results in the largest river delta in the world.

The Ganga basin is inhabited by 37 per cent of India's population. It effectively drains eight States of India. About 47 per cent of the total irrigated area in India is located in the Ganga basin alone. Today, one-third of the country's urban population lives in the towns of the Ganga basin. Out of the 2,300 towns in the country, 692 are located in this basin, and of these, 100 are located along the river bank itself. All the towns along its length contribute to the pollution load. It has been assessed that more than 80 per cent of the total pollution load (in terms of organic pollution expressed as biochemical oxygen demand (BOD)) arises from domestic sources, i.e. from the settlements along the river course.

There are also about 100 identified major industries located directly on the river, of which 68 are considered as grossly polluting. Fifty-five of these industrial units have complied with the regulations and installed effluent treatment plants (ETPs) and legal proceedings are in progress for the remaining units. The natural assimilative capacity of the river is severely stressed.

The principal sources of pollution of the Ganga River can be characterized as follows :

- Domestic and industrial wastes. It has been estimated that about 1.4 × 106 m^3 d-1 of domestic wastewater and 0.26 × 106 m^3 d-1 of industrial sewage are going into the river.
- Solid garbage thrown directly into the river.
- Non-point sources of pollution from agricultural run-off containing residues of harmful pesticides and fertilizers.
- Animal carcasses and half-burned and unburned human corpses thrown into the river.
- Defecation on the banks by the low-income people.
- Mass bathing and ritualistic practices.

Ganga Action Plan (GAP)

The Central Pollution Control Board (CPCB), which is India's national body for monitoring environmental pollution, undertook a comprehensive scientific survey in 1981-82 in order to classify river waters according to their designated best uses. This report was the first systematic document that formed the basis of the Ganga Action Plan (GAP). The plan was formally launched on 14 June, 1986. The main thrust was to intercept and divert the wastes from urban settlements away from the river. Treatment and economical use of waste, as a means of assisting resource recovery, were made an integral part of the plan.

The broad aim of the GAP was to reduce pollution and to clean the river and to restore water quality at least to Class B.

The GAP had a multi-pronged strategy to improve the river water quality. It was fully financed by the Central Government, with the assets created by the Central Government to be used and maintained by the State governments. The main thrust of the plan was targeted to control all municipal and industrial wastes. All possible point and non-point sources of pollution were identified. The control of point sources of urban municipal wastes for the 25 Class I towns on the main river was initiated from the 100 per cent centrally-invested project funds.

A total of 261 sub-projects were sought for implementation in 25 Class I (population above 100,000) river front towns. This would eventually involve a financial outlay of Rs 4,680 million. More than 95 per cent of the programme has been completed and the remaining sub-projects are in various stages of completion.

It is very important for the Ganga because the river water is used directly by millions of devout individuals for drinking and bathing.

(d) Soil Pollution

Soil Pollution is the presence of man-made chemicals or other alteration to the natural soil environment.

❖ Causes of Soil Pollution

Soil pollution typically arises from application of pesticides and herbicides, percolation of contaminated surface water to subsurface strata, leaching of wastes from landfills or direct discharge petroleum hydrocarbons, solvents, pesticides, lead and other heavy metals. The occurrence of this phenomenon is correlated with the degree of industrialization and intensity of chemical usage of industrial wastes to the soil. The most common chemicals involved are petroleum hydrocarbons, solvents, pesticides, lead and other heavy metals.

The concern over soil contamination stems primarily from health risks, both of direct contact and from secondary contamination of water supplies.

Microanalysis of Soil Contamination

To understand the fundamental nature of soil contamination, it is necessary to envision the variety of mechanisms for pollutants to become entrained in soil. Soil particulates may be composed of a gamut of organic and inorganic chemicals with variations in cation exchange capacity, buffering capacity, and poise capacity. For example, at the extremes, one has a sand component, a coarse grained, inert, and totally inorganic substance; whereas peat soils are dominated by a fine organic material, made of decomposing organic material and highly active. Most soils are mixtures of soil subtypes and thus have quite complex characteristics. There is also a great diversity of soil porosity, ranging from gravels to sands to silt to clay (in increasing order of porosity), pore size, and pore tortuosity (both in decreasing order). Finally, there is a wide spectrum of chemical bonding or adhesion characteristics: each contaminant has a different interaction or bonding mechanism with a given soil type.

On balance, some contaminants may literally drain through soils such as sand and gravel and move to other soils or deeper aquifers, while polar or organic chemicals discharged into a clay soil will have a very high adsorption. Thus most soil contamination is the result of pollutants adhering to the soil particle surface, or lodging in interstices of a soil matrix. Clearly, the equilibrium reached is a dynamic one, where new pollutants may lodge on new soil particles and the action of groundwater movement may over time transport some of the soil contaminants to other locations or depths.

➢ Control of Soil Pollution

- ☞ Effluents should be properly treated before discharging them on the soil.
- ☞ Solid waste shoud be properly collected and disposed of by appropriate method.
- ☞ From the waste, recovery of usefull products shoud be done. Biodegradable organic waste should be used for generation of biogas.
- ☞ Cattle dung should be used fore methane generation.

(e) Marine Pollution

Marine pollution is the harmful entry into the ocean of chemicals or particles. A big problem is that many toxins adhere to tiny particles which are taken up within a few days by plankton and benthos animals, most of which are filter feeders, concentrating upward within ocean foodchains. Because most animal feeds contain high fish meal and fish oil content, toxins can be found a few weeks later in commonly consumed food items derived from livestock and animal husbandry such as meat, eggs, milk, butter and margarine.

➢ Causes of Marine Pollution

- One common path of entry by contaminants to the sea are rivers. Many particles combine chemically in a manner highly depletive of oxygen, causing estuaries to become anoxic.
- Catchment area i.e. coastline where human settlement in the form of hotel, agriculture practices have been established.
- Oildrilling and shipment.
- Dumping of radioactive wastes into the sea.
- Huge amount of plastics and packing materials dumped in the sea.

Assessment of Pollution Load from Land Based Activities influencing the Coastal Marine Environment of Gujarat and Maharashtra

The marine ecosystem is considered as most complex and dynamic physical ecosystem existing on the earth. India is having the coastline of about 8,118 kilometres covering the littoral States and the union territories. The coastal area accommodates about 25 per cent of country's total population by virtue of its geographical location. The human intervention through the developmental activities like extensive urbanization, industrialization, construction of ports and harbours, development of cities and towns along the coast is drastically changing the coastal dynamics.

All these man made activities are directly or indirectly influencing the water quality coastal waters by way of generating some sort of waste in the form of liquid or solid, which is being discharged into the coastal waters, resulting in drastic change in water quality and depletion of marine productivity, etc. The domestic effluent or the municipal wastewater constitutes the largest single source of coastal pollution, followed by the discharges from the industries, ports and harbours, etc.

The Central Pollution Control Board has undertaken a study to assess the pollution load from land based activities influencing the coastal marine environment of Gujarat and Maharashtra States by way of collecting the dry data on industrial development, population of the cities and towns, water consumption, waste water generation, treatment systems provided from all the littoral States and union territories. The collected data will be used for the assessment of pollution load received by the sea.

The studies conducted in the littoral States of Gujarat and Maharashtra and Union Territories of Daman & Diu and Dadra & Nagar Haveli indicated that out of

27 metrocities in the country, 4 are located in the coastal areas of Gujarat and Maharashtra. The 19 Class-I cities including metrocities having population of 21,342,379 and 15 Class-II towns having a population of 993,228 are located in coastal areas of Gujarat and Maharashtra.

The quantity of treated/partially treated/ untreated domestic sewage reaching the coastal waters from these cities and towns is about 3,114 MLD. Besides there are about 220 industries including industrial estates discharging their treated/ partially treated/ untreated effluents of various dimensions to the coastal waters of these States. The activities like coastal aquaculture, salt pans, and ship building also affect the quality of the coastal waters to some extent.

❖ Control of Marine Pollution

- Toxic pollutants from industries and sewage treatment plants should not be discharged in the coastal waters.
- Sewer overflows should be prevented by having separate sewer and rain water pipes.
- Development activities on coastal areas should be minimized.
- Oil ballast should not be dumped into the sea.
- Drilling should be prohibited in the ecologically sensitive areas.

(f) Thermal Pollution

Thermal pollution is a temperature change in natural water bodies caused by human influence.

❖ Causes of Thermal Pollution

The main cause of thermal pollution is the use of water as a coolant, especially in power plants. Heat producing industries i.e., thermal power plants, nuclear power plants, refineries, steel mills, etc. are the major source of thermal pollution. Power plants utilize onlt 1/3 of the energy provided by fossil fuels for their operations. Remaining 2/3 is generally lost in the form of heat to the water used for cooling. Normal water, generallly drawn from some nereby water body , passed through the plant and returned to the same water body, with temperature 10 – 16 ^{0}C higher than the initial temperature. Excess of heat reaching such water bodies causes thermal pollution of water.

➢ Effects of Thermal Pollution

Water used as a coolant is returned to the natural environment at a higher temperature. Increases in water temperature can alter aquatic organisms by (a) decreasing oxygen supply, (b) killing fish juveniles which are vulnerable to small increases in temperature, and (c) affecting ecosystem composition.

Thermal pollution can decrease the level of dissolved oxygen in the water. The decrease in levels of dissolved oxygen can harm aquatic animals such as fish, amphibians and copepods.

Thermal pollution may also increase the metabolic rate of aquatic animals, as enzyme activity, meaning that these organisms will consume more food in a shorter time than if their environment was not changed. An increased metabolic rate may result in food source shortages, causing a sharp decrease in a population. Changes in the environment may also result in a migration of organisms to another, more suitable environment, and to in-migration of organisms that normally only live in cooler waters elsewhere. This leads to competition for lesser resources; the more adapted organisms moving in may have an advantage over organisms that are not used to the warmer temperatures. As a result one has the problem of compromising food chains of the old and new environments. Biodiversity can be decreased as a result.

It is known that temperature changes of even one to two degrees Celsius can cause significant changes in organism metabolism and in adverse cellular biology effects. Principal adverse changes can include rendering cell walls less permeable to necessary osmosis, coagulation of cell proteins, and alteration of enzyme metabolism. These cellular level effects can adversely affect mortality and reproduction.

Primary producers are affected by thermal pollution because higher water temperature increases plant growth rates, resulting in a shorter life span and species overpopulation. This can cause an algae bloom which reduces the oxygen levels in the water. The higher plant density leads to an increased plant respiration rate because the reduced light intensity decreases photosynthesis. This is similar to the eutrophication that occurs when water-courses are polluted with leached agricultural inorganic fertilizers.

A large increase in temperature can lead to the denaturing of life-supporting enzymes by breaking down hydrogen and disulphide bonds within the quaternary structure of the enzymes. Decreased enzyme activity in aquatic organisms can cause problems such as the inability to break down lipids, which leads to malnutrition.

It is prudent to add that in limited cases, thermal pollution has little deleterious effect and may even lead to improved function of the receiving aquatic ecosystem. This phenomenon is seen especially in seasonal waters and is known as thermal enrichment. An extreme case is derived from the aggregational habits of the manatee, which often uses power plant discharge sites during winter. FWC projections suggest that manatee populations would drastically reduce upon the removal or mitigation of these discharges.

❖ Control of Thermal Pollution

The following methods can be employed for the control of thermal pollution :

- Cooling Ponds,
- Spray Ponds, and
- Cooling towers.

Cooling Ponds

Water from condensers is stored in the ponds where natural evaporation cools the water which can then be recirculatedor discharged in nearby water body.

Spray Ponds

The water from condensers is receaved in the spray ponds. Here, the water is sprayed through nozzles where fine droplets are formed. Heat from these fine droplets is dissipated to the atmosphere.

Cooling Towers

Wet cooling towers : Hot water is sprayed over baffles.Cool air entering from the sides takes away the heat and cools the water. This cooled water can be recycled or discharged. Large amount of water is lost through evaporation and in the vicinity of wet cooling tower extensive fog is formed which is not good for environment and cause damage to the environment.

Dry cooling towers : The heated water flos in the system of pipes. Air is passed over these hot pipes and fans. There is no water loss in this method but installation and operation coast of dry cooling tower is many times higher than wet cooling tower.

(g) Nuclear Pollution

Radioactive subsistence is present in the nature. Nuclear energy has been recognized as a clean energy because it does not release pollutants such as CO_2 to the atmosphere after its reaction that could damage our environment. It is also known that nuclear energy has reduced the amount of greenhouse gas emission, reducing emissions of CO_2 for about 500 million metric tonnes of carbon.

Despite the advantage of nuclear as a clean energy, the big concern is the waste resulted from nuclear reaction, which is a form of pollution, called radioactivity. They undergo natural radioactive decay in which unstable isotopes spontaneously give out fast moving particles, high energy radiation or both, at a fixed rate until a new stable isotope is formed.

The isotopes release energy either in the form of gamma rays (high energy electromagnetic radiation) or ionization particles. The alpha particles are fast moving positively charged particles whereas beta particles are high speed negatively charged electrons. These ionization radiations have variable penetration power.

Alpha particles can be interrupted by a sheet of paper while beta particles can be blocked by a piece of wood or a few millimetres of aluminium sheet. The gamma rays can pass through paper and wood but can be stopped by concrete wall, lead slabs or water.

❖ Source of Radioactivity

Various sources of radioactivity can be categorized into two groups :

(i) *Natural Source* : Sources of natural radioactivity include cosmic rays from outer space, radioactive radon-222, soil, air, water and food, which contain one or more radioactive subsistence.

(ii) *Anthropogenic sources:* These sources are nuclear power plants, nuclear accidents, X-rays, diagnostics kits, test laboratories, etc. Where radio substances is used.

➢ Effects of Radiation

Radiation can affect living organism by causing harmful changes in the body cells and also changes at genetic level.

(i) *Genetic damages* are caused by radiation, which induce mutation in the DNA, thereby affecting genes and chromosomes. The damage is often seen in the offsprings and may be transmitted up to several generations.

(ii) *Somatic damage* includes burns, miscarriages, eye cataract and cancer of bones, thyroid, breast, lungs and skin.

➢ Control of Nuclear Pollution

Nuclear power plants should be carefully done after studying long-term and short-term affects.

Proper disposal of waste from laboratory involving the use of radioisotopes should be done.

IV. Critical Pollution Problem Areas in India

There are 24 problem areas identified in the country and action plans for pollution control in these areas have been under implementation since more than last one and half decade.

Problem areas include a wide spectrum of industrial activities starting from clusters of small-scale industries such as textile units in Pali (Rajasthan) and metal processing units in Govindgarh (Punjab) to large industrial estates of Ankleshwar and Vapi (Gujarat).

Pollution Problem Areas in India

Sl. No.		*NameState/ U.T.*
1.	Bhadravathi	Karnataka
2.	Chembur	Maharashtra
3.	Digboi	Assam
4.	Dhanbad	Bihar
5.	Durgapur	W.B.
6.	Gobindgarh	Punjab
7.	Greater Cochin	Kerala
8.	Howrah	W.B.
9.	Jodhpur	Rajasthan
10.	Kala Amb	H.P.
11.	Korba	M.P.
12.	Manali	T.N.
13.	Nagda-Ratlam	M.P.
14.	Najafgarh Basin	Delhi
15.	North Arcot	T.N.
16.	Pali	Rajasthan
17.	Parwanoo	H.P.
18.	Patancheru-Bollaram	A.P.
19.	Singrauli	U.P.
20.	Talcher	Orissa
21.	Vapi	Gujarat
22.	Visakhapatnam	A.P.
23.	Tarapur	Maharashtra
24.	Ankleshwar	Gujarat

Source: Annual Report CPCB, 2002- 2003.

The Central Pollution Control Board (CPCB) has taken a number of initiatives during this period for an effective implementation of these action plans. The initiatives include meeting with industries, coordination with SPCBs/ PCCs, review for implementation of action plans and their revision wherever necessary.

The first round of review at CPCB was done during 2000-01 for all 24 problem areas. Revised action plan was framed for each of these areas based on their pollution control status at that time. Implementation of these action plans has since been monitored by CPCB.

A Review Committee, under chairmanship of the Chairman, CPCB, was constituted in 2005 to take stock of overall status of efforts made in improving the environmental quality of the problem areas. Follow up action was initiated since 2005 and the problem areas are being inspected by the Zonal Offices of CPCB. Their status is being discussed on case to case basis by the Review Committee.

Based on the level of compliance of the original action plan and the present environmental issues in these areas, revised action plans are being framed wherever required.

The second round of review has so far covered 13 problem areas and is in progress in respect of the remaining 11 problem areas. The findings, which need attention of SPCBs/ PCCs, are :

1. Strict vigilance on compliance of environmental laws and CREP guidelines (wherever applicable) by industries located in the areas.
2. Proper treatment of municipal sewage.
3. Regular monitoring of ambient air, ground water and surface water quality for general and specific parameters.
4. Networking of ambient air quality monitoring stations (AAQMSs) where a large number of AAQMSs are being operated by individually by industries.
5. Ensuring proper collection and transportation of effluents to CETPs and proper operation of CETPs. Strict vigilance to prevent illegal/clandestine discharge of effluents by industries through underground drains or other means.
6. Ensuring proper upgradation and operation of hazardous waste disposal sites/common incinerators.
7. Flyash utilization/disposal by the concerned industries
8. Adoption of cleaner fuels/technologies by industries.

V. Role of Man in Prevention of Pollution

The role of every individual is very important to prevent pollution. It is the duty of human race, which is the supreme creature of Lord to save the earth from pollutants.

It is possible by adopting the following suggestions :

☞ Every individual should change his/her life style to reduce environmental pollution. It is possible with the following suggestions:

☞ Help more in pollution control and prevention.

☞ Use eco-friendly Products.

☞ Cut down the use of chlorofluorocarbons (CFCs) as they destroy the ozone layer.

☞ Reduce the dependency on fossil fuels especially coal and petroleum.

☞ Save electricity by not wasting it.

☞ Adopt the renewable sources of energy.

☞ Promote reuse and recycle.

☞ Minimize the use of automobiles by preferring mass transportation system. For shorter distances use bicycle or go on foot.

☞ Use rechargeable batteries; they will reduce the metal pollution.

☞ Use less hazardous chemicals.

☞ Do not put pesticides, paints, solvents, oils, or other harmful chemicals into the drain or groundwater.

- Use only minimum requirement of water for various activities.
- Plant more trees as they can absorb many toxic gases and can purify the air by releasing oxygen.
- Adopt one or two child family policy to reduce the demand of resources.

VI. Solid Waste

Waste, rubbish, trash, or garbage is unwanted or undesired material. Waste can exist in any phase of matter (solid, liquid, or gas). When released in the latter two States, gas especially, the wastes are referred to as emissions. It is usually strongly linked with pollution. Some types of waste can be recycled, e.g. plastic bottles or paper.

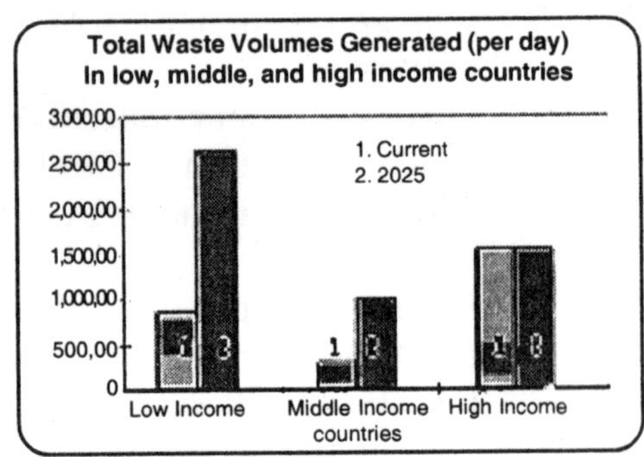

(a) Major types of Solid Waste

Solid waste can be classified into different types depending on their source :

1. Municipal solid waste (Household Waste)

Municipal solid waste consists of household waste, construction and demolition debris, sanitation residue, and waste from streets. This garbage is generated mainly from residential and commercial complexes.

2. Hazardous wastes (Industrial and hospital waste)

Hazardous waste is waste that owing to its toxic, infectious, radioactive or flammable properties poses an actual or potential hazard to the health of humans, other living organisms, or the environment.

In the 1989 Basel Convention on the Control of Transboundary Movements of Hazardous Wastes and their Disposal, 164 countries agreed to minimize the generation of hazardous waste, to assure sound management of hazardous wastes.

3. Hospital wastes (Biomedical waste)

Hospital waste is generated during the diagnosis, treatment, or immunization of human beings or animals or in research activities in these fields or in the production or testing of biologicals. This waste is highly infectious and can be a serious threat to human health if not managed in a scientific manner.

Categories of Solid Waste	
Organic waste	Kitchen waste, vegetables, flowers, leaves, fruits.
Toxic waste	Old medicines, paints, chemicals, bulbs, spray cans, fertilizer and pesticide containers, batteries, shoe polish.
Recyclable	Paper, glass, metals, plastics.
Soiled	Hospital waste such as cloth soiled with blood and other body fluids

(b) Health Impacts of Solid Waste

1. Exposure to hazardous waste can affect human health, children being more vulnerable to these pollutants. Many studies have been carried out in various parts of the world to establish a connection between health and hazardous waste.
2. Waste from agriculture and industries can also cause serious health risks. Waste dumped near a water source also causes contamination of the water body or the ground water source.
3. Disposal of hospital and other medical waste requires special attention since this can create major health hazards.
4. Waste treatment and disposal sites can also create health hazards for the neighbourhood. Improperly operated incineration plants cause air pollution and improperly managed and designed landfills attract all types of insects and rodents that spread disease
5. Recycling too carries health risks if proper precautions are not taken.
6. Direct handling of solid waste can result in various types of infectious and chronic diseases with the waste workers and the rag pickers being the most vulnerable.

(c) Solid Waste in India

➤ *Municipal solid waste*

As per an estimate, the present annual generation of solid waste in Indian cities has increased from 6 million tonnes (MT) in 1947 to 48 MT in 1997 and is expected to increase to 300 MT by 2047. Though it is difficult to give an exact estimate of the per capita rate of generation of solid waste because of the large variations both in quality and quantity, on an average it ranges between 400 and 500 g/capita/day.

Most surveys have found the organic component of the waste to be around 40 per cent. The share of recycled waste has increased over the years mainly due to the increased content of plastic. While the per capita waste generation in India is low as compared to western countries, the volume generated is enormous given the size of the population. Due to lack of awareness and absence of legislation, till recently medical wastes were also deposited and mixed with municipal waste collection. The Director General of Health Services estimates that 54,404 MT of medical wastes are generated in the country every year.

The average waste collection in Indian cities is 72 per cent and only 70 per cent of cities have adequate waste transport facilities. There is a lot of littering at collection centres and also during transportation. Unscientific disposal practices leaves waste unattended at the disposal site and this attracts birds, animals and microorganisms, which create a health hazard. Plastic contents of the waste are picked up by rag pickers for recycling. This recycling is carried out in small factories with no adequate technology, leading to the emission of toxic fumes.

The various initiatives taken to tackle this are :

- A National Waste Management Council (NWMC) was constituted in 1990 to suggest disposal of the municipal solid waste.
- The Recycled Plastic Use Rules, 1998 were issued based on the recommendations of the Plastic Management Task Board. This rule bans the use of recycled plastic for food items and also specifies standards for manufacturing recycled plastic bags.
- National Environmental Engineering and Research Institute (NEERI) have prepared a manual on solid waste management which highlights various critical issues relating to the task.
- Central Public Health Environmental Engineering Organization (CPHEEO) has prepared a policy paper on promoting the integrated provision of water, sanitation, solid waste management and drainage utilities in India.
- Master Plan for Municipal Solid Waste: The Ministry of Environment and Forests has organized an interaction meet in 1995 with municipal authorities to evolve a strategy for municipal solid waste.
- The National Programme on Energy Recovery from Urban Wastes scheme has been launched by the Ministry of Non-Conventional Energy Sources with many physical and financial incentives for energy recovery from wastes.
- Two high-powered committees were set up on Urban Waste, one in 1975 and again one in 1995. They made several recommendations like segregation, door-to-door collection, proper handling and transportation, waste composting and treatment and use of appropriate technologies for waste treatment and disposal.
- The Bio-medical Waste Management and Handling Rules, 1998, have been

formulated to take care of infectious bio-medical waste which can spread various diseases and create health problems.

☞ The Municipal Solid Waste Management and Handling Rules, 2000, has been introduced to bring in an element of urgency in the forests and environment waste management efforts by urban local bodies. Under the rules, municipalities would be required to submit annual reports on waste management in their areas to the CPCB.

Plastic and Waste Management Issues

It is estimated that approximately 4-5 per cent post-consumer plastics waste by weight of Municipal Solid Waste (MSW) is generated in India. The plastics waste generation is more i.e. 6-9 per cent in USA, Europe and other developed countries due to their consumption habits. As per data available on MSW, approximately, 4000-5000 tonnes per day post-consumer plastics waste is generated, however, pre-consumer waste or scrap is directly utilised in the industry itself.

The plastics waste constitutes two major category of plastics :

(1) Thermoplastics, and (2) Thermoset plastics.

Thermoplastics, constitutes 80 per cent and Thermoset constitutes approximately 20 per cent of total post-consumer plastics waste. The Thermoplastics are recyclable plastics which include; PET, LDPE, PVC, HDPE, PP, PS etc., however, Thermoset plastics contains Alkyd, Epoxy, Ester, Melamine Formaldehyde, Phenolic Formaldehyde, Silicon, Urea Formaldehyde, Polyurethane, Metalised and Multilayer Plastics etc.

The major problem in plastics waste management is of collection, segregation and disposal. At present, the plastics waste disposal is done through unorganised sectors i.e. Rag pickers and Kabariwalas. More importantly, the collection, segregation and to an extent disposal system is carried out through unscientific method which create environmental problem as well as an "Eyesore". Therefore, there is need to reorganise whole recycling process and in this context, CPCB has enlightened this issue to a extent by developing new recycling technique as well as developed innovative technologies for disposal of plastics waste such as "utilization of plastic waste in road construction" and "re-engineering the recycling process".

Recycled Plastics Manufacture and Usage Rules, 1999 (as amended 2003)

Features of the Rules:

- Rules are applicable in all the States/Union Territories;
- The prescribed authority for enforcement of these Rules in the States are State Pollution Control Boards and in the Union Territory, the Pollution Control Committees;
- No vendor shall use carry bags/containers made of recycled plastics for storing, carrying, dispensing, or packaging of foodstuffs;
- No person shall manufacture, stock, distribute or sell carry bags made of virgin; or recycled plastics which are < 8 feet 12 inches in size and < 20 micron in thickness; or recycled plastics which are <8 feet 12 inches in size and < 20 micron in thickness; Carry bags/containers made of virgin plastic shall be in natural shade or white; Every Plastics manufacturing and recycling Units shall be registered with concerned State Pollution Control Board/ Pollution Control Committee fulfilling consent conditions.

➢ Industrial and Hazardous Waste

Hazardous waste includes sludge contaminated with heavy metals, wastes from paints, dyes and organic chemical units and highly acidic and alkaline wastes. The relatively more industrialized States like Gujarat, Maharashtra, Tamil Nadu and Andhra Pradesh face problems relating to toxic and hazardous waste. The major hazardous waste generating industries are petroleum and petrochemicals, pharmaceuticals, pesticides, paint and dyes, fertilizers, inorganic chemicals and general engineering industries, etc. The presence of toxic chemicals in solid/liquid effluents from industries and other activities leads to groundwater contamination. Direct contact with and exposure to hazardous waste can also lead to diseases or chemical poisoning.

At present, around 7.2 MT of hazardous waste are generated in the country, out of which, according to one estimate, 1.4 MT are recyclable, 0.1 MT to be incinerated and 5.2 MT to be disposed on land. The hazardous waste of 5.3 MT would require about Rs. 1,600 crore a year for treatment and disposal at an estimated rate of Rs. 3,000/tonne. In addition, land required for disposal will be around 1 km^2, taking a depth of 4 m and density of disposal as 1.2 tonnes/m^3.

The Water Act (1974) and Air Act (1981) were not sufficient to regulate the disposal of hazardous waste and this called for the formulation of the Hazardous Waste Management and Handling Rules, 1989. Since then, efforts to make an inventory of hazardous waste were initiated.

The initiatives taken in this direction are :

- Estimate of the hazardous waste inventory in various States and identification of disposal sites based on environment impact assessment.
- CPCB has prepared a ready reckoner to provide information on the source of the hazardous waste, their characteristics and the method for recycling and disposal.
- Training programmes have been organized to deal with hazardous waste management.
- Import of hazardous waste containing toxic metals like beryllium, selenium, chromium, thallium, pesticides etc. have been restricted on the recommendations of an Expert Committee.
- Export and import of waste containing cyanide, mercury and arsenic have been prohibited since December 1996.
- The import of waste oil and metals such as brass, zinc and lead for processing to recover resources is fully regulated by the Ministry of Environment and Forests.
- The failure to implement existing legislation to check environmental damage by industrial units led to a public interest litigation being filed.

This resulted in orders for the closure/shifting of industrial units producing hazardous chemicals from Delhi, closure of 200 tanneries in Tamil Nadu and 35 foundries in Bengal.

- An Australian-aided Project (worth Australian $8.4 million) was taken up in 1996 for the management of hazardous waste generated from industries located in the Medak, Hyderabad and Ranga Reddy districts.
- The Karnataka Government is implementing a German Technical Cooperation Project relating to hazardous waste management at an estimated cost of DM 3 million for the creation of a hazardous waste disposal facility and DM 3 million for technical cooperation.

(d) Preventive Measures of Solid Waste at Household Level

At the household-level proper segregation of waste has to be done and it should be ensured that all organic matter is kept aside for composting, which is undoubtedly the best method for the correct disposal of this segment of the waste.

- Carry your own cloth or jute bag when you go for shopping.
- Say no to all plastic bags as far as possible.
- Reduce the use of paper bags also.
- Reuse the soft drinks polybottles for storing water.
- Segregate the waste in the house—keep two garbage bins and see to it that the biodegradable and the non-biodegradable is put into separate bins and dispose of separately.
- Dig a compost pit in your garden and put the entire biodegradable into it.
- See to it that all garbage is thrown into the municipal bin as the collection is generally done from there.
- When you go out do not throw paper and other wrappings or even leftover food here and there, make sure that it is put in the correct place, that is into a dustbin
- As far as possible try to sell all the recyclable items that are not required to the Kabariwala (person who trades in waste)

VII. Disasters

Disaster is a sudden adverse or unfortunate extreme event, which causes great damage to human beings as well as plants and animals. We cannot prevent/stop disaster, but we can minimize losses.

Frequently occurring Natural Disaster in India

Type	Location/ Area	Affected Population
Floods	Eight major river valleys in 40 million hectares of area.	260 million
Drought	Spread in 14 States – A. P., Bihar, Gujarat, Haryana, J&K., Karnataka, M.P., Maharashtra, Orissa, T.N., U.P., W.B. Rajasthan, and Himachal Pradesh covering a total of 116 districts and 740 blocks.	86 million
Earthquack	Nearly 55 per cent of the total area of the country falling in the seismic zone IV & V.	400 million
Cyclones	5700 km. long coast line of India covering 9 States viz. A.P. Gujarat, Karnataka, Maharashtra, Orissa, T.N., W.B., Goa, Kerala and Union Territory of Pondicherry.	10 million
Land Slides	Entire sub-Himalayan Region and Western Ghat.	10 million

Source : State of Environment, 1995, Ministry of Environment and Forest, India.

(a) Earthquake

An earthquake is caused by a sudden slip on a fault. Stresses in the earth's outer layer push the sides of the fault together. Stress builds up and the rocks slips suddenly, releasing energy in waves that travel through the earth's crust and cause the shaking that we feel during an earthquake. An earthquake occurs when plates grind and scrape against each other. The point on a fault at which the first movement occurs during an earthquake is called the **epicenter.** The sensitivity of an earthquake is generally measured by its magnitude on Richter Scale, as shown below.

Richter Scale	Severity of Earthquake
Less than 4	Insignificant
4 – 4.9	Minor
5 – 5.9	Damaging
6 – 6.9	Destructive
7- 7.9	Major
More than 8	Great

Earthquakes are part of a global tectonic process that generally occurs well beyond the influence or control of humans. The focus (point of origin) of earthquakes is typically tens to hundreds of miles underground. The scale and force necessary to produce earthquakes are well beyond our daily lives. We cannot prevent earthquakes, however, we can significantly mitigate their effects by identifying hazards, building safer structures, and providing education on earthquake safety.

The largest earthquake ever recorded occurred on May 22, 1960 in Chile with the estimated magnitude of 9.5 on Richter scale, affecting 90,000 squre miles and killing 6,000 people. The earthquack which hit Bhuj town in Gujarat had caused massive damage, killing 20,000 to 30,000 people and leaving many injured.

Anthropogenetic activities can also cause or enhance the frequency of earthquakes as construction of big dam, underground nuclear testing and deep well disposal of liquid waste.

Table : Number of Earthquakes Worldwide for 2000-2005

Magnitude	*2000*	*2001*	*2002*	*2003*	*2004*	*2005*
8.0 to 9.9	1	1	0	1	2	1
7.0 to 7.9	14	15	13	14	14	9
6.0 to 6.9	158	126	130	140	140	116
5.0 to 5.9	1345	1243	1218	1203	1509	1307
4.0 to 4.9	8045	8084	8584	8462	10894	10264
3.0 to 3.9	4784	6151	7005	7624	7937	5782
2.0 to 2.9	3758	4162	6419	7727	6317	3249
1.0 to 1.9	1026	944	1137	2506	1344	20
0.1 to 0.9	5	1	10	134	103	0
No Magnitude	3120	2938	2937	3608	2939	642
Total	22256	23534	27454	31419	* 31199	* 21390
Est. Deaths	231	21357	1685	33819	284010	1957

Source: US Geological Survey National Earthquake Information Centre

Table : Largest and Deadliest Earthquakes (World) by Year 1990 - 2005

	Largest Earthquakes				*Deadliest Earthquake*			
Year	*Date*	*Magnitude*	*Deaths*	*Country*	*Date*	*Magnitude*	*Deaths*	*Country*
2005	03/28	8.7	1,313	Indonesia	03/28	8.7	1,313	Indonesia
2004	12/26	9.0	283,106	Indonesia	12/26	9.0	283,106	Indonesia
2003	09/25	8.3	0	Japan	12/26	6.6	31,000	Iran
2002	11/03	7.9	0	USA	03/25	6.1	1,000	Afghanistan
2001	06/23	8.4	138	Peru	01/26	7.7	20,023	India
2000	11/16	8.0	2	Ireland	06/04	7.9	103	Indonesia
1999	09/20	7.7	2,297	Taiwan	08/17	7.6	17,118	Turkey
1998	03/25	8.1	0	Balleny	05/30	6.6	4,000	Afghanistan
1997	10/14	7.8	0	Fiji	05/10	7.3	1,572	Iran
1996	02/17	8.2	166	Indonesia	02/03	6.6	322	China
1995	07/30	8.0	3	Chile	01/16	6.9	5,530	Japan

Source : US Geological Survey National Earthquake Information Centre

Frequency of Occurrence of Earthquakes in the World

Descriptor	*Magnitude*	*Average Annually*
Great	8 and higher	1 [1]
Major	7 - 7.9	17 [2]
Strong	6 - 6.9	134 [2]
Moderate	5 - 5.9	1319 [2]
Light	4 - 4.9	13,000 (estimated)
Minor	3 - 3.9	130,000 (estimated)
Very Minor	2 - 2.9	1,300,000 (estimated)

Note - [1] Based on observations since 1900. [2] Based on observations since 1990.

INDIA : EARTHQUAKES

Seismic Zonation Map of India

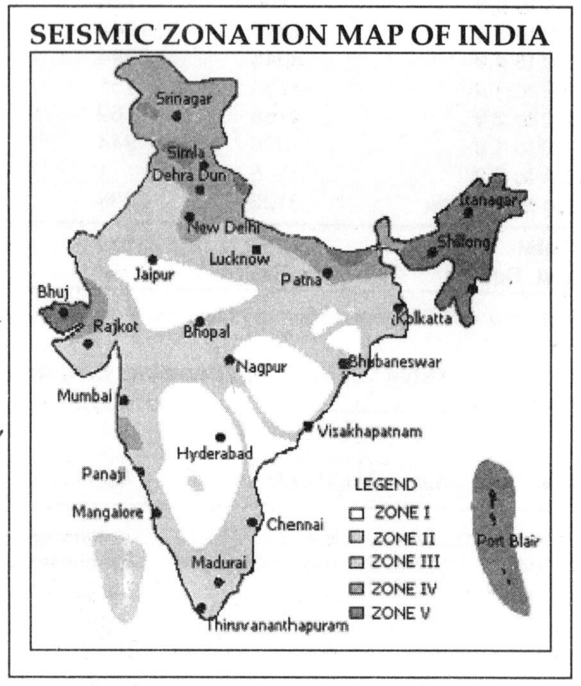

Seismic Zonation map of a country is a guide to the seismic status of a region and its susceptibility to earthquakes. India has been divided into five zones with respect to severity of earthquakes. Of these, Zone V is seismically the most active where earthquakes of magnitude 8 or more could occur.

Recent strong motion observations around the world have revolutionized thinking on the design of engineering structures, placing emphasis also on the characteristics of the structures themselves it should be realized that in the case of shield type earthquakes, historic data are insufficient to define zones because recurrence intervals are much longer than the recorded human history this may often give a false sense of security. Occurrence of the damaging earthquake at Latur, falling in Zone I is a typical example of this situation.

Tsunami

Tsunami is a Japanese word with the English translation, "harbour wave." Represented by two characters, the top character, "tsu," means harbour, while the bottom character, "nami," means "wave." In the past, tsunamis were sometimes referred to as "tidal waves" by the general public, and as "seismic sea waves" by the scientific community. The term "tidal wave" is a misnomer; although a tsunami's impact upon a coastline is dependent upon the tidal level at the time a tsunami strikes, tsunamis are unrelated to the tides. Tides result from the imbalanced, extraterrestrial, gravitational influences of the moon, sun, and planets. The term "seismic sea wave" is also misleading. "Seismic" implies an earthquake-related generation mechanism, but a tsunami can also be caused by a non-seismic event, such as a landslide or meteorite impact.

List of Some Significant Earthquakes in India

Date	Epicentre		Location	Magnitude
	Lat. N	Long. E		
1819 Jun 16	23.6	68.6	Kutch, Gujarat	8.0
1869 Jan 10	25	93	Near Cachar, Assam	7.5
1885 May 30	34.1	74.6	Sopor, J&K	7.0
1897 Jun 12	26	91	Shillong Plateau	8.7
1905 Apr 04	32.3	76.3	Kangra, H.P	8.0
1918 Jul 08	24.5	91.0	Srimangal, Assam	7.6
1930 Jul 02	25.8	90.2	Dhubri, Assam	7.1
1934 Jan 15	26.6	86.8	Bihar-Nepal Border	8.3
1941 Jun 26	12.4	92.5	Andaman Islands	8.1
1943 Oct 23	26.8	94.0	Assam	7.2
1950 Aug 15	28.5	96.7	Arunachal Pradesh-China Border	8.5
1956 Jul 21	23.3	7.0	Anjar, Gujarat	7.0
1967 Dec 10	17.37	73.75	Koyna, Maharashtra	6.5
1975 Jan 19	32.38	78.49	Kinnaur, HP	6.2
1988 Aug 06	25.13	95.15	Manipur-Myanmar Border	6.6
1988 Aug 21	26.72	86.63	Bihar-Nepal Border	6.4
1991 Oct 20	30.75	78.86	Uttarkashi, UP Hills	6.6
1993 Sep 30	18.07	76.62	Latur - Osmanabad, Maharashtra	6.3
1999 Mar 29	30.41	79.42	Champoli, UP	6.8
2001 Jan 26	23.40	70.28	Bhuj, Gujarat	6.9

(b) Landslides

A landslide is a geological phenomenon which includes a wide range of ground movement, such as rock falls, deep failure of slopes and shallow debris flows.

All earth and material on a slope has an "angle of repose," or an angle at which that material will remain stable. Loose dry rock remains in place at angles up to 30 degrees, but wet clay will start to slip at more than 1 or 2 degree inclinations. Landslides are the sudden downhill movements of earth or other solid material, and are usually caused by rain, thaws, or forces increasing the top material weight, lubricating the material layers, or making the slope too steep. They can be triggered by earthquakes, saturation with heavy rain, or crashing waves.

➢ Causes of Landslides

Natural Causes

- Erosion by rivers
- Glaciers melting
- Soil slopes are weakened through saturation by snowmelt or heavy rain

- Ocean waves create oversteepened slopes
- Earthquake create stresses that make weak slopes fail
- Volcanic eruption produces loose ash deposits, heavy rain, and debris flows.
- Excess weight from accumulation of rain or snow

Human Causes

- Vibration from machinery
- Traffic and road construction
- Blasting
- Mining
- Logging
- Overgrazing

❖ Landslide Types

Debris Flow

Slope material that becomes saturated with water may develop into a debris flow or mud flow. The resulting slurry of rock and mud may pick up trees, houses, and cars, thus blocking bridges and tributaries causing flooding along its path

Earth Flow

Earth flows are down slope, viscous flows of saturated, fine-grained materials, that move at any speed from slow to fast. Typically, they can move at speeds from 0.17 to 20 km/h. Though these are a lot like mudflows, overall they are slower moving and are covered with solid material carried along by flow from within. They are different from fluid flows in that flows in that they are more rapid.

Sturzstrom

A sturzstrom is a rare, poorly understood type of landslide. Often very large, these slides are unusually mobile, flowing very far over a low angle, flat, or even slightly uphill terrain. They are suspected of "riding" on a blanket of pressurized air, thus reducing friction with the underlying surface.

Shallow Landslide

Landslide in which the sliding surface is located within the soil mantle or weathered bedrock (typically to a depth from few decimetres to some metres). They usually include debris slides, debris flow, and failures of road cut-slopes. Landslides occurring as single large blocks of rock moving slowly down slope are sometimes called block glides.

Deep-seated Landslide

Landslides in which the sliding surface is mostly deeply located below the maximum rooting depth of trees (typically to depths greater than ten metres). Deep-seated landslides usually involve deep regolith, weathered rock, and/or bedrock and include large slope failure associated with translational, rotational, or complex movement.

(c) Cyclones

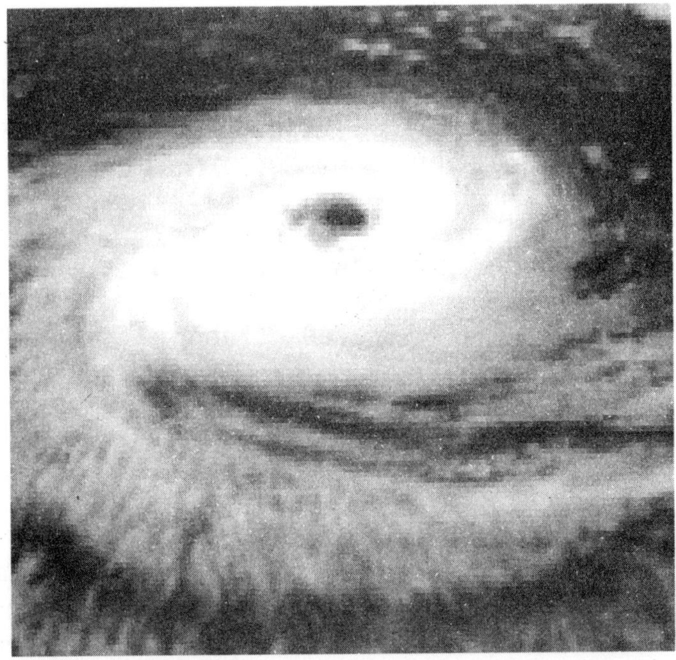

A "Cyclonic Storm" or a "Cyclone" is an intense vortex or a whirl in the atmosphere with very strong winds circulating around it in anti-clockwise direction in the Northern Hemisphere and in clockwise direction in the Southern Hemisphere.

The word "Cyclone" is derived from the Greek, word "Cyclos" meaning the coils of a snake. To Henri Peddington, the tropical storms in the Bay of Bengal and in the Arabian Sea appeared like the coiled serpents of the sea and he named these storms as "Cyclones".

Cyclones are intense low pressure areas from the centre of which pressure increases outwards. The amount of the pressure drop in the centre and the rate at which it increases outwards gives the intensity of the cyclones and the strength of winds.

The criteria followed by the Meteorological Department of India to classify the low pressure systems in the Bay of Bengal and in the Arabian Sea as adopted by the World Meteorological Organization (WMO) are in the following table :

Types of Low Pressure in India

Types of Disturbances	Associated wind speed in the Circulation
Low Pressure Area	Less than 17 knots (< 31 kmph)
Depression	17 to 27 knots (31 to 49 kmph)
Deep Depression	28 to 33 knots (50 to 61 kmph)
Cyclonic Storm	34 to 47 knots (62 to 88 kmph)
Severe Cyclonic Storm	48 to 63 knots (89 to 118 kmph)
Very Severe Cyclonic Storm	64 to 119 knots (119 to 221 kmph)
Super Cyclonic Storm	120 knots and above (222 kmph and above)

Note: 1 knot = 1.85 km per hour

A full-grown cyclone is a violent whirl in the atmosphere 150 to 1000 km across, 10 to 15 km high. Gale winds of 150 to 250 kmph or more spiral around the centre of very low pressure area with 30 to 100 hPa below the normal sea level pressure. The central calm region of the storm is called the "Eye". The diameter of the eye varies between 30 and 50 km and is a region free of clouds and has light winds. Around this calm and clear eye, there is the "Wall Cloud Region" of the storm about 50 km in extent, where the gale winds, thick clouds with torrential rain, thunder and lightning prevail. Away from the "Wall Cloud Region", the wind speed gradually decreases. However, in severe cyclonic storms, wind speeds of 50 to 60 kmph can occur even at a distance of 600 km from the storm centre. The gales give rise to a confused sea with waves as high as 20 metres, swells that travel a thousand miles. Torrential rains, occasional thunder and lightning flashes—join these under an overcast black canopy. Through these churned chaotic sea and atmosphere, the cyclone moves 300 to 500 km, in a day to hit or skirt along a coast, bringing with it storm surges as high as 3 to 12 metres, as if splashing a part of the sea sometimes up to 30 km inland leaving behind death and destructions.

❖ Cyclones in the Indian Ocean

Cyclones form in certain favourable atmospheric and Oceanic conditions. There are marked seasonal variations in their places of origin, tracks and attainment of intensities. These behaviours help in predicting their movements.

Cyclones affect both the Bay of Bengal and the Arabian Sea. They are rare in Bay of Bengal from January to March. Isolated ones forming in the South Bay of Bengal move west-north-westwards and hit Tamil Nadu and Sri Lanka coasts. In April and May, these form in the South and adjoining Central Bay and move initially northwest, north and then recurve to the northeast striking the Arakan coasts in April and Andhra-Orissa-West Bengal-Bangla Desh coasts in May. Most of the monsoon (June-September) storms develop in the central and in the North Bay and move west-north-westwards affecting Andhra-Orissa-West Bengal coasts. Post monsoon (October-December) storms form mostly in the south and the central Bay, recurve between 15^0 and 18^{0}N affecting Tamil Nadu-Andhra Orissa-West Bengal-Bangla Desh coasts.

Cyclones do not form in Arabian Sea during the months of January, February and March and are rare in April, July, August and September. They generally form in southeast Arabian Sea and adjoining central Arabian Sea in the months of May, October, November and December and in east-central Arabian Sea in the month of June. Some of the cyclones that originate in the Bay of Bengal travel across the peninsula weaken and emerge into Arabian Sea as low pressure areas. These may again intensify into cyclonic storms. Most of the storms in Arabian Sea move in west-north-westerly direction towards Arabian Coast in the month of May and in a northerly direction towards Gujarat Coast in the month of June. In other months, they generally move north-west-north and then recurve north-east affecting Gujarat-Maharashtra coasts; a few, however, also move west north westwards towards Arabian coast. Pre- and Post-monsoon storms are more violent than the storms of the monsoon season. Life span of a severe cyclonic storm in the Indian seas averages about 4 days from the time it forms until the time it enters the land.

❖ Destruction caused by Cyclones

There are three elements associated with a cyclone, which cause destruction. They are explained in the following paragraphs :

1. Cyclones are associated with high-pressure gradients and consequent strong winds. These, in turn, generate storm surges. A storm surge is an abnormal rise of sea level near the coast caused by a severe tropical cyclone; as a result, sea water inundates low lying areas of coastal regions drowning human beings and live stock, eroding beaches and embankments, destroying vegetation and reducing soil fertility.
2. Very strong winds may damage installations, dwellings, communication systems, trees., etc. resulting in loss of life and property.
3. Heavy and prolonged rains due to cyclones may cause river floods and submergence of low lying areas by rain causing loss of life and property. Floods and coastal inundation due to storm surges pollute drinking water sources causing outbreak of epidemics.

It may be mentioned that all the three factors mentioned above occur simultancously and, therefore, relief operations for distress mitigation become difficult. So it is imperative that advance action is taken for relief measures before the commencement of adverse weather conditions due to cyclones.

The most destructive element associated with an intense cyclone is storm surge. Past history indicates that loss of life is significant when surge magnitude is 3 metres or more and catastrophic when 5 metres and above.

❖ Surge Prone Coasts of India

Storm surge heights depend on the intensity of the cyclone, i.e., very high pressure gradient and consequent very strong winds and the topography of seabed near the point where a cyclone crosses the coast. Sea level also rises due to astronomical high tide. Elevation of the total sea level increases when peak surge occurs at the time of high tide.

Vulnerability to storm surges is not uniform along Indian coasts. The following segments of the east coast of India are most vulnerable to high surges :

- ☞ North Orissa and West Bengal coasts.
- ☞ Andhra Pradesh coast between Ongole and Machilipatnam.
- ☞ Tamil Nadu coast, south of Nagapattinam.

The West coast of India is less vulnerable to storm surges than the east coast of India in terms of both the height of storm surge as well as frequency of occurrence. However, the following segments are vulnerable to significant surges :

- ☞ Maharashtra coast, north of Harnai and adjoining south Gujarat coast and the coastal belt around the Gulf of Mumbai.
- ☞ The coastal belt around the Gulf of Kutch.

❖ Cyclone Accounts in India

The accounts of some of the cyclones that struck the coasts of India are given below :

- ☞ The oldest and the worst cyclone on record is that of October 1737 which hit Calcutta and took a toll of 3,00,000 lives in the deltaic region. It was accompanied by a 12 metres high surge. A violent earthquake coinciding with this storm enhanced the destruction.
- ☞ Midnapore Cyclone of October 1942 was accompanied by gale wind speed of 225 kmph
- ☞ Rameshwaram Cyclone of 17th to 24th December, 1964 wiped out Dhanuskodi in Rameshwaram Island from the map. A passenger train which left Rameshwaram Road Station near about the midnight of 22nd was washed off by the storm surges sometimes later, nearly all passengers travelling in the train meeting water graves. The Pamban Bridge connecting Mandapam and Rameshwaram Island was also washed away by the storm surges which could be 3-5 metres high.

- Andhra Cyclone of 14-20 November, 1977 that crossed coast near Nizampatnam in the evening of 19th took a toll of about 10,000 lives. The Ship Jagatswamini, which went right into the eye of the storm in the evening of 17th experienced maximum wind speed of 194 kmph. As the storm approached the coast, gale winds reaching 200 kmph lashed Prakasam Guntur, Krishna, East and West Godavari districts. Storm surge of 5 metres high inundated Krishna estuary and the coasts south of Machilipatnam.

❖ Prevention / Preparedness from Cyclones

World

The World Meteorological Organization (WMO) has established in 1972, a Tropical Cyclone Project (TCP) with the objective of assisting the member countries to increase their capabilities to detect and forecast the approach and landfall of the tropical cyclones, evaluate and forecast, the storm surges, forecast the flooding arising from the cyclones and to develop schemes to organize and execute disaster prevention and preparedness measures. One such plan that is in operation for assisting the countries adjoining the Bay of Bengal and the Arabian Sea is the panel on the tropical cyclones of World Meteorological Organization (WMO) and the Economic and Social Council for Asia and Pacific (ESCAP). The WMO/ESCAP panel has a technical support unit (TSU) and its office is rotated every four years and is at present located in Dhaka in Bangladesh. The present members of WMO/ ESCAP panel on Tropical cyclone are Bangladesh, Burma, India, Maldives, Pakistan, Sri Lanka and Thailand.

The panel co-ordinates the Co-operative activities among the member countries in facing the cyclone problems. Guidelines have also been drawn up for disaster prevention and preparedness jointly by the WMO/ESCAP, League of Red Cross Societies (LRCS) and the United Nations' Disaster Relief Organization (UNDRO), which are being, implemented by the concerned countries. Recently, a cyclone operational plan for the region has been formulated and accepted by member countries under this panel. RMC New Delhi is issuing advisory bulletin to the member countries, whenever, there is a cyclonic storm in North Indian Ocean.

India

The Government of India suggested in 1969 to the governments of the maritime States to set up "Cyclone Distress Mitigation Committee" (CDMC) in the respective States with the objective of preventing loss of life and minimizing damage to properties. CDMCs are to plan the communication systems in the State for quick dissemination of Meteorological warnings and prevention measures. Prevention measures include construction of storm shelters, connecting roads for evacuation of people, construction of wind breaks, dykes, bunds, flood storage reservoirs, afforestation along the coastal belts and improvement of drainage facilities. An advance warning will not be effective unless the public is enlightened about the destructive features and the actions to be taken by them to avoid sufferings. CDMCs have also, therefore, programmes for generating public awareness through information pamphlets, brochures, audiovisual materials, cyclone preparedness meetings, talks and discussions over the radio and television.

(d) Disaster Planning and Management in India

Government of India has taken several initiatives for strengthening disaster reduction strategies. Government of India constituted an Expert Group to examine the related issues and evolve recommendations for improving preparedness and prevention with respect to natural disasters caused by earthquakes, floods and cyclones.

The Expert Group appointed by the Government of India examined the current status of work being carried out in these areas :

- Monitoring of Hazards.
- Vulnerability Assessment.
- Prediction and Forecasting.
- Retrofitting of Existing Unsafe Structures and Buildings.
- Hazard Mapping.
- Disaster Risk Assessment and Mapping.
- Preparation of Building Guidelines.
- Assessing Gaps in the Above. Filling them as much as possible.

The Report has covered the following issues :

- Identification of various hazard prone areas.
- Vulnerability and Risk Assessment of Buildings.
- Disaster damage scenarios.
- Technical Guidelines for Hazard Resistant Construction of Buildings.
- Upgrading of Hazard Resistance of Existing Housing Stock by Retrofitting, and Techno-Legal Regime to be adopted.

Based on the findings as above, the Group has recommended strategies to be adopted and Action Plan for consideration of the Government. The Group feels strongly that these need to be urgently considered for **evolving a national policy** keeping in view of the Government of India's commitment to the Yokohama Strategy for Natural Disaster Reduction. The major issues are highlighted as follows :

1. The first and the foremost is to restructure the National Policy on Disaster Management reflecting the holistic approach involving *prevention, mitigation* and *preparedness* in *pre-disaster phase* with appropriate additional funding, along with the so far existent policy of the *post-disaster relief and rehabilitation* under crisis management.
2. *Creation of awareness* for disaster reduction is urgently needed amongst policy makers, decision-makers, administrators, professionals (architects, engineers and others at various levels) financial institutions (banks, insurance, house financing institutions) and NGOs and voluntary organizations.
3. *Creating awareness for improving preparedness amongst the communities,* using media, school education, and the network of the building centre.
4. *Appropriate amendments* in the legislative and regulatory instruments (State laws, master plans, development area plan rules, building regulations and bye-laws of local bodies) along with *strengthening of the enforcement mechanisms* at different levels.
5. *Capacity building at local and regional levels* for undertaking rapid-assessment surveys and investigations of the nature and extent of damage in post disaster situations.
6. *Conducting micro-zonation surveys of large urban areas* falling in the disaster prone regions and preparing appropriate preparedness and mitigation plans on an urgent basis.
7. *To ensure use of disaster resistant construction techniques in all housing and other buildings* to be undertaken under the Central and State schemes.
8. *Making mandatory, the use of disaster resistant codes and guidelines* related to disaster resistant construction in the houses and buildings in all sectors of the society by law and through incentives and disincentives.
9. *To create a suitable institutional mechanism at national/State level to advise and help the existing disaster relief set up in formulation and updating of short and long range action plans* for the preparedness, mitigation and prevention of natural disasters. (The mechanisms suggested are establishment of a National Scientific and Technical Committee at Central level and Natural Disaster Mitigation Centres at State levels).
10. To promote the study of natural disaster prevention, mitigation and preparedness as *subjects in architecture and engineering* curricula.
11. *To create detailed database* on hazard occurrences, damage caused to buildings and infrastructure and the economic losses suffered and ensure its

accessibility to interested researchers for effective analysis of costs of disasters and benefits of mitigative actions.

12. *To devise appropriate policy instrument and funding support* for urgent disaster preparedness and prevention actions in high risk areas including upgrading the resistance of existing housing and related structures and systems.
13. *To include R&D work in disaster preparedness, mitigation and prevention as a thrust area* so that adequate funds are earmarked for the schemes of R&D organizations as well as the concerned Central Ministries and State Governments.

Questions

Long answer type of questions

1. Define Pollution. Write down different types of pollutants.
2. What are the different types of Pollution?
3. What are the environmental damages caused by pollution?
4. What are the causes, effects and control measures of Air Pollution?
5. What are the causes, effects and control measures of Water Pollution?
6. What are the causes, effects and control measures of Noise Pollution?
7. What are the causes, effects and control measures of Soil Pollution?
8. What are the major types and effects of Solid Waste?
9. What are the measures taken to control Water Pollution in India?
10. Write down Disaster Planning and Management in India.
11. What are the types, causes and effects of landslides?
12. Give an account of cyclones in India.

Write short notes on the following :

1. Biodegradable pollutants
2. Non-degradable pollutants
3. Eutrophication
4. B.O.D.
5. Earthquake
6. Tsunami
7. Landslide
8. Cyclone

Fill in the blanks

1. The word Pollution is derived from Latin word ....
2. Noise intensity is measured in............... units.

3. An earthquake is caused by a sudden slip on a................
4. The intensity of an earthquake is measured on ....scale.
5. Urban air pollution is commonly known as...........
6. Cyclones are the centres of .... Pressure
7. The point on a fault at which the first movement occurs during an earthquake is called the.....................

   Keys : 1. "pollutionem". 2. decibel. 3. fault. 4. richter. 5. smog. 6. Low. 7. epicentre.

Tick the right answer

1. The World Health Organization estimates, how many people die each year from causes directly attributable to air pollution.
   (a) 3.6 million
   (b) 14.6 million
   (c) 74.6 million
   (d) 4.6 million
2. How many cities India has with populations of at least 1 million?
   (a) More than 20
   (b) More than 35
   (c) More than 60
   (d) More than 70
3. The saturation value of Dissolved Oxygen varies from
   (a) 18-25 mg/Litres.
   (b) 12-15 mg/Litres.
   (c) 8-15 mg/Litres.
   (d) 14-15 mg/Litres.
4. India's Supreme Court issued a ruling requiring all the city's buses to be run on compressed natural gas (CNG) by
   (a) May 31, 2004.
   (b) June 31, 2000.
   (c) March 31, 2005.
   (d) March 31, 2001.
5. At what decibels the ear registers pain.
   (a) 220
   (b) 75
   (c) 120
   (d) 320
6. How many towns have been considered under the National River Conservation Plan
   (a) 153
   (b) 183

(c) 253
(d) 173

7. Tsunami is a word
   (a) American
   (b) Japanese
   (c) Arabic
   (d) German

Keys : 1. d, 2. a, 3. c, 4. d, 5. c, 6. a 7. b.

True / False types of questions

1. The National Lake Conservation Plan was initiated in 2001.
2. The worst short term civilian pollution crisis in India was the 1984 Bhopal Disaster.
3. Subjected to 45 decibels of noise, the average person cannot sleep.
4. BOD is the amount of oxygen required by micro-organisms to decompose the organic substances in sewage.
5. Dissolved oxygen is an important factor that determines the quality of sand in water.
6. At present, around 7.2 MT of hazardous waste are generated in the country.
7. The World Meteorological Organization (WMO) has established in 1972.

Keys : 1. false, 2. true, 3. true, 4. true, 5. false, 6. true, 7. true

Unit - 6

Social Issues and Environment

I. Sustainable Development

(a) Concept of Sustainable Development

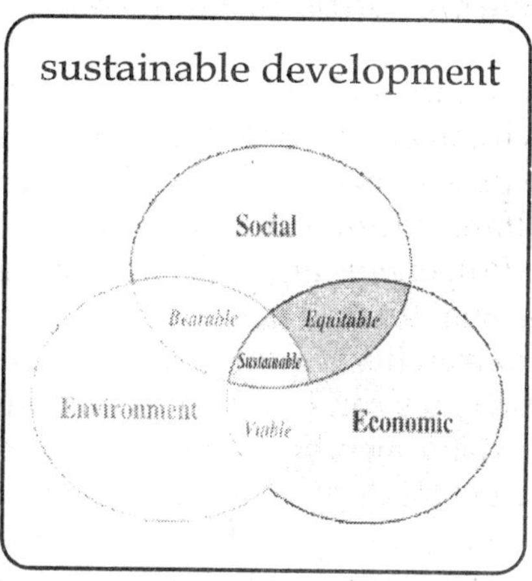

Sustainable development is defined as balancing the fulfilment of human needs with the protection of the natural environment so that these needs can be met not only in the present, but in the indefinite future. The term was used by the Brundtland Commission which coined what has become the most often-quoted definition of sustainable development as development that "meets the needs of the present without compromising the ability of future generations to meet their own needs."

Major areas as coming within the scope of Sustainable Development under Sustainable Development List of United Nations Division

Agriculture	Human Settlements	Science
Atmosphere	Indicators	Small Islands
Biodiversity	Industry	Sustainable tourism
Biotechnology	International Law	Technology
Demographics	International Cooperation	Toxic Chemicals
Desertification	Institutional arrangements	Trade
Education	Land management	Environment
Energy	Major Groups	Transport
Finance	Mountains	Waste (Hazardous)
Forests	Oceans and Seas	Waste (Radioactive)
Fresh Water	Poverty	Waste (Solid)
Health	Sanitation	Water, etc.

The Universal Declaration on Cultural Diversity (UNESCO,2001) elaborates further the concept by stating that "...cultural diversity is as necessary for humankind as biodiversity is for nature"; it becomes "one of the roots of development understood not simply in terms of economic growth, but also as a means to achieve a more satisfactory intellectual, emotional, moral and spiritual existence". In this vision, cultural diversity is the fourth policy area of sustainable development.

Sustainable Development is an ambiguous concept, as a wide array of views has fallen under its umbrella.

During the last ten years, different organizations have tried to measure and monitor the proximity to what they consider Sustainability by implementing what it has been called Sustainability metric and indices.

Environmental Sustainability

Environmental Sustainability is defined by its proponents as the ability of the environment to continue to function properly indefinitely. This involves meeting the present needs of humans as seen by the proponents without endangering the welfare of future generations.

Proponents argue that an "unsustainable situation" occurs when natural capital (the sum total of nature's resources) is used up faster than it can be replenished. Sustainability requires that human activity only uses nature's resources at a rate at which they can be replenished naturally.

Many environmentalists have criticized some interpretations of the term "sustainable development" as an oxymoron, claiming that economic policies based on concepts of growth and continued depletion of resources cannot be sustainable, since that term implies resources remain constant.

Many people prefer the term "developing sustainability", as it does not imply that something needs to be created.

(b) Sustainable Development in India

The 3,287,590 sq km of the country area characterized by upland plain in the South, flat to rolling plain along the Ganges, deserts in the West, the Himalayas in the North. The climate varies from temperate in the North to tropical monsoon in the South. The monsoon causes severe droughts, flash floods and flooding of large areas because of monsoon rains and thunderstorms.

Current environmental issues are deforestation, soil erosion, overgrazing, desertification, air pollution from industrial effluents and vehicle emissions, water pollution from raw sewage and runoff of agricultural pesticides. Tap water is not potable in some parts of the country. The huge and growing population is overstraining natural resources.

Even before India's independence in 1947, several environmental legislations existed. But only after the UN Conference on the Human Environment in Stockholm

1972, the Government began to install a first well-developed framework. Under the influence of this declaration, the National Council for Environmental Policy and Planning within the Department of Science and Technology was set up in 1972. This Council evolved into the new Ministry of Environment and Forest in 1985. (MoEF 2002a) After the UNCED, it developed a number of strategic environmental plans, ratified the Kyoto-Protocol and a number of other international treaties and paid strong attention to the implementation of Local Agenda 21.

India is signatory of many important international treaties in the field of environment, e.g. the International Convention for the Regulation of Whaling, the International Plant Protection Convention, the Antarctic Treaty, the Vienna Convention for the Protection of the Ozone Layer; the Basel Convention on Trans-boundary movement of hazardous substances, the Framework Convention on Climate Change; Convention on the Conservation of Biodiversity and the Montreal Protocol on the Substances that Deplete the Ozone Layer.

❖ Approaches to a National Sustainable Development Strategy

India presented its perspective on sustainable development before the World Summit for Sustainable Development (WSSD) in 2002 as detailed study "Empowering People for Sustainable Development" (EPSD). It was brought out by the Ministry of Environment and Forests (MoEF).

The Indian Government did not feel the need for a separate specific strategy for sustainable development. The Five Year Plans provide medium-term strategies for overall development. However, after the WSSD, the Indian Government initiated a process of preparing and implementing a national strategy for sustainable development by 2005. EPSD introduces the essential framework for sustainable development in India: democratic continuity, devolution of power, independent judiciary, and civilian control of the armed forces, independent media, transparency and people's participation. It follows multidimensional, sectoral and cross-sectoral approaches.

❖ National Five Years Planning and Sustainable Development

Planning is an important steering instrument of India's democracy. It is based on an iterative process involving interaction between the centre, the State and the local bodies. Multiple stakeholders participate in the planning process. Working groups and task forces are established to prepare plans and reports for various sectors. They are responsible for substantial participation of civil society.

Sustainability concerns have become a vital element in the planning process. The Planning Commission of India (PCI) is responsible for making the Five Year Plans. The PCI works under the overall guidance of the National Development Council (NDC), the highest decision-making authority in the country on development matters. In a preparatory meeting, the NDC directed the Planning Commission to prepare the Tenth Five Year Plan with a target growth rate of 8 per cent per annum along with significant improvements in social and environmental indicators. The PCI consults with the Central Ministries and the State Governments while formulating FYPs and Annual Plans for short-term development goals and also oversees their implementation. The Commission also functions as an advisory planning body at the highest level.

Targets of the Tenth Five Year Plan for Sustainable Development :

- Reduction of poverty ratio by 5 percentage points by 2007 and by 15 percentage points by 2012.
- All children to complete 5 Years in school by 2007.
- Reduction in gender gaps in literacy and wage rates by at least 50 per cent by 2007.
- Reduction in population growth between 2001 and 2011 to 16.2 per cent.
- Increase in literacy rate to 75 per cent by 2007.
- Reduction of Infant Mortality Rate (IMR) to 45 per 1000 live births by 2007 and to 28 by 2012.
- Reduction of Maternal Mortality Rate (MMR) to 2 per 1000 live births by 2007 and to 1 by 2012.
- Increase in forest cover to 25 per cent by 2007 and 33 per cent by 2012.
- All villages to have sustained access to potable drinking water by 2007.
- Cleaning of major polluted rivers by 2007 and other notified stretches by 2012.

❖ Integration of Sustainable Development Principles

The Five year planning includes all pillars of sustainable development. With regard to the poverty in the country, the main focus lies on economic growth and social development (especially employment and education) but with consideration of environmental aspects, too. For instance, a new approach in the Tenth Five Year planning is social mobilisation as key to self-employment. This process-oriented programme is for the poor with a focus on the formation of self help groups (SHGs). It is a holistic programme operating largely through SHGs, with the provision of micro-finance, training and capacity building. It is a holistic programme operating largely through SHGs, with the provision of micro-finance, training and capacity building.

"The economy is a sub-system of the finite regional ecosystem..." (MoEF 2002). In order to encourage regional authorities and institutions to apply sustainable development in their planning, the MoEF published a manual on "Carrying Capacity based Regional Developmental Planning" in 2002. It describes the content of sustainable development and the "carrying capacity" process, a scheme to analyse regions and case studies.

❖ Aspects of a National Sustainable Development Strategy

(1) Development and Institutional Aspects

The National Environmental Council (NEC) chaired by the Prime Minister and the Minister of Environment and Forests, advises the Ministry of Environment and Forest (MoEF) in its work in environment policy and planning matters of national concern. It consists of representatives of Ministries of Environment and Forests, Power, Surface Transport, Industry, Chemicals and Petrochemicals, Petroleum and Natural Gas, Urban Affairs, Non-conventional Energy Sources, and Mines and Members of Parliament, the Planning Commission, Central Pollution Control Board, Federation of Indian Chambers of Commerce and Industry, Associated Chambers of Commerce and Industries of India, Confederation of Indian Industry, Federation of Small Industries, National Consumer Federation and National Environmental Engineering Research Institute, the non-governmental Tata Energy Research Institute, World Wide Fund - India, Smt. Nandita Krishna, CPR Centre for Environment Education, INTACH, New Delhi and several individuals.

There are several institutions working on sustainable development issues. The Centre of Environment Education (CEE) is an autonomous agency and a Centre of Excellence under the MoEF. CEE organized the multi-stakeholder consultations and facilitated preparatory processes. The outcome of this process was prepared by CEE with support from MoEF and is called "Sustainable Development Learnings and Perspectives from India". With CEE's regional Cells, projects can be implemented with a strong local focus. It is an important partner within the Five Year Planning process by coordinating the education, awareness building and training for the Planning Commission, e.g. the Thematic Working Group of the National Biodiversity Strategy and the Action Plan. Additionally, it provides comprehensive information on key sustainable development issues to policy makers.

The Tata Energy and Resources Institute (TERI) is the largest research institution working on local, national and global sustainability issues in all developing countries. TERI hosts the Delhi Sustainable Development Summit (DSDS), an annual international event, and provides knowledge and stimulating debate on various aspects of sustainable development.

(2) Participation Aspects

In the run-up to WSSD, a number of initiatives were taken such as a review of policies in relation to Agenda 21 and a view towards a national strategy for sustainable development, multi-stakeholder consultations, a media campaign and websites to give information about India's preparations towards the Summit as well as a nationwide children's competition. Organized by the CEE and supported by the MoEF, seven Regional Consultations and several smaller, thematically specialized meetings were organized. By and large, these Consultations covered general sustainable development concerns and a few regional issues. These discussions were condensed into a draft document "Sustainable Development - Learnings and Perspectives from India". The draft was submitted for discussion at a National Consultation in May 2002. The National consultation brought together over 150 representatives from several central Ministries, State governments, NGOs, academic institutions and civil society organizations. The draft document was spread through well-targeted mailings and through a web forum. The document was finalized based on input received from various cross-sections of society before World Summit for Sustainable Development (WSSD) and contains listed requirements and suggestions, perspectives and approaches towards achieving a sustainable future. This process is seen as the beginning of continuing discussion and dialogue.

A large number of NGO's are actively discussing issues with the government. A few hundred NGO's called themselves environmental activists in the beginning of the 80's. Today, there are more than 10,000. Information technology provides also platforms to raise awareness, peoples' participation and increase transparency. The MoEF has set up a National Environmental Information System (ENVIS). The MoEF also led the implementation of the UNDP and IDRC (International Development Research Centre, Canada) assisted project, Sustainable Development Networking Programme (SDNP). It was launched worldwide in 1990. SDNP India facilitates the process of sustainable development by providing information for NGOs, government and research organizations, business establishments and civil society. SDNP provides a platform for debates and discussions as well. Currently, the SDNP homepage gives information about a research of a sectoral approach for sustainable development and a multidimensional indicators system worked out by the Indira Gandhi Institute of Development Research.

(3) Monitoring Aspects

India has developed specific sustainability indicators as well as the strategy for sustainable development. The commitment to principles of sustainable development is already reflected in the monitorable targets of human development and conservation of natural resources that were set up in the Tenth Five Year Plan.

The indicators became an instrument in the Tenth Five Year Plan relating the importance of human development with economic growth. Earlier Plans focused on many of these, but no specific targets and indicators were set. Additionally, the "Empowering People for Sustainable Development" (EPSD) introduced a few indicators to monitor social changes and named them India's Human Development Indicators.

The government reports the progress within the Tenth Five Year Plan and hence the sustainable development targets annually.

India's internet performance is worth mentioning. A web enabled system contains information on financial data of Annual plans and Five Year Plan. Planning Commission uses this information from various Public Sector Undertakings, Departments and Ministries.

The Information System for Forest, Wildlife and Environment is a web based application to provide information regarding forests, wildlife and environment of all States. It helps users in the Planning Commission to take decisions on future plans. A database has been implemented dealing with parliament questions and their answers, handled by the Parliament Section of the Planning Commission. The system with search facilities enables users to have easy access to the documents by means of search options according to year of parliament-session and related subjects.

The Environmental Information System (ENVIS) deals with 'Centres of Excellence' related to environment. Nearly 6,000 queries are received by the ENVIS network per year. The data bases are available in the internet to everybody.

(4) Implementation Aspects and Specific Initiatives

Principles of sustainable development passed the first bottleneck by being accepted in the Tenth Five Year Plan. New approaches and instruments like measurable national indicators improved the planning towards sustainable development even further.

A lot will depend on the performance on the State level and the progress in capacity building from there down to the municipal level, where objectives and plans have to be translated into practical action. The same applies to the citizens' participation and the influence that the new sustainable thinking will have on their lives. Poverty and inter-regional and inter-class conflicts remain a major challenge.

Concerning capacity building in the young generation, India set up a National Green Corps (NGC) programme several years ago. The programme aims to provide opportunities for children to understand the environment and environmental problems through school eco-clubs. The MoEF launched NGC with the main objective of creating environmental awareness through people's participation especially among school children. During the Tenth Plan it is expected that about 50,000 schools will participate in NGC related activities. In addition, 3,000 eco-clubs have been set up in schools with the Ministry's assistance.

The concept of sustainable development was cast into a law, the Biological Diversity Act, for the first time in 2002. According to the act, the Central government shall integrate the conservation, promotion and sustainable use of biological diversity into relevant sectoral or cross-sectoral plans, programmes and policies. "Sustainable use" is defined as the use of components of biological diversity in such manner and at such rate that does not lead to the long-term decline of the biological diversity thereby maintaining its potential to meet the needs and aspirations of present and future generations. Further national strategies, plans, programmes are to be developed to increase awareness with biodiversity.

Joint Forest Management (JFM) is a new style of governance. Similarly, in the case of environmental clearance all major projects have to go through the process of a public hearing. Both, the government and the local communities participate in managing the forest resources.

India has an ambitious development programme that reflects the importance of sustainable growth of the economy. But many projects and further steps will be successful only if financial support is given and international co-operation and transfer of knowledge strengthen. And of course there has to be an effective national monitoring.

Empowering people to participate substantially is one of the main objectives of the Five Year Plan. Special attention was paid to this objective in the "Programmatic Activities" of the Five Year Plan under the paragraph "Improving governance".

In the Tenth Five Year Plan, much attention was also given to an integrated approach to improve the agricultural sector in order to protect natural resources and combat poverty at the same time. This is quite a sustainable approach that has to be implemented in the next few years.

II. Global Warming

The term *global warming* is a specific example of the broader term climate change, which can also refer to global cooling. In principle, global warming is neutral as to the period or causes, but in common usage the term generally refers to recent warming and implies a human influence.

(a) History of Global Warming

Relative to the period 1860–1900, global temperatures on both land and sea have increased by 0.75 °C (1.4 °F), according to the instrumental temperature record. Since 1979, land temperatures have increased about twice as fast as ocean temperatures (0.25 °C/decade against 0.13 °C/decade) (Smith, 2005). Temperatures in the lower troposphere have increased between 0.12 and 0.22° C per decade since 1979, according to satellite temperature measurements. Over the one or two thousand years before 1850, world temperature is believed to have been relatively stable, with possibly regional fluctuations such as the Medieval Warm Period or the Little Ice Age.

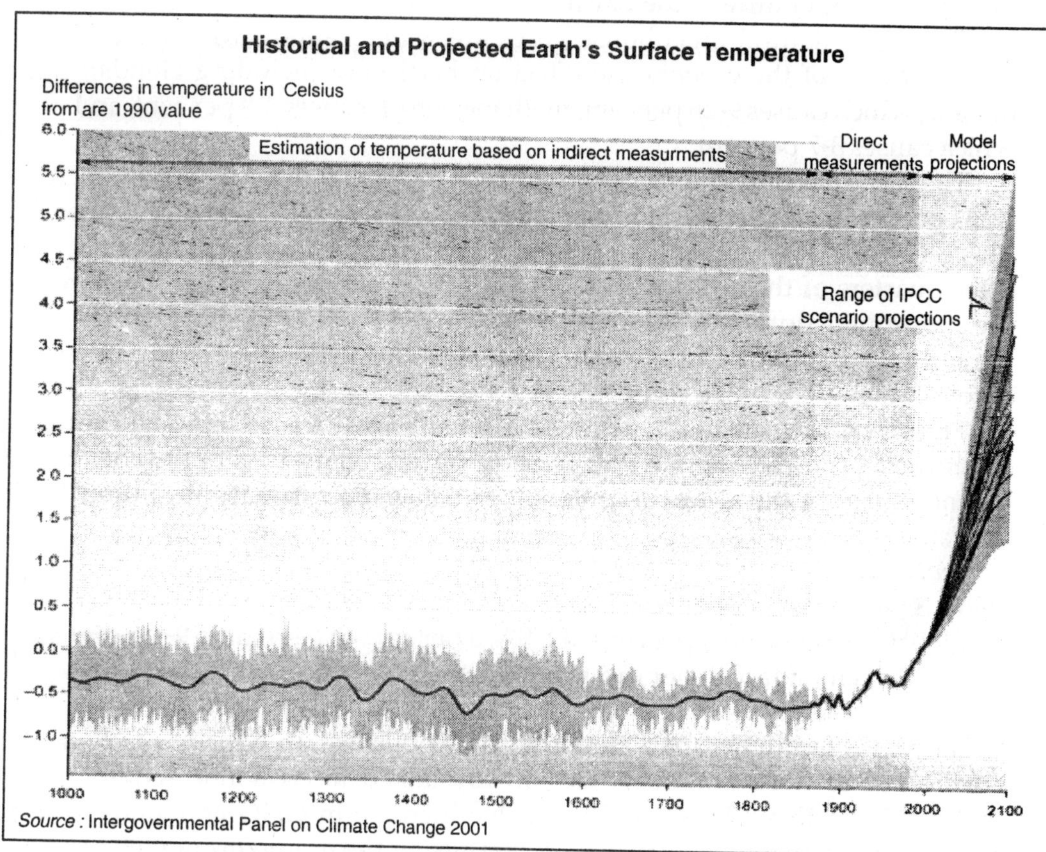

Source : Intergovernmental Panel on Climate Change 2001

(b) *Causes of Global Warming*

The climate system varies through natural, internal processes and in response to variations in external "forcing" from both human and natural causes. These forcing factors include solar activity, volcanic emissions, variations in the earth's orbit (orbital forcing) and greenhouse gases. The detailed causes of the recent warming remain an active field of research, but the scientific consensus identifies greenhouse gases as the main influence. The major natural greenhouse gases are water vapour, carbon dioxide, methane, and ozone.

Greenhouse gases in the atmosphere

Greenhouse gases are transparent to shortwave radiation from the sun, the main source of heat on the Earth. However, they absorb some of the longer infrared radiation emitted by the Earth, thereby reducing radiational cooling and hence raising the temperature of the Earth.

The major natural greenhouse gases are water vapour, which causes about 36-70 per cent of the greenhouse effect on Earth (not including clouds); carbon dioxide, which causes 9-26 per cent; methane, which causes 4-9 per cent, and ozone, which causes 3-7 per cent.

The atmospheric concentrations of carbon dioxide and methane have increased by 31 per cent and 149 per cent respectively above pre-industrial levels since 1750. This is considerably higher than at any time during the last 6,50,000, years. About three-quarters of the anthropogenic (man-made) emissions of carbon dioxide to the atmosphere during the past 20 years are due to fossil fuel burning. The rest of the anthropogenic emissions are predominantly due to land-use change, especially deforestation.

Future carbon dioxide levels are expected to rise due to ongoing burning of fossil fuels. The rate of rise will depend on uncertain economic, sociological, technological, natural developments, but may be ultimately limited by the availability of fossil fuels.

India's GHG emissions in 1994 was 1228 million tonne CO equivalent, which is below 3 per cent of global GHG emissions. In per capita terms, it is 23 per cent of the global average, and 4 per cent of USA, 8 per cent of Germany, 9 per cent of UK, and 10 per cent of Japan, per capita emissions in 1994. In terms of primary energy use, India's share of renewable energy (being a nonGHG emitting energy form) at 36 per cent is far higher than industrialized countries can hope to reach in many decades. Since GHG emissions are directly linked to economic activity, India's economic growth will necessarily involve increase in GHG emissions from the current extremely low levels. Any constraints on the emissions of GHG by India, whether direct, by way of emissions targets, or indirect, will reduce growth rates.

(c) Effects of Global Warming

Some effects on both the natural environment and human life are already being attributed at least in part to global warming. Glacier retreat, ice shelf disruption such as the Larsen Ice Shelf, sea level rise, changes in rainfall patterns, increased intensity and frequency of hurricanes and extreme weather events, are being attributed at least in part to global warming. While changes are expected for overall patterns, intensity, and frequencies, it is difficult or impossible to attribute *specific* events (such as Hurricane Katrina) to global warming.

Some anticipated effects include sea level rise of 110 to 770 mm by 2100, repercussions to agriculture, possible slowing of the thermohaline circulation, reductions in the ozone layer, increased intensity and frequency of hurricanes and extreme weather events, lowering of ocean pH, the spread of diseases such as malaria and dengue fever, and mass extinction events.

(d) Measures to Control Global Warming

The consensus among climate scientists that global temperatures will continue to increase has led nations, states, corporations and individuals to implement actions to try to curtail global warming. Some of the strategies that have been proposed for mitigation of global warming include development of new technologies; carbon offsets; renewable energy such as biodiesel, wind power, and solar power; nuclear power; electric or hybrid automobiles; fuel cells; energy conservation; carbon taxes; improving natural carbon dioxide sinks; deliberate production of sulfate aerosols, which produce a cooling effect on the Earth; population control; carbon capture and storage, and nanotechnology.

Many environmental groups encourage individual action against global warming, often aimed at the consumer, and there has been business action on climate change.

❖ Global Warming and Kyoto Protocol

The world's primary international agreement on combating global warming is the Kyoto Protocol. The Kyoto Protocol is an amendment to the United Nations Framework Convention on Climate Change (UNFCCC). Countries that ratify this protocol commit to reduce their emissions of carbon dioxide and five other greenhouse gases, or engage in emissions trading if they maintain or increase emissions of these gases. Developing countries are exempt from meeting emission standards in Kyoto. This includes China and India, the second and third largest emitters of CO_2, behind the United States.

III. Acid Rain

This is rain which has turned acidic because of the presence of sulphur dioxide (SO_2) and nitrogen oxides (NO_2) in the atmosphere. Sulphur dioxide is emitted from volcanoes, sea spra, rotting vegetation and plankton. But the large amount of coal and oil burning are the main cause of the pollution. Nitrogen dioxide, on the other hand, are from power stations and exhaust fumes. Acidity is measured on a pH scale. A substance with a pH value of less than 7 is acidic.

$$\text{Acid rain} = SO_2 + NO_2 + H_2O$$

Here is a little bit on the history of the acid rain problem. The problem of acid rain probably originated during the 1730's, at the height of the industrial revolution. It was discovered in the 1950's and started being noticed in the 1960's. Since the

1960's, the problem has gotten worse in rural areas because the tall chimneys on factories allow the wind to transport pollutants far away from their sources. In 1984 it was reported that almost half of the trees in the famous black forest in Germany had been damaged by acid rain. In 1988, as part of the United Nations sponsored Long Range Transboundary Air Pollution Agreement, the U.S.A. and 24 other nations agreed to some rules limiting nitrogen oxide emissions to 1987 levels. 1990 changes to the Clean Air Act set rules to cut down the release of sulphur dioxide from power plants down to 10 million tonnes by January 1, 2000.

(a) *Causes of Acid Rains*

Many things can cause acid rain. Industrial emissions from factories and power plants that burn fuels such as natural gas, coal or oil, emit smoke that gives off oxides of sulphur and nitrogen is one cause. Another cause is vehicles (e.g. cars, buses) that burn gasoline and diesel. The exhaust emitted by burning these fuels contains sulphur dioxide, an oxide of sulphur. Also, vehicles that have gas engines will produce oxides of nitrogen, another cause of acid rain. One other cause is home fires giving off smoke that contains sulfur dioxide. Some fairly minor causes are natural causes which are volcanoes, swamps and rotting plants giving off sulphur dioxide. Natural causes only account for 10 per cent of the pollution causing acid rain.

(b) *Effects and Problems of Acid Rains*

There are several places around the world affected by acid rain and here are the main ones. The Northeastern section of the United States where acid rain is caused by high number of factories and power plants is one affected area. Also in that same region, the Southeastern section of Canada is affected and the main cause is factories in the Toronto-Hamilton area. Central Europe and Scandinavia (Sweden, Norway and Finland) are also affected, here being the British and other European factories doing the damage. One more main area that is affected is parts of Asia, specifically India and China, where acid rain is caused by large number of factories.

There are many problems and effects caused by acid rain. Acid rain can cause buildings, statues and bridges to deteriorate faster than usual. Another problem is it harms thousands of lakes, rivers, and streams worldwide. It disrupts lake ecosystems and kills wildlife in affected lakes, rivers and streams. Acid rain also damages soil and the tree roots in it. When soil is acidified, tree roots are damaged, leaving them not able to draw in enough nutrients to support the tree. When acid rain falls on trees, it makes their leaves turn brownish-yellow and the tree can no longer carry out photosynthesis properly. Another problem is, it will harm people when they breathe in smog, acid rain in one of its many forms. Acid rain can also harm people indirectly. This happens when people eat fish caught in affected lakes or rivers. Also, if the water source is acidic enough, it will react with copper or lead pipes to harm humans. It also washes aluminium into the water supply. Birds can be harmed if they live in affected waters or feed on fish living in affected waters.

Acid rain causes lakes and rivers to become acidic, killing off fish— all the fish in 140 lakes in Minnesota have been killed, and the salmon and trout populations of Norway's major rivers have been severely reduced because of the increased acidity of the water. Short-term increases in acid levels kill lots of fish, but the greatest threat is from long-term increases, which stop the fish from reproducing. The extra acid also frees toxic metals which were previously held in rocks, especially aluminium, which prevents fish from breathing. Single-celled plants and algae in lakes also suffer from increased acid levels, with numbers dropping off quickly once the pH goes below 5, and by the time the pH gets down to 4.5, virtually everything is dead. A very highly publicised problem is the effect of acid rain on trees. Conifers appear to be particularly affected, with needles dropping off, and seedlings failing to produce new trees. The acid also reacts with many nutrients the trees need, such as calcium, magnesium and potassium, which starves the trees. The trees are then much more susceptible to other forms of damage, such as being blown down, or breaking under the weight of snow.

Rather surprisingly, the effects of acid rain on trees have overshadowed the effects on people. Many toxic metals are held in the ground in compounds. However, acid rain can break down some of these compounds, freeing the metals and washing them into water sources such as rivers. In Sweden, nearly 10,000 lakes now have such high mercury concentration that people are advised not to eat fish caught in them. As the water becomes more acidic, it can also react with lead and copper water pipes, contaminating drinking water supplies. In Sweden, the drinking water reached a stage where it contained enough copper to turn the hair green ! The worst part is that much copper can also cause diarrhoea in young children, and can damage livers and kidneys.

In Sweden, drinking water once contained enough water to make people's hair turn green. In the Czech Republic, many trees lost all their leaves as a result of acid rain. The Taj Mahal in India, one of the ten wonders of the world, is being constantly threatened by acid rain. Some famous statues, such as the Lincoln Memorial and Michaelangelo's statue of Marcus Aurelius, have started deteriorating because of acid rain. In London in 1952, very thick acid smog killed 4,000 people.

In India acid rain is recorded form certain places Kodaikanal (ph of rainwater = 5.18), Minicoy (ph = 5.52), Mohanbari (ph = 5.50).

(c) *Possible Solutions of Acid Rain*

The bottom line is that all things on earth are being affected by this problem and the good news is that something is being done to solve it. Pressure from the environmental groups and public has increased as the effects of the havoc caused by acid rain become more apparent. Governments all over the world have drawn up plans to tackle this problem.

Lakes that have become highly acidic can be treated by adding large quantities of alkaline substances like quicklime, in a process called liming. Although it has worked in several places, it has not been successful where the lake is very large, making this procedure economically unfeasible, or in other lakes where the flushing rate of the lake waters is too large resulting in the lake becoming acidic again.

The best approach seems to be in prevention. To this end environmental regulations have been enacted to limit the quantity of emissions released in the atmosphere. Several industries have added scrubbers to their smoke stacks to reduce the amount of sulphur dioxide dumped in the atmosphere. Specially designed catalytic converters are used to ensure that the gases coming out from exhaust pipes of automobiles are rendered harmless. Several industries which use coal as fuel have begun to wash the coal before using it thereby reducing the amount of Sulphur present in it, and consequently the amount of emissions. Usage of coal with a low Sulphur content also reduces the problem.

We as individuals can take several steps to alleviate the effects of this problem. A reduction in use of vehicles will reduce the amount of emission caused by our vehicles. So do not use the car unless it is absolutely required. For going short distances, walk or try to use a bicycle. This will not only protect the environment but also improve your health. If the distance is greater, try using public transportation. If you must use your vehicle try forming a car pool and share your vehicle with someone else. Ensure that your vehicle is properly tuned, and fitted with a catalytic converter, to reduce the emissions.

Reduce use of electric power. Switch off lights, and other electrical appliances when not required. Do not leave your televisions, VCRs, microwave ovens or music systems on stand-by when not required. Switch them off.

Reducing power consumption will reduce the amount of coal burnt to produce electricity, and thus reduce the amount of pollution. This is true even if your electricity company does not use coal for producing electricity, but some other more environmentally friendly way. This is because the electricity you have saved can now be used elsewhere, thus benefiting nature.

Speak to others about this problem. Increasing awareness is one way of ensuring that things are done to solve this global problem. Find out what fuel is being used by your electricity company to produce electricity. If they use coal, ask what methods they use to contain, if not eliminate, the problem of sulphur emissions. Washing the coal used, or using coal having a low sulphur content, is costly and, therefore, some companies try to avoid this. If you have the option, switch to a utility that shows more concern for the environment.

Write to your representative in Government. Pressure from people can make governments enact suitable legislation, to ensure that industries keep their emissions within limits. Join some group which works to protect the environment. When people get together and speak with one voice they are more likely to be heard.

IV. Ozone Depletion

Ozone (O_3) is a triatomic molecule, consisting of three oxygen atoms. It is an allotrope of oxygen that is much less stable than the diatomic species O_2. Ozone is a pale blue gas at standard temperature and pressure, and one of the most toxic inorganic compounds known. It forms a dark blue liquid below—112°C and a dark blue solid below—193° C. Ozone is a powerful oxidizing agent.

O_3 is present in low concentrations throughout the Earth's atmosphere: ground level ozone is an air pollutant with harmful effects on lung function and in the upper atmosphere it prevents damaging ultraviolet light from reaching the Earth's surface. It is also formed from O_2 by electrical discharges such as lightning, and by action of high energy electromagnetic radiation. Certain electrical equipment generate significant levels of ozone. This is especially true of devices using high voltages, such as laser printers, photocopiers, and arc welders. Electric motors using brushes can generate ozone from repeated sparking inside the unit. Large motors, such as those used by elevators or hydraulic pumps, will generate more ozone than smaller motors.

Ozone was discovered by Christian Friedrich Schonbein in 1840, who named it after the Greek word for smell (*ozein*), from the peculiar odour in lightning storms. The odour from a lightning strike is from electrons freed during the rapid chemical changes, not the ozone itself. Sax's Dangerous Properties of Industrial Materials, 8th. ed. indicates that ozone is colorless (perhaps pale blue) in gas but dark blue as a liquid. In concentrations of 0.015ppm, ozone has a barely detectible odour.

(a) Ozone Layer

The highest levels of ozone in the atmosphere are in the stratosphere, in a region also known as the ozone layer. Here it filters out the shorter wavelengths (less than 320 nm) of ultraviolet light (270 to 400 nm) from the Sun that would be harmful to most forms of life in large doses. These same wavelengths are also responsible for the production of vitamin D, which is essential for human health. The standard way to express total ozone amounts in the atmosphere is by using Dobson units. Ozone used in industry is measured in ppm , and percent by mass or weight.

(b) Industrial Production of Ozone

Industrially, ozone is produced with short wavelength ultraviolet radiation from a mercury vapour lamp or the application of a high voltage electrical field in a process called *cold or corona discharge*. The cold discharge apparatus consists of two metal plates separated by an air gap and a high dielectric strength electrical insulator such as borosilicate glass or mica. A high voltage alternating current is applied to the plates and the ozone is formed in the air gap when O_2 molecules disassociate

Note : nm = nanometers.

and recombine into O_3. A faint corona may be present in the air gap, but the voltage is maintained below that which would cause punch-through of the insulator with subsequent arcing and plasma formation. In the laboratory ozone can be produced by electrolysis using a 9 volt battery, a pencil graphite rod cathode, a platinium wire anode and a 3'M' sulphuric acid electrolyte.

(c) Applications of Ozone

1. Industrial Applications

Ozone can be used for bleaching substances and for killing bacteria. Many municipal drinking water systems kill bacteria with ozone instead of the more common chlorine.

Ozone does not form organochlorine compounds, but it also does not remain in the water after treatment, so some systems introduce a small amount of chlorine to prevent bacterial growth in the pipes, or may use chlorine intermittently, based on results of periodic testing. Where electrical power is abundant, ozone is a cost-effective method of treating water, as it is produced on demand and does not require transportation and storage of hazardous chemicals. Once it has decayed, it leaves no taste or odour in drinking water.

Industrially, ozone or ozonated water is used to :

- disinfect water before it is bottled,
- deodorize air and object, such as after a fire
- kill bacteria on food-contact surfaces
- scrub yeast and mould spores from the air in food processing plants
- wash fresh fruits and vegetables to kill yeast, mould and bacteria
- chemically attack contaminants in water (iron, arsenic, hydrogen sulphide, nitrites, and complex organics lumped together as "colour"),
- provide an aid to flocculation (a process of agglomeration of molecules, which aids in filtration... this is where the iron and arsenic are removed),
- clean and bleach fabrics (the latter use is patented)
- assist in processing plastics to allow adhesion of inks,
- age rubber samples to determine the useful life of a batch of rubber.
- Used in surface water treatment plants to eradicate bacteria such as *Giardia* and *Cryptosporidium*. This process is known as ozonation.

Ozone is a reagent in many organic reactions in the laboratory and in industry. Ozonolysis is the cleavage of an alkene to carbonyl compounds.

2. Consumer Applications

Ozonated water can be used to sanitize food, water, and surfaces in the home. According to the FDA, it is "amending the food additive regulations to provide for the safe use of ozone in gaseous and aqueous phases as an antimicrobial agent on food, including meat and poultry." Ironically, while ozone is considered an atmospheric pollutant, it can actually reduce pollutants like pesticides in fruits and vegetables.

3. Pharmaceutical Applications

Ozone, along with hypochlorite ions, is naturally produced by white blood cells and the roots of marigolds as a means of destroying foreign bodies. When ozone breaks down it gives rise to oxygen free radicals, which are highly reactive and damage or destroy most organic molecules.

Ozone, along with hypochlorite ions, is naturally produced by white blood cells and the roots of marigolds as a means of destroying foreign bodies. When ozone breaks down it gives rise to oxygen free radicals, which are highly reactive and damage or destroy most organic molecules.

Ozone therapy has blossomed into a thriving field of alternative medicine, and there are a host of claimed applications above and beyond what has actually been verified by studies.

In the United States ozone therapy is illegal, as the Food and Drug Administration (FDA) has not approved its use on humans. Medical ozone therapy is recognized in Bulgaria, Cuba, Czech Republic, France, Germany, Israel, Italy, Mexico, Romania and Russia. It is currently used legally in 16 nations.

4. Other Uses

Ozone is also popularly used in spas or hot tubs instead of chlorine or bromine for keeping the water free of bacteria.

Ozone gas is created by an ultraviolet light bulb or corona discharge chip and injected into the plumbing system.

Ozone is also widely used in treatment of water in aquaria and fish ponds. Its use can minimise bacterial growth control parasites and removes or reduce "yellowing" of the water. As the ozone rapidly decomposes, at correctly controlled levels the application has no effect on the fish.

(d) Ozone as a Pollutant

Ozone is not directly emitted by car engines or by industrial operations. These sources emit hydrocarbons and nitrogen oxides that react with sunlight to form ozone directly at the source of the pollution being emitted and in the atmosphere's boundary layer (1 to 3 km altitude).

The mix of hydrocarbons, nitrogen oxides, and ozone are the major components of smog that frequently occurs in urban and suburban areas. Recent satellite maps of nitrogen dioxide (NO_2) clearly show the worldwide distribution of polluted regions associated with industrial activity (automobiles, factories, and fossil fuel power generation).

There is a great deal of evidence to show that ozone at the earth's surface can harm lung function and irritate the respiratory system. Ozone has been found to convert cholesterol in the blood stream to plaque (which causes hardening and narrowing of arteries). This cholesterol product has also been implicated in Alzheimer's disease, suggesting a link between the inflammatory response associated with head injury and Alzheimer's. Air quality guidelines such as those from the World Health Organization are based on detailed studies of what levels can cause measurable health effects.

There is also evidence of significant reduction in agricultural yields due to increased ground-level ozone which interferes with photosynthesis and stunts overall growth of some species of plant.

Although ozone was present at ground level before the industrial revolution, peak concentrations are far higher than the pre-industrial levels and even background concentrations well away from sources of pollution are substantially higher.

Ozone reacts directly with some hydrocarbons such as aldehydes and thus begins their removal from the air, but the products of ozonolysis are themselves key components of smog. Ozone photolysis by UV light leads to production of the hydroxyl radical and this plays a part in the removal of hydrocarbons from the air, but is again a step in the creation of components of smog such as peroxyacyl nitrates which are powerful eye irritants.

Ultimately, ozone is one component of smog which is harmful in itself and contributes both to the production and ultimate removal of other air pollutants.

V. Environment and Consumerism

Ecolabelling

The label indicates the ecofriendly nature of the product. Many countries like India, Germany, U.S.A., Sweden, Canada, and Japan have adopted this method. Motives behind eco-labelling are :

- To compel manufactures to make the product more environment friendly.

- To create awareness among the people about the effects of the products.
- To influence the behaviour of the consumers.

Green marketing

This aims at production and marketing in a more enviroment friendly material.

Ecomark

Eco labelling scheme called ecomark was launched by Government of India in 1991 for easy identification of environment friendly product and is repersented by an earthen pot. Objectives are as follows :

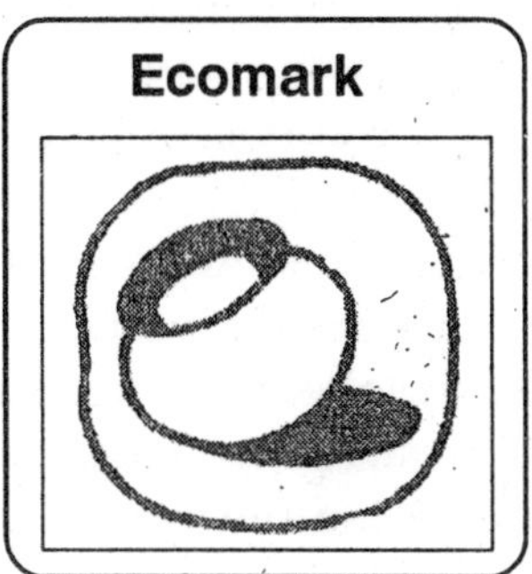

- Reduces adverse environmental impact of the products.
- It acts as a reward for companies.
- It improve the quality of the environment and promote the sustainable development.
- Encourages people to buy environment friendly products.
- Make consumer environmentally responsible.

VI. Environmental Laws in India

Laws and regulations are a major tool in protecting the environment. To put those laws into effect, government agencies create and enforce regulations.

In India even before independence (1947), several environmental legislations existed. But only after the UN Conference on the Human Environment in Stockholm 1972, the Government began to install a first well-developed framework. Under the influence of this declaration, the National Council for Environmental Policy and Planning within the Department of Science and Technology was set up in 1972. This Council evolved into the new Ministry of Environment and Forest in 1985. After the UNCED, it developed a number of strategic environmental plans, ratified the Kyoto Protocol and a number of other international treaties and paid strong attention to the implementation of Local Agenda 21.

India is signatory of many important international treaties in the field of environment, e.g. the International Convention for the regulation of Whaling, the International Plant Protection Convention, the Antarctic Treaty, the Vienna Convention for the protection of the Ozone Layer; the Basel Convention on Trans-boundary movement of hazardous substances, the Framework Convention on Climate Change; Convention on the Conservation of Biodiversity and the Montreal Protocol on the Substances that Deplete the Ozone Layer.

Following is the brief description of how laws and regulations come to be, what they are, and where to find them, with an emphasis on environmental laws and regulations. The Constitution of Indian is amongst the few in the world that contains specific provisions on environment protection.

(a) Forest Laws

- Forest Conservation Act, 1980;
- Forest (Conservation) Rules, 1981; and
- National Forest Policy, 1988.

The Forest Act is administered by forest officers who are authorized to compel the attendance of witness and the production of documents, to issue search warrants and to take evidence in an enquiry into forest offences. The Forest Act is administered by forest officers who are authorized to compel the attendance of witness and the production of documents.

(b) Laws to Protect the Wild Life

The Wildlife Act of 1972 was passed to make provision for control of wild life by formation of Wild Life Advisory Board, regulation on hunting and establishment of sanctuaries, national parks.

- The Wildlife (Transaction and Taxidermy) Rules, 1973.
- The Wildlife (Stock Declaration) Central Rules, 1973.
- The Wildlife (Protection) Licensing (Additional Matters for Consideration) Rules, 1983.
- Recognition of Zoo Rules 1992 Wild life (Protection) Rules, 1995.
- Wildlife (Specified Plants— Conditions for Possession by Licensee) Rules, 1995.
- Wildlife (Specified Plant Stock Declaration) Central Rules, 1995.

(c) Water Pollution Prevention Laws

- The Water (Prevention and Control of Pollution) Act of 1974.
- The Water (Prevention and Control of Pollution) Act, as amended up to 1988.
- The Water (Prevention and Control of Pollution) Rules, 1975.
- The Water (Prevention and Control of Pollution) (Procedure for Transaction of Business) Rules, 1975.

- The Water (Prevention and Control of Pollution) Cess Act, 1977, as amended by Amendment Act, 1991.
- The Water (Prevention and Control of Pollution) Cess Rules, 1978.

The Water Act of 1974 was the result of discussions over a decade between the Centre and States and was passed by the Parliament. The Act vests regulatory authority in the State boards and empowers these boards to establish and enforce effluent standards for factories discharging pollutants into bodies of water.

The Water Cess Act of 1977 was passed to help meet the expenses of the Central and State water boards. The Act creates economic incentives for pollution control through a differential tax structure (higher rates applicable to defaulting units) and requires local authorities and certain designated industries to pay a cess (tax) for water consumption. To encourage capital investment in the pollution control, the Act gives a polluter a 25 per cent rebate of the applicable cess upon installing effluent treatment equipment and meeting the applicable norm.

The 1988 amendment strengthened the Acts implementation provisions and a board may take decisions regarding closure of a defaulting industrial plant. The water act is comprehensive and applies to streams, inland waters, subterranean waters, sea or tidal waters. The legislation establishes a Central Pollution Control Board, and State Pollution Control Boards for Assam, Bihar, Gujarat, Haryana, Himachal Pradesh, Jammu and Kashmir, Karnataka, Kerala, Madhya Pradesh, Rajasthan, Tripura and West Bengal, as well as the Union Territories. Each Board, Central or State, consists of a chairman and five members, with agriculture, fisheries and government-owned industry all having representation.

(d) Air Prevention and Control of Pollution

- The Air (Prevention and Control of Pollution) Act of 1981.
- The Air (Prevention and Control of Pollution) Rules, 1982.
- The Air (Prevention and Control of Pollution) (Union Territories) Rules, 1983.

The Air Act of 1981, States that all industries operating within designated air pollution control areas must obtain a permit from the State Board. The States are also required to provide emission standards for industry and automobiles after consulting the Central Board.

(e) The Environmental Protection Act (EPA) of 1986

The EPA was passed to protect and improve human environment and to prevent hazards to human beings, other than plants and property. The EPA was passed to protect and improve human environment and to prevent hazards to human beings, other than plants and property. In the wake of Bhopal Gas tragedy, the Government of India enacted the Environmental (Protection) Act of 1986 (EPA) under Article 253 of the Constitution. The purpose of the Act is to implement the decisions of the United Nations Conference on Human Environment of 1972. The EPA is an umbrella legislation designed to provide a framework for Central Government coordination of the activities of various Central and State authorities established under previous laws, such as Water Act and Air Act. The scope of the EPA is broad, with "environment" defined to include water, air, land and the inter-relationships which exists among water, air and land and human beings and other living creatures, plants, micro-organisms and property. The law also promulgates rules on hazardous waste management and handling.

(f) Noise Pollution (Regulation and Control) Rules, 2000

This rule aims at controlling noise levels in public places from various sources, *interalia,* industrial activity, construction activity, generator sets, loudspeakers, public address systems, music systems, vehicular horns and other mechanical devices have deleterious effects on human health and the psychological well being of the people.

The objective of the rule is to regulate and control noise producing and generating sources with the objective of maintaining the ambient air quality standards in respect of noise.

(g) Coastal Zone

- Coastal Regulation Zone — Notification dated May 21, 2002
- Coastal Regulation Zone—Notification
- Aquaculture Authority —Notifications
- Coastal Zone Management Authority Notifications

India's lengthy coast stretches over 6,000 kilometres, supporting numerous fishing communities and driving the economies of coastal villages, towns and cities. The legislative framework for controlling marine pollution is provided by the Territorial Waters, Continental Shelf, Exclusive Economic Zone and Other Maritime Zones Act of 1976.

Development along coastal stretches is severely restricted under a regime comprising the Coastal Regulation Zone (CRZ) notification of 1991, the approved Coastal Zone Management Plans (CZMPs) for each State or region.

(h) Hazardous Substances Act

- Hazardous Wastes (Management and Handling) Rules, 1989.

- Manufacture, Storage and Import of Hazardous Chemical Rules, 1989.
- Manufacture, Use, Import, Export and Storage of Hazardous Microorganisms, Genetically Engineered Organisms or Cells Rules, 1989.
- Bio-Medical Waste (Management and Handling) Rules, 1998.
- Recycled Plastics Manufacture and Usage Rules, 1999.
- Dumping and Disposal of Fly Ash Notification.
- Hazardous Wastes (Management and Handling) Amendment Rules, 2000 — Draft Notification.
- Municipal Solid Wastes (Management and Handling) Rules, 2000.
- Batteries (Management and Handling) Rules, 2001.
- Recycled Plastics Manufacture and Usage Amendment Rules, 2002.
- Manufacture, Storage and Import of Hazardous Chemical (Amendment) Rules, 2000 — Draft Notification.
- Hazardous Wastes (Management and Handling) Amendment Rules, 2002.
- The laboratories were allowed the use of pathogenic micro organism or genetically engineered organisms or cells for the purpose of research, 2000— Draft Notification.

Hazardous substances pervade modern industrialized societies. Indian industry generates, uses, and discards toxic substances. Hazardous substances include flammables; explosives; heavy metals such as lead, arsenic and mercury; nuclear and petroleum fuel by- product; dangerous microorganism; and scores of synthetic chemical compounds like DDT and dioxins. Exposure to Toxic substances may cause acute or chronic health effects. Toxic substances are extensively regulated in India.

The first comprehensive rules to deal with one segment of the toxics problem, namely hazardous wastes, were issued by the Central Government in July, 1989. Radioactive wastes, covered under the Atomic Energy Act of 1962, and wastes discharged from ships, covered under the Merchant Shipping Act of 1958, are explicitly excluded from the Hazardous Wastes Rules.

VII. Major Environmental Treaties

(a) ASEAN Agreement on Transboundary Haze Pollution

The ASEAN Agreement on Transboundary Haze Pollution is an environmental agreement signed in 2002 between all ASEAN nations to bring haze pollution under control in South East Asia. Malaysia, Singapore, Brunei, Myanmar, Vietnam, Thailand and Laos are the parties to this agreement. Indonesia has yet to ratify the treaty, however.

(b) Antarctica Treaty

The Antarctica Treaty System (ATS) regulates international relations with respect to Antarctica. The treaty has been signed by 46 countries and set aside Antarctica as a scientific preserve, established freedom of scientific investigation. The treaty was opened for signature on December 1, 1959, and officially entered into force on June 23, 1961.

(c) Basel Convention

It is an international treaty that was designed to reduce the movements of hazardous waste between nations and specifically to prevent transfer of hazardous waste from developed countries to Less Developed Countries (LDCs) which, was opened for signature on March 22, 1989, and officially entered into force on May 05, 1992. Out of the166 parties to the convention, Afghanistan, Haiti, and the U.S.A have signed the convention, but have not yet ratified it.

(d) Convention on Biological Diversity

The Convention on biological diversity was adopted at the Earth Summit in Rio de Janeiro in 1922. The convention has three goals: 1. Conservation of biological diversity; 2. Sustainable use of its components; 3. Fair and equitable sharing of benefits arising from genetic resources.

It was opened for signature on 5 June, 1992 and entered into force on 29 December, 1993. 193 countries are the parties to the convention. The only country that has signed the convention but not ratified is USA.

(e) Convention on Long Range Transboundary Air Pollution

Its main objective is to protect he human environment against the air pollution and to gradually reduce the air pollution, including long range transboundary air pollution. It was opened for signature on 13 November, 1979 and entered into force on 16 March, 1983. 51 countries are the parties to the convention.

(f) The Convention on the Conservation of Migratory Species of Wild Animals

It is also known as Bonn convention. Its main objective is to protect terrestrial, marine and avian migratory species throughout their range. It was opened for signature on 1979 and entered into force on 1983. 100 countries are the parties to the convention.

(g) The Convention on the Prevention of Marine Pollution by Dumping of Wastes

It is commonly known as "London Convention" or "LC 72", is an agreement to control pollution of the sea by dumping and to encourage regional agreements supplementary to the convention. The convention was called for by the US Stockholm Conference on Human Environment in June 1972 and the treaty was drafted at the inter-governmental conference on the convention on the dumping of the wastes at sea (November 13, 1972, London.)

(h) ENMOD Convention

The convention on the prohibition of Military or any other hostile use of Environmental Modification Techniques (ENMOD Convention) is a 1976 international treaty prohibiting the military or other hostile use of environmental modification techniques. It was opened for signature at Geneva on 18 May, 1977 and entered into force on 5 October, 1978. There are 67 countries to the convention including India and Pakistan.

(i) Ramsar Convention

It is an international treaty for the conservation and sustainable utilization of wetlands. The convention was developed and adopted by participating nations at a meeting in Ramsar, Iran on February 2, 1971 and came into force on December 21, 1975. The headquarters is located in Gland, Switzerland.

Presently there are 153 contracting parties, grown up from 119 in 2000 and from 18 initial signatory nations in 1971.

The Ramsar List of wetlands of international importance now includes over 1,616sites (Ramsar sites) covering around 1,455,000 km^2 grown up from 1,021 sites in 2000.

(j) International Convention for Regulating of Whaling

It is an international Convention, signed in 1946 designated to make whaling sustainable. It was signed by 42 nations in Washington D.C. on December 2, 1946 and took effect on November 10, 1948.

(k) International Treaty on Plant Genetic Resources for Food and Agriculture

Also known as international seed treaty is a comprehensive international agreement in harmony with convention on biological diversity, which aim at guaranteeing food security through the conservation, exchange and sustainable use of the world's plant genetic resources for food and agriculture, as well as the fair and equitable benefit share arising from its use.

The Treaty came into force on 29th June 2004 at that time there were more than 54 ratifications by countries.

(l) Kyoto Protocol

The Kyoto Protocol to the United Nations framework convention on climate change is an amendment to the international treaty on climate change, assigned mandatory emission limitation for the reduction of their emission of carbon dioxide and five other green house gases to the signatory nations. Under the protocol industrialized countries will reduce their collective emission of greenhouse gases by 5.2 per cent compared to the year 1990. The objective of the protocol is the stabilization of greenhouse gas concentrations in the atmosphere at a level that would prevent dangerous anthrop genetic interferences with the climatic system.

The treaty was negotiated in Kyoto, Japans in December 1997, opened for signature on March 16, 1998, and closed on March 15, 1999. The agreement came into the force on 16 February, 2005, a total of 169 countries and other governmental entities have ratified the agreement. India signed and ratified the protocol in August, 2002.

(m) Montreal Protocol

The Montreal Protocol on substances that deplete the ozone layer is an international treaty designed to protect the ozone layer from depletion. The treaty was opened for signature on September 16, 1987 and entered into force on January 1, 1989.

(n) Stockholm Convention

Stockholm Convention is an international legally binding agreement on Persistent Organic Pollutants (POPs). The negotiations for the Stockholm convention on persistent organic pollutants were completed on May 23, 2001 in Stockholm, Sweden. The conventions entered into force on May 17, 2004 with ratification by an initial 128 parties and 151 signatories.

(o) Comprehensive Nuclear-Test Ban Treaty

The Comprehensive Nuclear Test Ban Treaty (CTBT) bans all nuclear explosions in all environments, for military or civil purposes. The treaty was opened for signature in New York on 24th September, 1996, when it was signed by 71 States, including five of the eight then nuclear capable States. The CTBT has now been signed by 177 States and ratified by 138. On 16 January, 2007, Moldova ratified the CTBT, completing the ratification of the treaty by all the States of the Europe.

India and Pakistan, though not nuclear weapon states as defined by the Nuclear Nonproliferation Treaty (NPT), did not sign; neither did the North Korea. India and Pakistan conducted back to back nuclear test in 1998, while North Korea withdrew from the NPT in 2003 and tested a nuclear device in 2006. Fifteen other nations have not signed.

(p) United Nations Conventions on the Law of the Sea

It is an international agreement that sets rules for the use of world's oceans. It came into force in 1994, and to date, 154 countries and the European countries have joined the convention. The USA has not.

VIII. Public Environmental Awareness

Enhancing environmental awareness is essential to harmonize patterns of individual behaviour with the requirements of environmental conservation. Awareness relates to the general public, as well as specific sections, e.g. the youth, adolescents, urban dwellers, industrial and construction workers, municipal and other public employees, etc. The Government of India as well as our Parliament is increasingly supportive of stringent environmental legislations and Regulations. Various legislations have been enacted by Indian Parliament in last about 30 years to tackle the problem of environmental protection. Various Rules and Regulations have also been framed. Despite these legislations, Rules and Regulations, protection and preservation of environment is still a pressing issue. Today, the necessity of environmental awareness and enforcement is more demanding and urgent than ever before.

Every person, organization and institution has an obligation and duty to protect it. Environmental consciousness deserves to be propagated at all levels. Environmental conservation can be achieved if we all share a single thought, the thought of creating a better world to live in, the thought to give a better deal to everyone, human or otherwise, to the present as well as to the future generation who all have to share the Almighty's great gifts of clean environment and abundant natural resources on this planet earth. Environmental protection encompasses not only pollution but also sustainable development and conservation of natural resources and the eco-system. Environmental degradation can be either localized such as the depletion of a nation's forest resources, or global, such as destruction of the ozone layer.

The environmental problems of today whether it is air and water pollution, ozone depletion, land degradation, deforestation, destruction of ecosystem or mismanagement of waste all damage our natural environment and life on earth. There is tremendous pressure on forests and unsustainable removals and threat of massive destruction and wild life habitat. Every person and institution has to play the assigned role to the best of one's capability to save India's forest and wild life.

It is necessary to stress on the relationship between destruction of environment on one hand and social as well as health problems on the other. It is especially the poor and illiterate who are most exposed to environmental pollution. It is necessary to enlighten them of the link between social and environmental problems. This realization can propel environmentalism to the top of national agenda. Who has suffered the most whether it be Bhopal Gas Tragedy or any other similar disaster? It is the poor and illiterate. It is this class which is exploited most; whether in case of illegal felling of trees or of killing of animals; vested interest mislead them or misguide them. This class has to be educated about the need to protect environment for their self-preservation as well.

❖ Methods to Propagate Environmental Awareness

➢ *Environmental Education*

Environmental education is the principal means of enhancing such awareness, both among the public at large, and among focused groups. Such education may be formal, or informal, or a combination of both. It may rely on educational institutions at different levels. Environmental education became an integral component of the National Policy on Education in 1986. It was declared that there is a need to create consciousness of the environment which must permeate all ages and all sections of the society beginning with the child. Environmental consciousness should inform teaching in schools and colleges and should be integrated in the entire education process.

➢ *Mass Media*

It can be done by medium of *Television, Radio and Print Media.* They can increase environmental awareness or even help remedying environmental problems. The communication media can play a positive role in the protection and preservation of environment. They can play an active role in alerting people about environmental damages, corporate failure to meet its legal obligations and truthful analysis of new legislations.

The emergence of the *Internet* as a source of information, with its vast reach and accessibility, has been an extremely important development.

Further, the radio has a large audience in the rural areas. Issues such as forestry, nutrition, women's health, children's rights, overall development, could occupy a top slot on a regular basis. Audio-visual media could rely on various documentaries on the environmental abuses, and facilitate awareness by interviews with environmental activists.

➢ *Stakeholders*

Companies should commit themselves to reducing their environmental impact and should create a set of environmental principles and standards and should have environmental audit. Companies should recognize that to be effective, an environmental policy needs to be adopted by employees throughout the organization, not just by those whose work is related to the environment.

Towards that end companies should engage in a variety of activities, especially education, to help employees understand the environmental impact of their jobs and to support their efforts to make positive changes. To help ensure that their products and processes are environmentally responsible, companies should buy greener products and materials from their suppliers. Products themselves may be made more environmental friendly, with regard to the control of emissions, noise, reduced health and safety risks, and reduced energy requirements.

➢ *Non Governmental Organisations (NGOs)*

The importance of Public Awareness and NGOs involvement in environmental protection is acknowledged worldwide. It was also highlighted in Rio Conference in 1992. UNCED supported NGO involvement in an unprecedented manner.

NGOs have been taking a number of steps to promote discussion and debate about environmental issues, outside the broad spheres of popular media and the educational system. Advocacy and awareness is especially crucial in promoting concepts such as sustainable development, natural resource conservation and the restoration of ecosystems. NGOs can sensitize policy makers about the local needs and priorities. They can often intimate the policy makers about the interests of both the poor and the ecosystem as a whole.

In providing training facilities, both at community and government levels, NGOs can play a significant role. They can also contribute significantly by undertaking research and publication on environment and development related issues. It is necessary to support and encourage genuine, small, local level NGOs in different parts of the country which can provide much needed institutional support specific to the local needs.

The "Chipko Movement" for conservation of trees by Dasholi Gram Swarajya Mandal in Gopeshwar or the "Narmada Bachao Andolan" organized by Kalpavriksh, are some of the instances where NGOs have played a landmark role in the society for conservation of environment.

Finally, it is necessary to emphasise that problem of environmental degradation can be tackled only by concerted efforts by every person, organization and institution and by extremely stringent enforcement of the laws. We have to educate, spread awareness, involve and motivate every child, woman and man in the country to conserve the local flora and fauna, soil and water resources and all other gifts of God which are national properties and belong to all and to none individually.

Questions

Long answer type of questions

1. What do you mean by Sustainable Development? Write down its scope.
2. Aspects of a National Sustainable Development Strategy.
3. Discuss the causes and effects of Global warming.
4. What are the causes and consequences of acid rain?
5. What is Ozone? Write down its applications.
6. Discuss the Environmental Laws in India.
7. What are the Water Pollution Prevention Laws.
8. Discuss Hazardous Substances Act.

Write short notes on the following:

1. Environmental Sustainability
2. Ecolabelling
3. Ecomark
4. Air (Prevention and Control of Pollution) Act
5. Water (Prevention and Control of Pollution) Act
6. Wild Life Protection Act
7. Forest Conservation Act

Fill in the blanks

1. Sustainable development is defined as balancing the fulfilment of human needs with the protection of the natural.......................
2. The Planning Commission of India (PCI) is responsible for making the..............
3. Water vapour, causes about..............of the greenhouse effect on Earth
4. The atmospheric concentrations of carbon dioxide have increased by ....per cent above pre-industrial levels since 1750.
5. The world's primary international agreement on combating global warming is the.................
6. Ozone (O_3) is a triatomic molecule, consisting of three.................. atoms.
7. The Forest Act is administered by ....

Keys : 1. environment; 2. Five Year Plans; 3. 36-70 per cent; 4. 31 5. Kyoto Protocol; 6. oxygen; 7. forest officers.

Tick the right answer

1. India presented its perspective on sustainable development before the World Summit for Sustainable Development (WSSD) in

(a) 2005
(b) 1995
(c) 2000
(d) 2002

2. UN Conference on the Human Environment was held in
(a) Stockholm
(b) New Delhi
(c) Paris
(d) Japan
3. The concept of sustainable development was cast into a law, the Biological Diversity Act, for the first time in
(a) 1999
(b) 1991
(c) 2002
(d) 2006
4. Relative to the period 1860–1900, global temperatures on both land and sea have increased by
(a) 2.75° C
(b) 1.95° C
(c) 0.25° C
(d) 0.75° C
5. Ozone was discovered by Christian Friedrich Schonbein in
(a) 1940
(b) 1740
(c) 1840
(d) 1951
6. The highest levels of ozone in the atmosphere are in the
(a) Stratosphere
(b) Troposphere
(c) Mesosphere
(d) Ionosphere
7. India's sea coast stretches over
(a) 3,000 kilometres
(b) 6,000 kilometres
(c) 9,000 kilometres
(d) 4,000 kilometres

Keys : 1. d, 2. a, 3. c, 4. d, 5. c, 6. a, 7. b.

True / False types of questions

1. *India's* GHG emissions in 1994 was 1228 million tonne CO equivalent, which is below 3 per cent of global GHG emissions.

2. Ground level ozone is an air pollutant with harmful effects on lung function and in the upper atmosphere it prevents damaging ultraviolet light from reaching the Earth's surface.
3. Ozone is directly emitted by car engines or by industrial operations.
4. Ozone can be used for bleaching substances and for killing bacteria.
5. The Wildlife Act of 1972 was passed to make provision for control of wild-life by formation of Wildlife Advisory Board.
6. Narmada Bachao Andolan organized by Kalpavriksh.
7. Environmental education became an integral component of the National Policy on Education in 1986.

   Keys : 1. true, 2. true, 3. false, 4. true, 5. true, 6. true, 7. true.

Unit - 7

Human Population and Environment

Population is the collection of people living in a given geographic area or space, usually measured by a census.

According to estimates published by the United States Census Bureau, the world population hit 6.5 billion (6,500,000,000) on February 25, 2005. On October 18, 2012, the Earth will be home to 7 billion. The United Nations Population Fund designated October 12, 1999 as the approximate day on which world population reached six billion. This was about 12 years after world population reached five billion, in 1987.

I. Population Growth

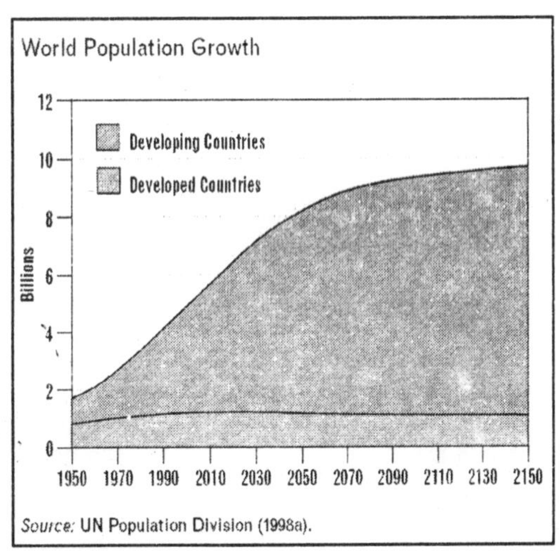

Source: UN Population Division (1998a).

Population growth is change in population over time. It also can be quantified as the change in the number of individuals in a population per unit time.

Population growth stresses resources because it contributes to increases in both consumption and conversion. Each year, the human population grows by approximately 80 million. Although global fertility rates decreased since the 1950s from 5.0 to 2.7 births per woman, the population will continue to grow. Past high fertility rates created today's pool of more than 1.5 billion people at the prime reproductive age between 15 and 29 years old; another 1.9 billion are younger than 15. An adjunct to population growth is the significant decrease in mortality. Since the 1950s the global mortality rate has dropped from about 20 to fewer than 10 deaths per year per 1,000 people. In contrast, the seven African countries hardest hit by the AIDS epidemic have actually experienced a decrease in life expectancy because of the high number of deaths caused by the disease (UN Population Division 1998a).

India : Population Density/Growth

Year	1901	1911	1921	1931	1941	1951	1961	1971	1981	1991	2001
Density	77	82	81	90	103	117	142	177	216	267	324
Growth	23.83	25.20	25.12	27.89	31.86	36.10	43.92	54.79	68.33	84.33	102.7

India : Population—2001

India/States/Union Territories	Population	Pop. Rank	Density (Person/ km^2)	Literacy	Area km^2
INDIA	**1,027,015,247**	—	**324**	**65.38**	**3,166,414**
Jammu & Kashmir	10,069,917	19	99	54.46	101,387
Himachal Pradesh	6,077,248	21	109	77.13	55,673
Punjab	24,289,296	15	482	69.95	50,362
Chandigarh	900,914	29	7,903	81.76	114
Uttaranchal	8,479,562	20	159	72.28	53,483
Haryana	21,082,989	16	477	68.59	44,212
Delhi	13,782,976	18	9,294	81.82	1,483
Rajasthan	56,473,122	8	165	61.03	342,239
Uttar Pradesh	166,052,859	1	689	57.36	240,928
Bihar	82,878,796	3	880	47.53	94,163
Sikkim	540,493	31	76	69.68	7,096
Arunachal Pradesh	1,091,117	27	13	54.74	83,743
Nagaland	1,988,636	25	120	67.11	16,579
Manipur	2,388,634	23	107	68.87	22,327
Mizoram	891,058	30	42	88.49	21,081
Tripura	3,191,168	22	304	73.66	10,486
Meghalaya	2,306,069	24	103	63.31	22,429
Assam	26,638,407	14	340	64.28	78,438
West Bengal	80,221,171	4	904	69.22	88,752
Jharkhand	26,909,428	13	338	54.13	79,714
Orissa	36,706,920	11	236	63.61	155,707
Chhattisgarh	20,795,956	17	154	65.18	135,191
Madhya Pradesh	60,385,118	7	196	64.11	308,245
Gujarat	50,596,992	—	258	69.97	196,022
Daman & Diu	158,059	34	1,411	81.09	112
D & Nagar Haveli	220,451	33	449	60.03	491
Maharashtra	96,752,247	2	314	77.27	307,713
Andhra Pradesh	75,727,541	5	275	61.11	275,069
Karnataka	52,733,958	9	275	67.04	191,791
Goa	1,343,998	26	363	82.32	3,702
Lakshadweep	60,595	35	1,894	87.52	32
Kerala	31,838,619	12	819	90.92	38,863
Tamil Nadu	62,110,839	6	478	73.47	130,058
Pondicherry	973,829	28	2,029	81.49	480
Andaman & Nicobar Islands	356,265	32	43	81.18	8,249

Source: Census Report, Government of India, 2001.

Growth is fastest in less developed nations, where populations are most dependent on ecosystems for a subsistence living. Demographers expect 97 per cent of all population growth in the next 5 decades to occur in developing countries.

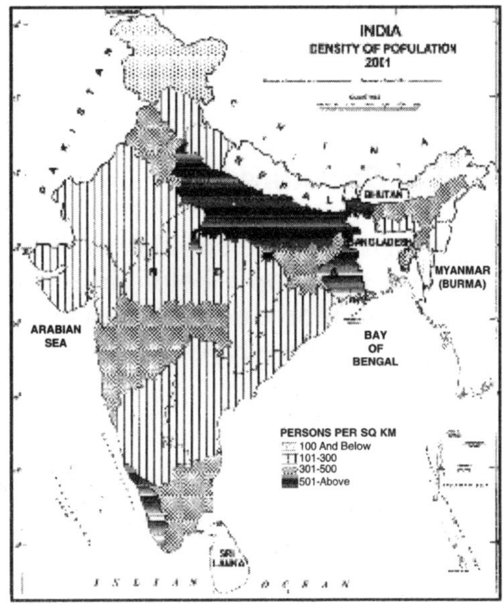

As the population grows in the next quarter century, pressures will increase, especially in countries where arable land is in short supply. In 14 countries, arable land per capita is expected to be less than 0.07 ha, equivalent to an area about 0.25 km^2, to sustain each human life (WHO 1997:59). Richer countries may supplement their food resources with imports, but poorer countries will have a more difficult time following such a strategy to feed their hungry populations.

II. Population Characteristics and Variations among Nations

The population of any place could not be studied only with the number of people. There are also other features as follows :

(a) Exponential Growth

When a quantity increases by a fixed percentage it is known as exponential growth e.g. 10, 10^2, 10^3, 10^4 or 2, 4, 8, 16, 32, etc. Population growth takes place exponentially and that explains the dramatic increase in world population in the last century.

(b) Doubling Time

The time needed for a population to double its size at a constant annual rate is known as doubling time. It is calculated as follows :

$$Td = 70/r \quad \text{(Where Td = Doubling time in a year, r = annual growth rate)}$$

If a nation has 2 per cent annual growth rate, its population will double in 35 years.

(c) Total Fertility Rate (TFR)

It indicates the population growth of a nation. It is defined as the average number of children that would be born to a woman in her life time if the age specific birth rates remain constant. The value of TFR varies from 1.9 in developed nations to 4.7 in developing nations. Comprehensive development decreases the TFR.

(d) Infant Mortality Rate

It indicates the future growth of a population. It is the percentage of infants died out of those born in a year.

(e) Age Structure

Age structure of the population of a nation can be represented by age pyramids, based on the people belonging to different age classes like pre-reproductive (0-14 years), reproductive (15 - 44 years), Post- reproductive (45 years and above).

There are three types of age pyramids.

➤ *Pyramid Shaped*

In such type of shape the young population is more, making a broad base and old people are less. India, Pakistan, Bangladesh, Nigeria are examples of this type. The large number of individuals in very young age will soon enter into reproductive age, thus causing an increase in the population.

➤ *Bell Shaped*

People of age group 0 - 35 years almost remain in equal number. Consequently, in the next ten years, the people entering into reproductive age are not going to change much and such type of pyramid indicates stable population. It occurs in the countries like USA, France and Canada.

➤ *Urn Shaped*

Here number of individuals in very young class is smaller than the middle reproductive age class. Consequently, in the next 10 years the number in reproductive age class will thus become less than before resulting decline in the population growth. Germany, Italy, Hungary, Sweden and Japan are examples of this type.

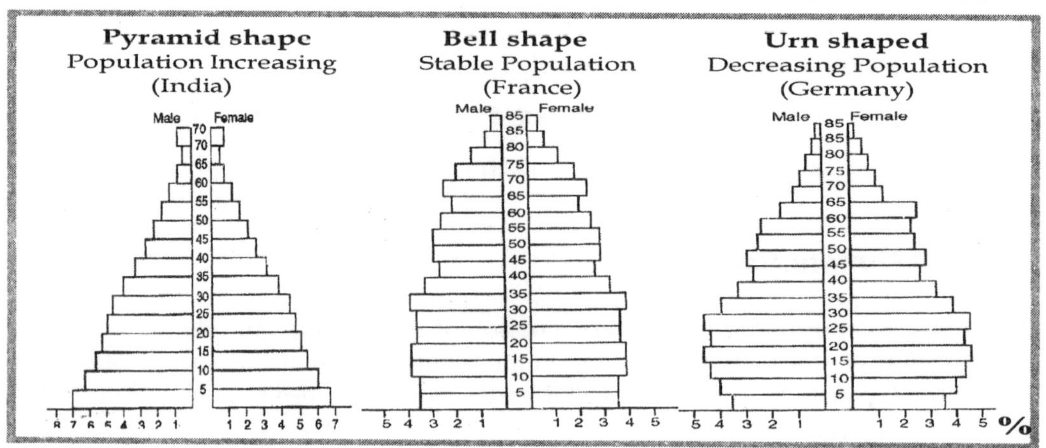

(f) Zero Population Growth (ZPG)

When birth plus immigration in a population are just equal to death plus emigration, it is said to be zero population growth.

(g) Life Expectancy

It is the average age that a new born infant is expected to attain in a given country. The average life expectancy, over the world, has risen from 40 to 65.5 years over the past century. In India, life expectancy of male and female was only 22.6 years and 23.3 years, respectively in 1900. In the last 100 years improved medical facilities and technological advances has increased the life expectancy to 60.3 years and 60.5 years, respectively for the Indian males and females. In Japan and Sweden, life expectancy is quite higher, being 82.1—84.2 for females and 77—77.4 for males.

(h) Urbanization

In both more and less developed nations, cities are drawing people into ever greater concentrations. Urban regions tend to offer more opportunities for economic development as well as better education and health resources.

Although urban areas occupy only about 4 percent of the Earth's land area, they are home to nearly half the world's population.

Currently cities are expansive consumers of ecosystem goods and services and prolific generators of ecosystem-damaging wastes—essentially concentrated centres of ecosystem pressures. By 2030, more than 60 per cent of all people are likely to be living in urban areas. In industrial countries and Latin America, the share is expected to exceed 80 per cent (UN Population Division 1998a).

Top 15 Urban Agglomeration of the World Estimates for mid-2005

Rank	*City*	*Population (millions)*	*Country*	*Area (km²)*
1.	Tokyo	35.19	Japan	13,500
2.	Mexico City	19.41	Mexico	7,815
3.	New York-Newark	18.71	U.S.A.	8,680
4.	Sao Paulo	18.33	Brazil	8,050
5.	Mumbai	18.19	India	4,360
6.	Delhi	15.04	India	1,480
7.	Shanghai	14.50	China	3,920
8.	Kolkata	14.27	India	1,780
9.	Jakarta	13.21	Indonesia	1,360
10.	Buenos Aires	12.55	Argentina	3,680
11.	Dhaka	12.43	Bangladesh	1,600
12.	Los Angeles-Long Beach-Santa Ana	12.29	U.S.A.	4,320
13.	Karachi	11.60	Pakistan	3,530
14.	Rio de Janeiro	11.46	Brazil	5,000
15.	Osaka-Kobe	11.26	Japan	2,070

Source : Statistics Division, U.N.O, 2005.

Box—India's Human Development Indicators

- Infant mortality — 72 per thousand live births
- Literacy rates — 65.2%
- Households with access to safe drinking water — 62.3%
- Households with access to proper sanitation facilities — 49.32%
- Households with electricity connection — 42.37%
- Households with electricity, safe drinking water and proper sanitation facilities — 16.1%
- Households with permanent houses — 41.61%
- Households with semi-permanent houses — 30.95%
- Households with temporary shelters — 27.44%

Source: MoEF (2002)

(i) Demographic Transition

In demography, the term *demographic transition* is a theory describing a possible transition from high birth rates and death rates to low birth and death rates as part of the economic development of a country from a pre-industrial to an industrialized economy. Usually it is described through the "Demographic Transition Model" *(DTM)* that describes the population changes over time. It is based on an interpretation begin in 1929 by the American demographer Warren Thompson of prior observed changes, or transitions, in birth and death rates in industrialized societies over the past two hundred years.

Demographic Transition Model

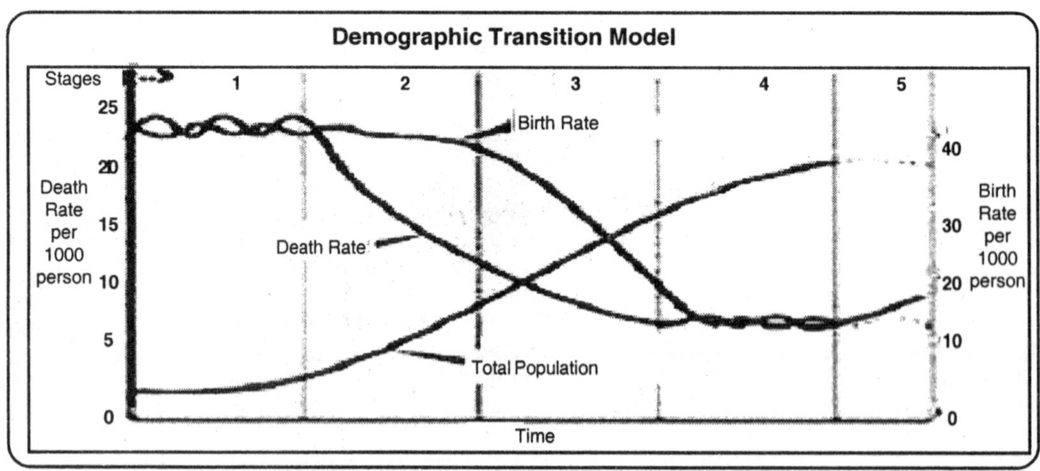

In *stage one*, pre-industrial society, death rates and birth rates are high and roughly in balance.

In *stage two*, that of a developing country, the death rates drop rapidly due to improvements in food supply and sanitation, which increase life spans and reduce disease. These changes usually come about due to improvements in farming techniques, access to technology, basic healthcare, and education. Without a corresponding fall in birth rates this produces an imbalance, and the countries in this stage experience a large increase in population. Countries in this stage include Yemen, Afghanistan, Palestine, Bhutan and Laos and much of Sub-Saharan Africa.

In *stage three* birth rates fall due to access to contraception, increases in wages, urbanization, a reduction in subsistence agriculture, an increase in the status and education of women, a reduction in the value of children's work, an increase in parental investment in the education of children and other social changes. Population growth begins to level off.

Countries that have experienced a fertility decline of over 40 per cent from their pre-transition levels include: Costa Rica, El Salvador, Panama, Jamaica, Mexico, Colombia, Ecuador, Guyana, Surinam, Philippines, Indonesia, Malaysia, Sri Lanka, Turkey, Azerbaijan, Turkmenistan, Uzbekistan, Egypt, Tunisia, Algeria, Morocco, Lebanon, South Africa and many Pacific islands.

Countries that have experienced a fertility decline of 25-40 per cent include: Honduras, Guatemala, Nicaragua, Paraguay, Bolivia, Vietnam, Myanmar, India, Bangladesh, Tajikistan, Iran, Jordan, Qatar, United Arab Emirates, Zimbabwe and Botswana.

Countries that have experienced a fertility decline of 10-25 per cent include Nepal, Pakistan, Syria, Iraq, Saudi Arabia, Libya, Sudan, Kenya, Ghana and Senegal.

During *stage four* there are both low birth rates and low death rates. Birth rates may drop to well below replacement level as has happened in countries like Italy, Spain and Japan, leading to a shrinking population, a threat to many industries that rely on population growth. The large group born during stage two ages and creates an economic burden on the shrinking working population. Death rates may remain consistently low or increase slightly due to increases in lifestyle diseases due to low exercise levels and high obesity and an ageing population in developed countries.

Countries that are at this stage (Total Fertility Rate of less than 2.5 in 1997) include: United States, Canada, Australia, New Zealand, most of Europe, Bahamas, Puerto Rico, Trinidad and Tobago, Brazil, Sri Lanka, South Korea, Singapore, China, North Korea, Thailand and Mauritius.

Fifth stage: The original Demographic Transition model has just four stages, but it is now widely accepted that a fifth stage is needed to represent countries that have undergone the economic transition from manufacturing based industries into service and information based industries called deindustrialization. Countries such as Germany, Italy, Spain, Portugal, Greece and most notably Japan, whose populations are now reproducing well below their replacement levels, that is they are not producing enough children to replace their parent's generation. China, South Korea, Singapore, Thailand and Cuba are also below replacement, but this is not producing a fall in population yet in these countries, because their populations are relatively young due to strong growth in the recent past.

The population of southern Europe is already falling and Japan and some of western Europe will soon begin to fall without significant immigration. However, many countries that now have sub-replacement fertility did not reach this stage gradually but rather suddenly as a result of economic crisis brought on by the post-Communist transition in the late 1980's and the 1990's. Examples include Russia, Ukraine, and the Baltic states. The population of these countries is falling due to fertility decline, emigration and, particularly in Russia, increased male mortality.

III. Overpopulation/Population Explosion

The problem of overpopulation is worlwide, India also has enormous problems with overpopulation. The current population is over a billion, but India does not have the large land mass that China has. Overpopulation has had a major impact on the environment of Earth starting at least as early as the twentieth century. Many posit that the human population has expanded, enabled by over-exploiting natural resources, with resultant adverse impacts upon biodiversity, aquifer sustainability, climate change and even human health.

Some problems associated with human overpopulation are as follows :

1. Inadequate fresh water for drinking and other use as well as sewage treatment and effluent discharge.
2. Depletion of natural resources, especially fossil fuels.
3. Increased levels of air pollution, water pollution, soil contamination and noise pollution.
4. Deforestation and loss of ecosystems that sustain global atmospheric oxygen and carbon dioxide balance; about eight million hectares of forest are lost each year.
5. Changes in atmospheric composition and consequent global warming.
6. Irreversible loss of arable land and increases in desertification, Deforestation and desertification can be reversed by adopting property rights, and this policy is successful even while the human population continues to grow.
7. Mass species extinctions from reduced habitat in tropical forests is due to slash-and-burn techniques that sometimes are practiced by shifting cultivators, especially in countries with rapidly expanding rural populations; present extinction rates may be as high as 140,000 species lost per year. The IUCN Red List lists a total of 698 animal species having gone extinct during recorded human history.

8. High infant and child mortality. High rates of infant mortaltity are caused by poverty.
9. Increased incidence of hemorrhagic fevers and other infectious diseases from crowding, lack of adequate sanitation and clean potable water, and scarcity of available medical resources.
10. Starvation, malnutrition or poor diet with ill health and diet-deficiency diseases (e.g. rickets). Famine is aggravated by poverty.
11. Poverty coupled with inflation in some regions and a resulting low level of capital formation. Low birth rate due to the inability of mothers to get enough resources to sustain a foetus from fertilization to birth.
12. Low life expectancy in countries with fastest growing populations.
13. Unhygienic living conditions for many based upon water resource depletion, discharge of raw sewage and solid waste disposal.
14. Elevated crime rate due to drug cartels and increased theft by people stealing resources to survive.
15. Conflict over scarce resources and crowding, leading to increased levels of warfare.
16. Over-utilization of infrastructure, such as mass transit, highways, and public health systems.
17. Higher land prices

(a) Increasing Human Consumptions

Humans consume goods and services for many reasons: to nourish, clothe, and shelter, certainly. But we also consume as part of a social compact, since each community or social group has standards of dress, food, shelter, education, and entertainment that influence its patterns of consumption beyond physical survival.

Consumption is a tool for human development that opens opportunities for a healthy and satisfying life, with adequate nutrition, employment, mobility, and education. Poverty is marked by a lack of consumption, and thus a lack of these opportunities. At the other extreme, wealth can and often does lead to excessive levels of material and non-material consumption. In spite of its human benefits, consumption can lead to serious pressure on ecosystems. Consumption harms ecosystems directly through overharvesting of animals or plants, mining of soil nutrients, or other forms of biological depletion. Ecosystems suffer indirectly through pollution and wastes from agriculture, industry, and energy use, and also through fragmentation by roads and other infrastructure that are part of the production and transportation networks that feed consumers.

Consumption of the major commodities ecosystems produce directly grains, meat, fish, and wood increased substantially in the last four decades and will continue to do so as the global economy expands and world population grows.

Plausible projections of consumer demand in the next few decades suggest a marked escalation of impacts on ecosystems.

- World cereal consumption has more than doubled in the last 30 years, and meat consumption has tripled since. Some 34 percent of the world's grain crop is used to feed livestock raised for meat. A crucial factor in the rise in grain production has been more than fourfold increase in fertilizer use since. By 2020, demand for cereals is expected to increase nearly 40 percent, and meat demand will surge nearly 60 per cent.
- The global fish catch has grown more than six fold since 1950 to 122 million metric tonnes in 1997. Three fourths of the global catch is consumed directly by humans as fresh, frozen, dried, or canned fish and shellfish. The remaining 25 per cent is reduced to fish meal and oil, which is used for both livestock feed and fish feed in aquaculture. Demand for fish for direct consumption is expected to grow some 20 per cent by 2010.

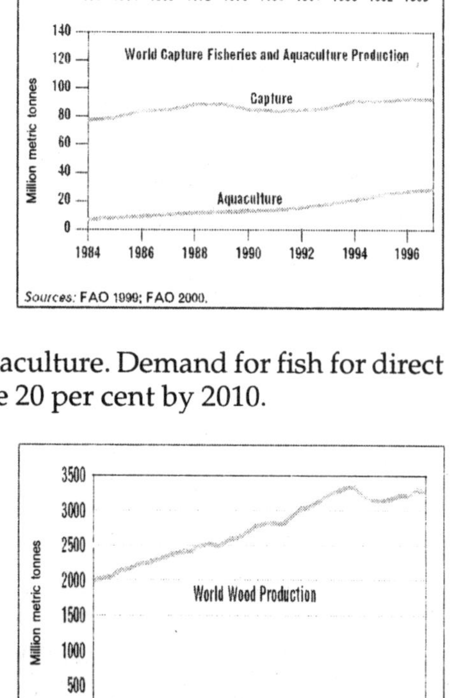

Sources: FAO 1999; FAO 2000.

- Global wood consumption has increased 64 per cent since 1961. More than half of the 3.4 billion m^3 of wood consumed annually is burned for fuel; the rest is used in construction and for paper and a variety of other wood products. Demand for lumber and pulp is expected to rise between 20 and 40 per cent by 2010. Forest plantations produce 22 percent of all lumber, pulp, and other industrial wood; old-growth and secondary growth forests provide the rest.

(b) Future Food Problems

The United Nations indicates that about 850 million people are malnourished or starving, and 1.1 billion people do not have access to safe drinking water. Thus some argue that the Earth may support 6 billion people, but only on the condition that many live in misery.

Water deficits, which are already spurring heavy grain imports in numerous smaller countries, may soon do the same in larger countries, such as China or India. The water tables are falling in scores of countries (including Northern China, the US, and India) due to widespread overpumping using powerful diesel and electric pumps. Other countries affected include Pakistan, Iran, and Mexico. This will eventually lead to water scarcity and cutbacks in grain harvest. Even with the overpumping of its aquifers, China is developing a grain deficit. When this happens, it will almost certainly drive grain prices upward. Most of the 3 billion people projected to be added worldwide by mid-century will be born in countries already experiencing water shortages. Unless population growth can be slowed quickly by investing heavily in female literacy and family planning services, there may not be a humane solution to the emerging world food shortage.

After China and India, there is a second tier of smaller countries with large water deficits — Algeria, Egypt, Iran, Mexico, and Pakistan. Four of these already import a large share of their grain. Only Pakistan remains self-sufficient. But with a population expanding by 4 million a year, it will also likely soon turn to the world market for grain.

Hunger and malnutrition kill nearly 6 million children a year, and more people are malnourished in sub-Saharan Africa this decade than in the 1990s, according to a report released by the Food and Agriculture Organization.

According to a 2007 article form the BBC, scientists at Columbia University have theorized that in the future, densely populated cities such as New York City may use vertical farming to grow food on each floor of 30 storey skyscrapers.

CASE STUDY

Population as a Function of Food Availability

Growth in food production has been greater than population growth. Food per person increased during the 1961-2005 period.

The amounts of natural resources in this context are not necessarily fixed, and their distribution is not necessarily a zero-sum game. For example, due to the green revolution and the fact that more and more land is appropriated each year from wild lands for agricultural purposes, the worldwide production of food has steadily increased faster than population growth. World food production per person was considerably higher in 2005 than 1961.

As world population doubled from 3 billion to 6 billion, daily calorie consumption in poor countries increased form 1,932 to 2,650, and the percentage of people in those countries who were malnourished fell from 45 per cent to 18 per cent. This suggests that third world poverty and famine are caused by underdevelopment, not overpopulation. However others question this kind of Data.

Worldwide, the number of people who are overweight has surpassed the number who are malnourished. In a 2006 news story, MSNBC reported, "There are an estimated 800 million undernourished people and more than a billion considered overweight worldwide."

Thinkers such as David Pimentel, a Professor from Cornell University, Virginia

Abernethy, Alan Thornhill, Russell Hopffenberg and author Daniel Quinn propose that like any animals, human populations predictably grow and shrink according to their available food supply – populations grow in an abundance of food, and shrink in times of scarcity.
Proponents of this theory argue that every time food production is increased, the population grows. Some human populations throughout history support this theory. Populations of hunter-gatherers fluctuate in accordance with the amount of available food. Population increased after the Neolithic Revolution and an increased food supply. This was followed by subsequent population growth after subsequent agricultural revolutions.
Critics of this idea point out that birth rates are lowest in the developed nations, which also has the highest access to food. In fact, some developed countries have both a diminishing population and an abundant food supply. The United Nations projects that the population of 51 countries or areas, including Germany, Italy, Japan and most of the successor States of the former Soviet Union, is expected to be lower in 2050 than in 2005. This shows that human populations do not always grow to match the available food supply; also, many of these countries are major exporters of food.

IV. Family Welfare Programmes

India is the first country in the world to formulate a National Family Planning Programme in 1952. The objective of the policy was *"reducing birth rate to the extent necessary to stabilize the population at a level consistent with requirement of national economy"*.

The First Five-Year Plan Stated that "the main appeal for family planning is based on considerations of health and welfare of the family. Family limitation or spacing of children is necessary and desirable in order to secure better health for the mother and better care and upbringing of children. Measures directed to this end should, therefore, form part of the public health programme".

(a) Evolution of India's Family Welfare Programme

The 1950s

At the time of Independence, health care services were predominantly urban, hospital based and curative. The majority of the population, especially those belonging to the poorer sections and those residing in rural areas, did not have access to health care, as a result of which morbidity and mortality rates among them were quite high. Many women died while seeking illegal induced abortion to get rid of unwanted pregnancy because they did not have access to contraceptive methods.

Thus, in the 1950s, good quality integrated maternal and child health care, and family planning services were available to those who were aware, had access and could afford the services of physicians. There were efforts to improve coverage and extend the services to rural areas as a part of the Block development programme. However, resource and manpower constraints were responsible for the slow progress on this front.

The 1960s

In the 1960s, safe, effective vaccines for the prevention of six childhood diseases and effective contraceptives for birth spacing such as Lippe's loop became available. In order to make these available to people, effective programmes for delivery of identified priority services were drawn up by professionals and implemented through the limited health care infrastructure available in rural areas and supplemented by camps.

The 1961 census showed a rising decadal population growth rate due to declining death rates and unchanged birth rates. The health infrastructure is still predominantly urban-based. During the 1960s, sterilization remained the focus of the National Family Planning Programme. Efforts were made to popularize vasectomy and to provide services in rural areas through camps. Tubectomy services, however, remained predominantly in urban hospitals.

1970s

The 1970s witnessed many initiatives to improve the health and nutritional status of women and children. The Massive Dose Vitamin A programme, the National Anemia Prophylaxis Programme and food supplementation to pregnant and lactating women and pre-school children through the Integrated Child Development Services (ICDS) programme were major initiatives to tackle micronutrient deficiencies and under-nutrition and its adverse consequences in women and children. With the improvement in primary health care infrastructure, access to health care improved. Sterilization, especially vasectomy services were made widely available. Intra-Uterine Devices (IUD) and condoms were made available through the PHCs. The hospital based postpartum programme provided contraceptive care to women coming for delivery.

The Medical Termination of Pregnancy (MTP) Act, 1972, enabled women with unwanted pregnancy to seek and obtain safe abortion services.

The massive sterilization drive of 1976 did result in eight million persons undergoing sterilization, but this did not have any perceptible impact on the birth rate, as the cases were not appropriately chosen.

There was a steep fall in acceptance in the very next year. In 1978, the Expanded Programme of Immunization was initiated to improve coverage for the six vaccine preventable diseases. In 1979, the Programme was renamed as the National Family

Welfare Programme and increasing integration of family planning services with those of maternal and child health and nutrition was attempted.

The 1980s

The major thrust during the 1980s was to operationalise the WHO's Alma Ata declaration of Health for All by 2000 A.D. (1978) by establishing a network of centres in urban and rural areas to provide essential primary health care. The network of post partum centres was expanded to improve access to family welfare services. In 1983, the National Health Policy was formulated and provided comprehensive framework for planning, implementation and monitoring of health care services. The Universal Immunization Programme (UIP), started in 30 districts in 1986, was extended to cover 448 districts by the end of the Seventh Plan.

The 1990s

The 1991 Census showed that India was entering the opportunity window in demographic transition, when larger proportion of the population is in the age group of 20-40 years, when it will be possible to achieve a rapid decline in fertility and mortality.

During the Eighth Plan, efforts were made under the Child Survival and Safe Motherhood initiative and the Social Safety Net programme to improve the access to maternal and child health services.

In view of the massive inter-State and intra-State differences in access to services and health indices, the Department of Family Welfare abolished the practice of setting centrally defined, method-specific targets for contraception. It was replaced by decentralized area-specific need assessment (community needs assessment approach), planning and implementing programmes aimed at fulfilling these needs.

In 1997, the Department of Family Welfare initiated the Reproductive and Child Health (RCH) programme aimed at providing integrated health and family welfare services to meet health care needs of women and children.

The components of the comprehensive RCH care are indicated as follows :

- Effective maternal and child health care.
- Increased access to contraceptive care.
- Safe management of unwanted pregnancies.
- Nutritional services to vulnerable groups.
- Prevention and treatment of RTI/ STD.
- Reproductive health services for adolescents.
- Prevention and treatment of gynecological problems.
- Screening and treatment of cancers, especially uterine, cervical and breast cancer.

These services are available in secondary and tertiary care centres in the country. Efforts are being made to improve the content, quality and coverage of care.

(b) National Population Policy and Family Welfare

The immediate objective of the National Population Policy is to meet all the unmet needs for contraception and health care for women and children. The medium-term objective is to bring the TFR to replacement level (TFR of 2.1) by 2010 and, the long-term objective is to achieve population stabilization by 2045. The Policy has set the following goals for 2010 :

- Universal access to quality contraceptive services in order to lower the TFR to 2.1 by adopting the small family norm;
- Universal registration of births and deaths, marriages and pregnancies;
- Universal access to information/counselling and services for fertility regulation and contraception with a wide basket of choices;
- To reduce the IMR to below 30 per 1,000 live births and a sharp reduction in the incidence of low birth weight (below 2.5 kg.);
- Universal immunization of children against vaccine preventable diseases;
- Promote delayed marriage for girls, not earlier than the age of 18 and preferably after 20 years;
- Achieve 80 per cent institutional deliveries and increase the percentage of deliveries conducted by trained persons to 100 per cent;
- Reduction in MMR to less than 100 per 100,000 live births;
- Universalisation of primary education and reduction in the drop-out rates at the primary and secondary levels to below 20 per cent for both boys and girls.

Several States/districts have demonstrated that the steep reduction in mortality and fertility envisaged in the National Population Policy are technically feasible within the existing infrastructure and manpower. All efforts are being made to provide essential supplies, improve efficiency and ensure accountability – especially in the States where performance is currently suboptimal—so that there is incremental improvement in performance. An Empowered Action Group attached to the Ministry of Health and Family Welfare has been constituted in 2001 to facilitate capacity building in poorly performing States/districts so that they attain the goals set in the Policy. If all these efforts are vigorously pursued it is possible that the ambitious goals set for 2007/2010 may be achieved.

One Child Policy of China

China's present population is approximately 1.2 billion, which is about one fifth of the earth's entire population. China has to feed 22% of the world's people on 7% of the world's arable land, which is a considerable task. Therefore, it is to China's interest as well as the world's that some form of population control is implemented. Although today the urban population density per square kilometre is about 360, China was not always such a major chunk of the world population. In 1949, the population on the mainland was a lot less—about 541.67 million people. However, due to improvements in living standards, by 1969 the population was 806.71 million. The birth rate then was very high—about 34.11 per thousand. The family planning programme had begun already, but due to a lack of understanding about the seriousness of the problem and a lack of a clear policy, there were no major effects. It was not until after the peak birth period, 1962-1972, that a stronger programme was made to control the ever increasing population. That programme is basically what is followed today.

One child policy is not really a one child per person sort of policy at all. Family planning advocates delayed marriage and child bearing, fewer and healthier births, and one child per couple in the extremely urbanized areas, such as Beijing and Shanghai. A couple in agricultural and pastoral areas may have a second child, and an even more flexible policy is held for farmers and herdsmen with difficulties such as a shortage of labour power. In such areas that are inhabited by a small population of ethnic minorities, there are no restrictions at all. There are also no specific requirements in Tibet for family planning. So in reality, the "one child policy" really applies to only the already densely populated coastal areas.

(c) Child Welfare

Infant and under-five mortality rates are excellent indicators of the health status of children. In India there is no system for collection and analysis of data on morbidity during childhood. In the absence of this, available mortality data and analysis of causes of death have been utilized for drawing up priority interventions for improving child health.

Components of child health care include :

- Essential newborn care;
- Immunisation;
- Nutrition :
  - Exclusive breast-feeding for six months;
  - Timely introduction of complementary feeding;
  - Detection and management of growth faltering;
  - Massive dose Vitamin-A supplementation; and
  - Iron supplementation, if needed.

- Early detection and appropriate management of :
  - Acute respiratory infections;
  - Diarrhoea; and
  - Other infections.

Essential New Born Care

India has the dubious distinction of having a very high prevalence of low birth weight. Currently nation-wide data on birth weight in different States and districts is not available because a majority of births occur at home and these infants are not weighed soon after birth. Estimates based on available data from institutional deliveries and smaller community- based studies suggest that nearly one-third of all Indian infants weigh less than 2.5 kg at birth. There are differences between States and between economic groups, with incidence of low birth rate being the highest among the low income groups. There has hardly been any change in birth weight trends in the past three decades. A gender difference has been noted in mean birth weights, with female infants tending weight lesser than male infants.

Birth weight is influenced by the nutritional and health status of the mother. Some factors, which have significant influence on birth weight, such as the parent's build, are not amenable to short term corrective interventions.

Immunisation

The Universal immunization programme which was taken up in 1986 as a National Technology Mission, became a part of the Child Survival and Safe Motherhood (CSSM) programme in 1992 and the RCH programme in 1997. Under the programme, infants are immunised against tuberculosis, diphtheria, pertussis, poliomyelitis, measles and tetanus.

There has not been any decline in the immunisation coverage in the 1990s. However, none of the States have achieved coverage levels of over 80 per cent; coverage level in States like Bihar, Uttar Pradesh and Rajasthan were very low.

One of the main reasons for not achieving 100 per cent routine immunisation is the focus on campaign mode programmes in health and family welfare. The Department of Family Welfare has now taken up a scheme for strengthening of routine immunisation. A pilot project on Hepatitis B immunisation has also been initiated.

Pulse Polio Immunisation

Under the Pulse Polio initiative, launched in 1995-96, all children under five years of age are to be administered two doses of oral polio vaccine in December and January every year until polio is eliminated. Coverage under the programme has been reported to be over 90 per cent in all States, with over 120 million children taking the vaccine every year.

Confirmed polio cases reported in the last four years is shown in the Table. Uttar Pradesh and Bihar account for most of the reported cases.

Number of Polio Cases in India

Year	*No. of cases of confirmed polio*
1998	1931
1999	1126
2000	265
2001	268

Source : Department of Family Welfare.

The medical goal of polio eradication is to prevent paralytic illness due to polio viruses by the elimination of wild poliovirus so that children need not be immunised perpetually. If there are no more cases over the next three years, the country will be declared polio free. When this is achieved, steps will have to be taken to ensure that the disease does not return, by continuing to ensure 100 per cent coverage under routine immunisation for another decade.

Diarrhoeal Disease Control Programme

Diarrhoea is one of the leading causes of death among children. Most of these deaths are due to dehydration caused due to frequent passage of stools and can be prevented by the timely and adequate replacement of fluids. The Oral rehydration programme was started in 1986-87 in order to prevent such deaths.

The use of fluids available at home and oral rehydration solution (ORS) has resulted in a substantial decline in the mortality associated with diarrhoea, from an estimated one million to 1.5 million children every year prior to 1985 to 600,000 to 700,000 deaths in 1996.

Control of Acute Respiratory Infections

Pneumonia accounts for around 30 per cent of under five deaths in the country. Mothers and community members are being informed about the symptoms of ARI, which would require antibiotic treatment or referral.

The ICMR is the nodal research agency for funding basic, clinical and operational research in contraception and maternal and child health. In addition, the Council for Scientific and Industrial Research (CSIR), Delhi, Department of Biotechnology (DBT) and the Department of Science and Technology (DST) fund research pertaining to the Family Welfare Programme.

V. Planning to reduce Fertility, Mortality and Population Growth in India

Reduction in fertility, mortality and population growth rate are major objectives of the Government Planning. These will be achieved through meeting all the felt needs for health care of women and children. The focus will be on improving access to services to meet the health care needs of women and children by :

- A decentralized area-specific approach to planning, implementation and monitoring of the performance and effective mid-course corrections.
- Differential strategy to achieve incremental improvement in performance in all States/districts.
- Special efforts to improve access to and utilization of the services in States/districts with high mortality and/or fertility rates.
- Filling the critical gaps, in existing infrastructure through appropriate reorganization and restructuring of the primary health care infrastructure.
- Ensuring that post of specialists in health centres does not remain vacant; upgrading skills and redeploying existing manpower to fill other critical gaps.
- Streamlining the functioning of the primary health care system in urban and rural areas; providing good quality integrated RCH services at the primary, secondary and tertiary care levels and improving referral services.
- Providing adequate supply of essential drugs, diagnostics and vaccines; improving the logistics of supply.
- Well coordinated activities for delivery of services by public, private and voluntary sectors to improve coverage.
- Involvement of PRIs in planning, monitoring and mid-course correction of the programme at the local level.
- Involvement of industry in the organized and unorganized sectors, agriculture workers and labour representatives in improving access to RCH services.
- Effective use of social marketing to improve access to simple over the counter (OTC) products such as ORT and condoms.
- Effective IEC and motivation programmes.
- Effective inter-sectoral coordination.

VI. Environment and Human Health

According to W.H.O. health is a state of complete physical, mental and social well being and not merely an absence of disease or infirmity.

Human health is influenced by many factors like nutritional, biological, chemical or psychological. These factors may cause harmful changes in the body's conditions called disease.

The State of health of the people does not depend on number of doctors and hospitals only but also on clean environment. Ecological changes have the direct impact on human health. Certain changes in the human environment increases the incidence of many diseases. These changes include socio-economic and cultural changes leading to stress of mankind on human health, e.g. urbanization, industrial stress, population stress and mechanization and modernization of agriculture ultimately bring about changes in the human environment making it a paradise for infectious agents. Such stress on environment contaminates our air, land, water, food etc. thus affecting our health.

Approximately 80 per cent of the world's diseases particularly in developing world can be linked with water.

The important aspects of environment health includes diarrhoeas, malaria, filarial, Japanese encephalitis and Kalazar. All these diseases are in increasing trends and their spread have direct correlation with water and pesticides. These are the negative aspects of modern agriculture.

➢ Human Health is influenced by following factors

☞ *Infectious Organisms*

High temperature and moisture along with malnutrition help many diseases in tropical countries. Microbes especially bacteria can cause food poisoning by producing toxins in the contaminated food. Some moulds grow on food and produce poisonous toxins.

Infectious organisms can also cause respiratory diseases (pneumonia, tuberculosis, influenza, etc.) and gastrointestinal diseases (diarrhoea, dysentery, cholera, etc.)

There are various types of parasites that cause diseases like malaria, schistosomiasis, and filariasis, etc. Most of these infections take place when the environmental conditions are unclean and unhygienic.

Chemicals

A large number of chemicals are introduced in the environment by anthropogenètic activities. Chemicals can be divided into two categories i.e. hazardous and toxic chemicals. Hazardous chemicals are dangerous like explosives, inflammable chemicals, etc. Toxic chemicals are poisonous which kill cells and can cause death. Many other chemicals can cause cancer affect genetic material (DNA) in cells, while there are others that affect nervous system and reproductive system.

Many chemicals present in the fresh water like heavy metals (mercury, cadmium, lead, etc.) fluoride and nitrate can affect human health. Metals can contaminate food while cooking in various types of utensils including alloys like steel. Containers for canned food, especially which are acidic in nature, contaminated the food with lead. Lead also comes in water from water pipes. Various alcoholic beverages contain lead while tobacco contain cadmium that goes in the body and affect.

Various chemicals, gases and particulates laden with chemicals, spewed into the environment from various industries cause air pollution and affect human health :

- *Noise* : The details of the effects of noise pollution are given in the chapter 5.
- *Radiation* : The details of the effects of radiations are given in the chapter 5.
- *Diet* : Diet has a very important role in maintaining health. Malnutrition makes humans prone to the other diseases. There is a strong relation between cardiovascular diseases and the amount of the salt and fat in one's diet. Food contamination can cause various ill effects.
- *Settlement* : Pure environment, availability of basic necessities of the life like water, sanitation, etc. are essential for healthy living. Improper settlement and poor physical environment may cause various health problems.

10 Facts on preventing Disease through Healthy Environments given by World Health Organisation (WHO)

1. Worldwide, 13 million deaths could be prevented every year by making our environments healthier.
2. In children under the age of five, one-third of all disease is caused by the environmental factors such as unsafe water and air pollution.
3. Every year, the lives of four million children under 5 years – mostly in developing countries – could be saved by preventing environmental risks such as unsafe water and polluted air.
4. In developing countries, the main environmentally caused diseases are diarrhoeal disease, lower respiratory infections, unintentional injuries, and malaria.
5. Better environmental management could prevent 40% of deaths from malaria, 41% of deaths from lower respiratory infections, and 94% of deaths from diarrhoeal disease – three of the world's biggest childhood killers.
6. In the least developed countries, one-third of death and disease is a direct result of environmental causes.
7. In developed countries, healthier environments could significantly reduce the incidence of cancers, cardiovascular diseases, asthma, lower respiratory infections, musculoskeletal diseases, road traffic injuries, poisonings, and drownings.
8. Environmental factors influence 85 out of the 102 categories of diseases and injuries listed in *The World Health Report.*
9. Much of this death, illness and disability could be prevented through well targeted interventions such as promoting safe household water storage, better hygiene measures and the use of cleaner and safer fuels.
10. Other interventions that can make environments healthier include: increasing the safety of buildings; promoting safe, careful use and management of toxic substances at home and in the workplace; and better water resource management.

VII. HIV/ AIDS

Human immunodeficiency virus (HIV) is a retrovirus that is the cause of the disease known as AIDS (*Acquired Immunodeficiency Syndrome*), a syndrome where the immune system begins to fail, leading to many life-threatening opportunistic infections.

HIV primarily infects vital components of the human immune system. HIV also directly attacks organs such as the kidneys, heart and brain.

HIV is transmitted through direct contact of a mucous membrane with a bodily fluid containing HIV, such as blood, semen, vaginal fluid, preseminal fluid or breast milk. This transmission can come in the form of: penetrative sex; blood transfusion; contaminated needles; exchange between mother and infant during pregnancy, childbirth, or breastfeeding; or other exposure to one of the above bodily fluids.

(a) Origin and Discovery

The AIDS epidemic was discovered on June 5, 1981, when the U.S. Centers for Disease Control and Prevention reported a cluster of *Pneumocystis carinii* pneumonia (now classified as Pneumocystis jiroveci pneumonia) in five homosexual men in Los Angeles. In 1982, the CDC introduced the term AIDS to describe the newly recognized syndrome, though it was still casually referred to as GRID.

Three of the earliest known instances of HIV-1 infection are as follows :

- A plasma sample taken in 1959 from an adult male living in what is now the Democratic Republic of Congo.
- HIV found in tissue samples from a 15 years old African-American teenager who died in St. Louis in 1969.
- HIV found in tissue samples from a Norwegian sailor who died around 1976.

The first symptoms of HIV infection often include moderate and unexplained weight loss, recurrent respiratory tract infections (such as sinusitis, bronchitis, otitis media, pharyngitis), herpes zoster and recurrent oral ulcerations.

UNAIDS and the WHO estimate that AIDS has killed more than 25 million people since it was first recognized in 1981, making it one of the most destructive epidemics in recorded history. Despite recent, improved access to antiretroviral treatment and care in many regions of the world, the AIDS epidemic claimed an estimated 2.8 million (between 2.4 and 3.3 million) lives in 2005 of which more than half a million (570,000) were children.

Globally, between 33.4 and 46 million people currently live with HIV. In 2005, between 3.4 and 6.2 million people were newly infected and between 2.4 and

3.3 million people with AIDS died, an increase from 2004 and the highest number since 1981.

Sub-Saharan Africa remains by far the worst-affected region, with an estimated 21.6 to 27.4 million people currently living with HIV.

South and South East Asia are second worst affected with 15 per cent. AIDS accounts for the deaths of 500,000 children in this region. Two-thirds of HIV/AIDS infections in Asia occur in India, with an estimated 5.7 million infections (estimated 3.4—9.4 million) (0.9% of population), surpassing South Africa's estimated 5.5 million (4.9-6.1 million) (11.9% of population) infections, making it the country with the highest number of HIV infections in the world.

In the 35 African nations with the highest prevalence, average life expectancy is 48.3 years—6.5 years less than it would be without the disease. In the United States, the number of persons with AIDS increased from about 35,000 in 1988 to over 220,000 in 1996.

The development of HAART as effective therapy for HIV infection and AIDS has substantially reduced the death rate from this disease in those areas where it is widely available. This has created the misperception that the disease has gone away. In fact, as the life expectancy of persons with AIDS has increased in countries where HAART is widely used, the number of persons living with AIDS has increased substantially.

(b) HIV/AIDS in India

India has had a sharp increase in the number of its people living with HIV, from a few thousand in the early 1990s to around 5.7 million adults and children in 2005. With a population of over one billion, the HIV epidemics in India will have a major impact on the overall spread of HIV in Asia and the Pacific and indeed worldwide.

The spread of HIV within the country is as diverse as the societal patterns between its different regions, States and metropolitan areas. In fact, HIV in India exists in a number of epidemics, and in some places they occur within the same State. The epidemics vary, from States with mainly heterosexual transmission of HIV, to some States where injecting drug use is the main route of HIV transmission. Tracking these epidemics and implementing effective responses poses a serious challenge to the authorities and communities in India.

It would be easy to underestimate the challenge of HIV/AIDS in India. The country has a large population and population density, low literacy levels and consequently low levels of awareness, and HIV/AIDS is one of the most challenging public health problems ever faced by the country.

The first case of HIV infection in India was diagnosed among commercial sex workers in Chennai, Tamil Nadu, in 1986. Soon after, a number of screening centres were established throughout the country. Initially the focus was on screening foreigners, especially foreign students. Gradually, the focus moved on to screening blood banks. By early 1987, efforts were made up to set up a national network of HIV screening centres in major urban areas.

A National AIDS Control Programme was launched in 1987 with the programme activities covering surveillance, screening blood and blood products, and health education. In 1992 the National AIDS Control Organization (NACO) was established. NACO carries out India's National AIDS Programme, which includes the formulation of policy, prevention and control programmes.

The same year that NACO was established, the Government launched a Strategic Plan for HIV/AIDS prevention under the National AIDS Control Project. The Project established the administrative and technical basis for programme management and also set up State AIDS bodies in 25 States and 7 Union Territories. The Project was able to make a number of important improvements in HIV prevention such as improving blood safety.

(c) Current Estimates and Future Projections

According to UNAIDS, India has 5.7 million people living with HIV—more than any other country in the world.

- NACO estimates there were 5.21 million Indians living with HIV at the end of 2005 (compared to 4.58 million in 2002), of whom 39 per cent were female.
- By the end of July 2005, the total number of AIDS cases reported in India was 111,608, of whom 32,567 were women. 37 per cent of reported AIDS cases were diagnosed among people under 30. Many more AIDS cases go unreported.
- The UN Population Division projects that India's adult HIV prevalence will peak at 1.9 per cent in 2019. The UN estimates there were 2.7 million AIDS deaths in India between 1980 and 2000. It has also projected that India will suffer 12.3 million AIDS deaths during 2000-15, and 49.5 million deaths during 2015-50.
- A 2002 report by the CIA's National Intelligence Council predicted 20 million to 25 million AIDS cases in India by 2010, more than any other country in the world.

(d) Care and Support of People living with HIV/AIDS

Since the launch of the second phase of the National AIDS Control Programme in 1999, the Government of India has established 25 community HIV/AIDS care centres across the country. But the standard of care that NACO supports is limited to the provision of drugs for the treatment of opportunistic infections. And the distribution of these drugs is limited to those institutions that qualify through a NACO State-level selection process. Many people living with HIV only have access to centres not selected to receive drugs, so cannot have access to treatment for most opportunistic infections. Just as importantly, a major obstacle to the provision of care for HIV positive people is the stigma surrounding the disease as described earlier.

With regard to antiretroviral drugs, India is a major producer of cheap generic copies of many HIV/AIDS drugs that are being sold to many countries all over the world. Despite that antiretroviral drugs are affordable to a tiny fraction of people in need of treatment in India.

> *"It is a sad irony that India is one of the biggest producers of the drugs that have transformed the lives of people with AIDS in wealthy countries. But for millions of Indians, access to these medicines is a distant dream"*
>
> — Joanne Csete, Director of the HIV/AIDS Programme at Human Rights Watch.

VIII. Human Rights

Human rights, which inhere in every human being by virtue of his birth as a member of the human family, are demands to protect our only common identity as human beings. These rights flow from the common humanity and inherent dignity of every human being. No compromise with violations of the same is permissible in any civilized society. These rights, which are non-negotiable, non-alienable, indivisible and recognize an essential worth of a human being, are ethical norms for the treatment of individuals. Human Rights are, thus, certain rights which have come to be recognized as basic conditions of civilized living for full development of a human being.

The aim of human rights is empowerment of people through human development. These rights are inter-dependent and inter-related and have a direct relationship with human development. Universality of human rights demands eradication of global inequities and to achieve this end the importance of "Right to Development" cannot, but, be emphasized.

The wide global disparities in different parts of the world are shown to be linked with varying levels of human development. Global disparities must be minimized to ensure that the minimum needs of everyone throughout the world are met. Strategies must be developed to achieve this result. It is only when the potential of all human beings is fully realized that we can talk of true human development.

❖ Universal Declaration of Human Rights by UNO

On 10th December, 1948, the Universal Declaration of Human Rights was adopted by the General Assembly of UNO as "a common standard of achievement of all peoples and nations". Article 1 to 30 of the declaration are as follows :

1. All human beings are born free and equal in dignity and rights. They are endowed with reason and conscience and should act towards one another in a spirit of brotherhood.
2. Everyone is entitled to all the rights and freedoms set forth in this Declaration, without distinction of any kind, such as race, colour, sex, language, religion, political or other opinion, national or social origin, property, birth or other status.
   Furthermore, no distinction shall be made on the basis of the political, jurisdictional or international status of the country or territory to which a person belongs, whether it be independent, trust, non-self-governing or under any other limitation of sovereignty.
3. Everyone has the right to life, liberty and the security of person.
4. No one shall be held in slavery or servitude; slavery and the slave trade shall be prohibited in all their forms.
5. No one shall be subjected to torture or to cruel, inhuman or degrading treatment or punishment.
6. Everyone has the right to recognition everywhere as a person before the law.
7. All are equal before the law and are entitled without any discrimination to equal protection against any discrimination in violation of this Declaration and against any incitement to such discrimination.
8. Everyone has the right to an effective remedy by the competent national tribunals for acts violating the fundamental rights granted him by the Constitution or by law.
9. No one shall be subjected to arbitrary arrest, detention or exile.
10. Everyone is entitled in full equality to a fair, and public hearing by an independent and impartial tribunal, in the determination of his rights and obligations and of any criminal charge against him.
11. (a) Everyone charged with a penal offence has the right to be presumed innocent until proven guilty according to law in a public trial at which he has had all the guarantees necessary for his defence. (b) No one shall be held guilty of any penal offence on account of any act or omission which did not constitute a penal offence, under national or international law, at the time when it was committed. Nor shall a heavier penalty be imposed than the one that was applicable at the time the penal offence was committed.
12. No one shall be subjected to arbitrary interference with his privacy, family, home or correspondence, nor to attacks upon his honour and reputation.

Everyone has the right to the protection of the law against such interference or attacks.

13. (a) Everyone has the right to freedom of movement and residence within the borders of each State. (b) Everyone has the right to leave any country, including his own, and to return to his country.
14. (a) Everyone has the right to seek and to enjoy in other countries asylum from persecution. (b) This right may not be invoked in the case of prosecutions genuinely arising from non-political crimes or from acts contrary to the purposes and principles of the United Nations.
15. (a) Everyone has the right to a nationality. (b) No one shall be arbitrarily deprived of his nationality nor denied the right to change his nationality.
16. (a) Men and women of full age, without any limitation due to race, nationality or religion, have the right to marry and to found a family. They are entitled to equal rights as to marriage, during marriage and at its dissolution. (b) Marriage shall be entered into only with the free and full consent of the intending spouses. (c) The family is the natural and fundamental group unit of society and is entitled to protection by society and the State.
17. (a) Everyone has the right to own property alone as well as in association with others. (b) No one shall be arbitrarily deprived of his property.
18. Everyone has the right to freedom of thought, conscience and religion; this right includes freedom to change his religion or belief, and freedom, either alone or in community with others and in public or private, to manifest his religion or belief in teaching, practice, worship and observance.
19. Everyone has the right to freedom of opinion and expression; this right includes freedom to hold opinions without interference and to seek, receive and impart information and ideas through any media and regardless of frontiers.
20. (a) Everyone has the right to freedom of peaceful assembly and association. (b) No one may be compelled to belong to an association.
21. (a) Everyone has the right to take part in the government of his country, directly or through freely chosen representatives. (b) Everyone has the right of equal access to public service in his country. (c) The will of the people shall be the basis of the authority of government; this will shall be expressed in periodic and genuine elections which shall be by universal and equal suffrage and shall be held by secret vote or by equivalent free voting procedures.
22. Everyone, as a member of society, has the right to social security and is entitled to realization, through national effort and international co-operation and in accordance with the organization and resources of each State, of the economic, social and cultural rights indispensable for his dignity and the free development of his personality.

23. (a) Everyone has the right to work, to free choice of employment, to just and favourable conditions of work and to protection against unemployment. (b) Everyone, without any discrimination, has the right to equal pay for equal work. (c) Everyone who works has the right to just and favourable remuneration ensuring for himself and his family an existence worthy of human dignity, and supplemented, if necessary, by other means of social protection. (d) Everyone has the right to form and to join trade unions for the protection of his interests.
24. Everyone has the right to rest and leisure, including reasonable limitation of working hours and periodic holidays with pay.
25. (a) Everyone has the right to a standard of living adequate for the health and well-being of himself and of his family, including food, clothing, housing and medical care and necessary social services, and the right to security in the event of unemployment, sickness, disability, widowhood, old age or other lack of livelihood in circumstances beyond his control. (b) Motherhood and childhood are entitled to special care and assistance. All children, whether born in or out of wedlock, shall enjoy the same social protection.
26. (a) Everyone has the right to education. Education shall be free, at least in the elementary and fundamental stages. Elementary education shall be compulsory. Technical and professional education shall be made generally available and higher education shall be equally accessible to all on the basis of merit. (b) Education shall be directed to the full development of the human personality and to the strengthening of respect for human rights and fundamental freedoms. It shall promote understanding, tolerance and friendship among all nations, racial or religious groups, and shall further the activities of the United Nations for the maintenance of peace. (c) Parents have a prior right to choose the kind of education that shall be given to their children.
27. (a) Everyone has the right freely to participate in the cultural life of the community, to enjoy the arts and to share in scientific advancement and its benefits. (b) Everyone has the right to the protection of the moral and material interests resulting from any scientific, literary or artistic production of which he is the author.
28. Everyone is entitled to a social and international order in which the rights and freedoms set forth in this Declaration can be fully realized.
29. (a) Everyone has duties to the community in which alone the free and full development of his personality is possible. (b) In the exercise of his rights and freedoms, everyone shall be subject only to such limitations as are determined by law solely for the purpose of securing due recognition and respect for the rights and freedoms of others and of meeting the just

requirements of morality, public order and the general welfare in a democratic society. (c) These rights and freedoms may in no case be exercised contrary to the purposes and principles of the United Nations.

30. Nothing in this Declaration may be interpreted as implying for any State, group or person any right to engage in any activity or to perform any act aimed at the destruction of any of the rights and freedoms set forth herein.

❖ INDIA

The Constitution of India envisages establishment of a welfare State at the federal level as well as at the State level. In a welfare State, it is the primary duty of the Government to secure welfare of the people.

Part III of the Constitution of our Republic dealing with Fundamental Rights. They are :

Right to Equality

- Article 14, which stipulates that the State shall not deny to any person equality before the law or the equal protection of laws within the territory of India. This also applies to non-citizens.
- Article 15, which expressly declares that the State shall not discriminate against any citizen on grounds only of religion, race, caste, sex, place of birth or any of them. It specifically adds that no citizen shall be subjected to any disability, liability, restriction or condition with regard to access to shops, public restaurants, hotels, and places of public entertainment; or to the use of wells, tanks, bathing ghats, roads and places of public resort maintained wholly or partly out of State Funds or dedicated to the use of the general public. In addition, Article 15(4) permits the State to make special provision for the advancement of any socially and educationally backward class of citizens as well as Scheduled Castes and Scheduled Tribes. It is under this provision that the States of the Union are permitted to make reservations in educational institutions for these groups of citizens.
- Article 16, which provides for equality of opportunity in matters of public employment. It also stipulates that no citizen shall on grounds only of religion, race, caste, sex, descent, place of birth, residence or any of them, be ineligible for, or discriminated against in respect of employment or office under the State. This Article further provides for affirmative action, through the reservation of appointments or posts, in favour of any backward class of citizens which, in the opinion of the State, is not adequately represented in the services of the State. It also covers promotions and provides further for the carry forward of unfilled vacancies of the quota for succeeding years.

- Article 17, which abolishes "Untouchability", and forbids its practice in any form.
- Article 18, which abolishes "Titles"

Right to Freedom

- Article 19—Protection of certain rights regarding freedom of speech, etc.
- Article 20—Protection in respect of conviction for offences.
- Article 21—Which protects life and personal liberty.
- Article 22—Protection against detention in certain cases.

Right against Exploitation

- Article 23—Which prohibits trafficking in human beings and forced labour.
- Article 24—Prohibition of employment of children in factories, etc.

Right to Freedom of Religion

- Article 25—Freedom of conscience and free pursuit of profession, practice and propagation of religion.
- Article 26—Freedom to manage religious affairs
- Article 27—Freedom as to payment of taxes for promotion of any particular religion
- Article 28—Freedom as to attendance at religious instruction or religious worship in certain educational institutions.

Cultural and Educational Rights

- Article 29—Protection of interests of minorities
- Article 30—Right of minorities to establish and administer educational institutions.

Right to Constitutional Remedies

- Article 32—Right to Constitutional remedies : The Supreme Court of India, through judicial interpretation, has widened the horizon of human rights in India.

❖ National Human Rights Commission

The National Human Rights Commission was established on 12th October, 1993 under the legislative mandate of the Protection of Human Rights Act, 1993. It extends to the whole of India.

The Commission has endeavoured to give a positive meaning and a content to the objectives set out in the Protection of Human Rights Act, 1993. It has moved vigorously and effectively to use the opportunities provided to it by the Act to promote and protect human rights in the country.

Functions of the Commission

Commission shall perform all or any of the following functions, namely :

(a) Inquire, *suo motu* or on a petition presented to it by a victim or any person on his behalf or on a direction or order of any court into complaint of :
(i) The Violation of human rights or abetment thereof; or
(ii) Negligence in the prevention of such violation, by a public servant;

(b) Intervene in any proceeding involving any allegation of violation of human rights pending before a court with the approval of such court;

(c) Visit, notwithstanding anything contained in any other law for the time being in force, any jail or other institution under the control of the State Government, where persons are detained or lodged for purposes of treatment, reformation or protection, for the study of the living conditions of the inmates thereof and make recommendations thereon to the Government;

(d) Review the safeguards provided by or under the Constitution or any law for the time being in force for the protection of human rights and recommend measures for their effective implementation;

(e) Review the factors, including acts of terrorism that inhibit the enjoyment of human rights and recommend appropriate remedial measures;

(f) Study treaties and other international instruments on human rights and make recommendations for their effective implementation;

(g) Undertake and promote research in the field of human rights;

(h) Spread human rights literacy among various sections of society and promote awareness of the safeguards available for the protection of these rights through publications, the media, seminars and other available means;

(i) Encourage the efforts of non-governmental organizations and institutions working in the field of human rights;

(j) Such other functions as it may consider necessary for the protection of human rights.

❖ Human Rights in India : Challenges

1. Poverty

Poverty is the biggest violator of human rights. Statistics provided by The Human

Development Reports demonstrate that there exist massive inequalities, more particularly in the developing countries. Political freedom would not have much significance or meaning for millions of poverty stricken people in various countries who suffer the social evils flowing from poverty. Eradication of poverty is, therefore, a big challenge. According to UNDP Report of 2003, Indian society is a highly inequitable society where the richest 10 per cent consume 33.5 per cent of resources and the poorest 10 per cent get only 3.5 per cent of resources. Around 233 million people are chronically hungry. Official figures State that in our country 26 per cent people are living Below Poverty Line.

2. Social, Economic and Cultural Rights

In our Constitution civil and political rights are contained as "fundamental rights" in Part-III, while social,economic and cultural rights are contained in Part IV as Directive Principles. The mandate of Article 37 of the Constitution, however, is that even though directive principles are not justiciable or enforceable by the courts, the same are "fundamental in the governance of the country" and it shall be the "duty" of the State to apply these principles. Unfortunately, the Governments at the Centre and the States, as statistics tell us, never whole-heartedly pursued the implementation of Directive Principles. The government dilly-dallied implementation of each principle generally citing the reasons of resource crunch. Governments have so far contented themselves by chalking out only strategies for promotion of economic and social rights.

The State must realize the importance of Economic, Social and Cultural Rights and should not content itself by only chalking out strategies for promotion of the same. The neglect of Economic, Social and Cultural Rights like right to food, health care, education, etc. gives rise to internal conflicts, which are caustic factors of conflict and terrorism. They pose a threat not only to human rights but also to peace. Where hunger persists, peace cannot prevail.

3. Corruption

It directly contributes to inequalities in income, status and opportunities. It remains one of the biggest threats to 'full human development' and 'human rights for all'. It undermines the rule of law. It distorts the development process and also poses a grave threat to human security. Corruption is not a new phenomenon. What is new and worrying is the magnitude and size of corruption. It has spread its tentacles to every sphere of national life. It is one of the biggest threats to development. It can tear the very fabric of the society and, in fact, it is doing so. Corruption benefits the rich and the well-to-do. It enriches the rich and disproportionally affects the poor, unprotected and the underprivileged and thereby it deepens their deprivation. Unless it is checked, the governments and people will have to pay a very heavy price in the consequent result of lower incomes, lower investments and lower developments resulting in volatile economic swings. It is unfortunate, but true, that growing politicization of public services and criminalization of politics have contributed in no small measure to let corruption flourish and the corrupt not only go scot-free but even earn a position of false respectability ! Zero tolerance to corruption by We the People of India, would go a long way to check the menace. To have corruption free governance is a basic human right and the need to recognize it as such and to take steps to eradicate it, is the need of the hour.

4. Sexual Exploitation of Women and Children

Sexual exploitation of women and children is also posing a big challenge for protection of human rights. Trafficking in women and children is a gross violation of their human rights and an affront to the supreme dignity of the females, apart from being a serious crime. It is a problem of Human Rights. It is a problem which should make the heads of the civil society fall in shame because here we are treating human beings as chattels, commodities, saleable items—the price tag varying with age, class, colour and sex.

IX. Information Technology and Environment

Information technology play direct role in creation, preservation and dissemination of ideas in the field of environmental protection.

Development of INTERNET facilities, World Wide Web, Geographical Information System (GIS) and information through satellites has generated a wealth of up-to-date information on various aspects of environment and health. A number of software has been developed for environment and health studies.

1. Computer

In the computers the information is arranged in a systemic manner that is easily manageable and can be very quickly retrieved. The Ministry of environment and forest has taken up the task of compiling the database on environment. Data base is available on forest, wildlife, resources, diseases, population, conservation and various contemporary issues.

The Information System for Forest, Wildlife and Environment is a web based application to provide information regarding forests, wildlife and environment of all States. It helps users in the Planning Commission to take decisions on future plans. A database has been implemented dealing with Parliament questions and their answers, handled by the Parliament Section of the Planning Commission. The system with search facilities enables users to have easy access to the documents by means of search options according to year of Parliament session and related subjects.

The Environmental Information System (ENVIS) deals with 'Centres of Excellence' related to environment. Nearly 6,000 queries are received by the ENVIS network per year. The data bases are available in the internet to everybody.

2. Remote Sensing

Remote sensing is one of the areas of rapidly advancing technology very useful in ecosystem and environmental management.

➢ Indian Remote Sensing Satellite (IRS)

Following the successful demonstration flights of Bhaskara 1 and Bhaskara 2 launched in 1979 and 1981, respectively, India began development of an indigenous IRS (Indian Remote Sensing Satellite) programme to support the national economy in the areas of "agriculture water resources, forestry and ecology, geology, watersheds, marine fisheries and coastal management". The Indian Remote Sensing satellites are the main-stay of National Natural Resources Management System (NNRMS), for which Department of Space (DOS) is the nodal agency, providing operational remote sensing data services. Data from the IRS satellites is received and disseminated by several countries all over the world. With the advent of high resolution satellites new applications in the areas of urban sprawl, infrastructure planning and other large scale applications for mapping have been initiated.

Remote sensing applications in the country, under the umbrella of NNRMS, now cover diverse fields such as crop acreage and yield estimation, drought warning and assessment, flood control and damage assessment, land use/land cover information, agro-climatic planning, wasteland management, water resources management, underground water exploration, prediction of snow-melt run-off, management of water-sheds and command areas, fisheries development, under development, mineral prospecting forest resources survey, Active involvement of the user ministries/departments has ensured in an effective harnessing of the potential of space-based remote sensing. An important application of IRS data is in the Integrated Mission for Sustainable Development (IMSD) initiated in 1992. IMSD, under which 174 districts have been identified, aims at generating locale-specific action plans for sustainable development.

The first-two IRS spacecraft, IRS-1A (March 1988) and IRS-1B (August, 1991) were launched.

IRS-1A and IRS-1B were to be joined in 1993 with IRS-1E. The spacecraft was lost, however, when its PSLV launch vehicle failed to reach Earth orbit. Thirteen months later, in October 1994, the PSLV functioned correctly, allowing IRS-P2 to assume an 820-km, sun-synchronous orbit. This spacecraft continued in operations until September 1997.

As of late 1999, five IRS satellites were operating, and more were scheduled for launch by the year 2000. IRS-1C, successfully launched on December 28, 1995, while IRS-1D was orbited by India's PSLV. IRS-P3 was launched by PSLV in 1996.

Upcoming launches include IRS-P5 in 1998, IRS-2A in 2000, and IRS-2B in 2004, all with the new sensor suite.

IRS-P4 (OCEANSAT-1) will have payloads, specifically tailored for the measurements of physical and biological oceanography parameters.

IRS-P5 (CARTOSAT-1) has an improved sensor system that provides 2.5 m resolution with fore-aft stereo capability. This mission caters to the needs of cartographers and terrain modelling applications. The satellite will provide cadastral level information up to 1 : 5000 scale and will be useful for making 2-5 m contour maps.

IRS-P6 (RESOURCESAT-1) will be a State-of-art satellite mainly for agriculture.

The IRS-2 series (OCEANSAT-2/CLIMATSAT-1/ATMOS-1) will be an integrated mission that will cater to global observations of climate, ocean and atmosphere.

IRS-3, beyond 2002, will have all-weather capabilities with multi-frequency and multi-polarisation microwave payloads and other passive instruments.

Questions

Long answer type of questions

1. What is Population? Describe the characteristics of the population.
2. What is demographic transition? Describe its stages.
3. What do you mean by overpopulation? Discuss the problems associated with overpopulation?
4. Describe the Family Welfare Programmes of India.
5. Discuss various issues and measures for women and child welfare in India.
6. Discuss the population policy of India.
7. What are the components of child health?
8. Discuss the planning to reduce fertility, mortality and population growth in India.
9. What are the factors which affect human health?
10. What is AIDS? What are the symptoms and mode of infection of HIV ? Describe the current status if the disease in India.
11. What is Universal Declaration of Human Rights? What is its importance in achieving the goals of equity and justice?
12. Write the fundamental rights given in the Constitution of India.
13. What are the functions of National Human Rights Commission in India?
14. How Information Technology play direct role in the field of environmental protection.

Write short notes on the following:

1. Exponential Growth
2. Doubling Time
3. Total Fertility Rate (TFR)
4. Infant Mortality Rate
5. Age Structure
6. Life Expectancy
7. Urbanization
8. AIDS
9. Human Rights

Fill in the blanks

1. According to estimates published by the United States Census Bureau, the world population hit ....on February 25, 2005.
2. During **stage four** of Demographic Transition model there are both low birth rates and low..................
3. Approximately 80 per cent of the world's diseases particularly in developing world can be linked with............
4. Diet has a very important role in maintaining...............
5. Malnutrition makes humans prone to the................
6. HIV is a retrovirus that is the cause of the disease known as ....
7. The National Human Rights Commission was established on 12th October..............,

   Keys : 1. 6.5 billion; 2. death rates; 3. water; 4. health; 5. diseases; 6. AIDS; 7. 1993.

Tick the right answer

1. On October 18, 2012, the Earth will be home for :
   (a) 3 billion
   (b) 5 billion
   (c) 9 billion
   (d) 7 billion
2. Each year, the human population grows by approximately :
   (a) 80 million
   (b) 60 million
   (c) 20 million
   (d) 120 million
3. Urban areas occupy only about of the Earth's land area :
   (a) 8 per cent

   (b) 6 per cent
   (c) 4 per cent
   (d) 10 per cent
4. By 2030, of all people are likely to be living in urban areas :
   (a) More than 10 per cent
   (b) More than 90 per cent
   (c) More than 70 per cent
   (d) More than 60 per cent
5. The original Demographic Transition model has just
   (a) Seven stages
   (b) Three stages
   (c) Four stages
   (d) Two stages
6. The AIDS epidemic was discovered
   (a) June 5, 1981
   (b) July 5, 1991
   (c) January 8, 1961
   (d) August 5, 1951
7. The first case of HIV infection in India was diagnosed among commercial sex workers in Chennai, Tamil Nadu, in :
   (a) 1976
   (b) 1986
   (c) 1966
   (d) 1996

Keys : 1. d, 2. a, 3. c, 4. d, 5. c, 6. (a), 7. (b)

True / False types of questions

1. The United Nations Population Fund designated October 12, 1999 as the approximate day on which world population reached nine billion.
2. The average life expectancy, over the world, has risen from 40 to 65.5 years over the past century.
3. In India, life expectancy of male and female was only 22.6 years and 23.3 years, respectively in 1900.
4. In Japan and Sweden, life expectancy is quite higher, being 82.1- 84.2 for females and 77- 77.4 for males.
5. World cereal consumption has become more than triple in the last 30 years.
6. Environmental factors influence 85 out of the 102 categories of diseases.
7. A National AIDS Control Programme was launched in 1987.

Keys : 1. false, 2. true, 3. true, 4. true, 5. false, 6. true, 7. true

Unit - 8

Field Work (Practical)

Visit to a local area to report environmental assets

Field experience is one of the most useful learning gear for environmental concerns. This moves out of the range of the text book method of teaching into the realm of real knowledge in the field, where the professor simply acts as a means to interpret what the student observes or discovers in his/her own environment.

Visit may be planned to any nearby river, forest, grassland, hill or mountain, depending upon easy access and regional importance. Students have to write a report based on their observation and understanding about various aspects of environment. The units from 1 to 7 provide the required information for the study and arriving at some important conclusion about the system.

I. Study of River/Forest/Grassland/Hill/Mountain

A. Study of the River Environment

Rivers are recognized as flowing fresh water ecosystem since the water keeps on flowing.

1. General Information

Note down the name of the river or tibutary/distributary. Its place of origin and its course or route. Mention the nature of the river as weather it is perennial or non-perennial (seasonal).

2. Water Quality Observations

- ❖ Mention whether the water of the river is clear or turbid (muddy).

- If it is clear, then penetration of the light into the waterbody will be more, consequently green aquatic plants will grow more and primary produtivity will be high.
- If it is turbide, how would it affect the primary productivity of the river because sunlight penetration is obstructed by turbidity.

- Note the temperature of water and air.

  - If the temperature of the river water is more than 5^0 C than the surrounding water of the same river, what could be the reason? Find out if any thermal pollution is occurring in the river due to discharge of effluents from some industries.
  - Write down the probable impacts of thermal pollution on aquatic life.

- Do you observe any foam or dark coloured or greasy substances in the rver. If yes, then find out the source.
- If there is any influx of municipal/industrial sewage into the river then differentiate the water quality at the upstream and downstream sites.
- Determine the pH of water using a portable pH–scan. The pH would normally range between 6.5 to 8.5. If pH is quite low i.e. acidic water, it indicates pollution by industries, If pH is quite high i.e. alkaline, it indicates contimination by municipal sewage.

3. Observations on Aquatic Life

- Look for different type of lifeforms. Do you find some free-floating small plants (phytoplankton) or small animals (zooplanktons) ? Are there some rooted plants seen underneath? Do you observe aquatic animal like different fishes, turtle, crocodile/ alligator, water snake etc.? What are the important aquatic birds seen by you.
- Draw a food-web diagram that wood be present in the river.

4. Uses

- How the water of river is used? Prepare a list of the uses.

5. Human Impacts

- What are the major impacts caused by human being in your area on the river? Have you learnt of any major incident e.g. massive fish death or cattle death or skin problems to human beings consuming the water? Try to interpret.

B. Study of the Forest Environment

1. General Information

Note down the name of the forest. What type of the forest is? i.e. a tropical rain forest/desiduous forest etc.? Is the present forest is the part of some Biosphere reserve or National Park or sanctuary? If yes, then what are the special features associated with it?

2. Forest Structure

Note down the salient features of the forest.

- What are the dominant trees? Is the forest having a close canopy or has open spaces.
- Is there an under storey of the shrubs, herbs and grasses of lower height?
- Is there a thick or thin forest floor consisting of leaf litter (dry dead leaves), algae, fungi, etc. What is the use of stratified structure i.e. multi-layered structure of vegetation in the forest ?

3. Commercial Uses

Prepare a list of the different uses of the present forest.

4. Ecological Utility

- Distinguish the differences in the air temperature and moisture present in the forest are and outside of it.
- How many birds, animals and insects do you see around ?
- Make a list of the ecological uses of the forest based on your observations.

5. Human Impacts

- Do you observe any anthropogenic activities in the forest e.g. mining, quarrying, deforestation, dam building, grazing, timber extraction, etc.

C. Environmental Aspects of Grassland

1. General Information

Note down the type of grassland, is this pasture or meadows? Is it perennial or Seasonal. Are there tall grasses or short grasses? Is it dominated by just a few species or is it a mixed type of grassland? Is it protected i.e. fenced or disturbed?

2. Grass Quality Observations

- Try to find out the names of some of the dominated grasses or plants. Are these dominated plants having a soft, delicate, juicy nature with green colour showing good palatability? Or dominated plant have a course, hard texture with spines/ thorns?
- Take out few plants to see what type of roots do they have. Are they adventure types, running types, having rhizomes or there is a single, longtap roots?
- If the roots are adventurous, they tend to bind the soil particles firmly and help in conserving the soil. If the root is tap root, then it cannot help in binding the soil particles firmly. What is the condition prevailing in the present grassland? Do you observe the soil erosion?

3. Grazing and Overgrazing

Find out if there is managed grazing on the grassland i.e. only a limited number of livestock (cattle) is being allowed to graze or there is unmanaged grazing.

Normal grazing is useful for increasing the overall productivity/ yield of the grassland. Overgrazing has several far reaching consequences. Make your own observations in the present grassland i.e. whether there is limited grazing or overgrazing?

- If you find that good quality grasses/herbs are growing then it is rightly grazed.
- If you see a denuded areas with little grasses, it shows overgrazing.
- If you observe thorny, hard, prickly plants occupying some areas, it indicates degradation of the grassland due to overgrazing.

4. Uses

- Prepare a list of the utilities of the grassland.

D. Study of the Mountain/Hilly area

1. General Information

Note down the name and type of mountain ranges or the hills. Note down the altitude of the hill region. Find out the average annual rainfall and temperature in the area.

2. Observations on Natural Vegetation

Make your observations on the forests present on the hill slopes. Do you find dense forests on the hills or deforestation is observed in some areas? Look for some dominated tree species and find out their names and uses from the local people.

3. Landslides

You might have come across some region, where landslide would have occurred recently in the past. Do you observe any anthropogenetic activity in the area? Can you establish some links between these aspects? You can gather some information about such aspects from the native people.

4. Watersheds

Try to look for some springs, rivers and channels coming out from the mountains. The land areas from which water drains under gravity to a common drainage channel is called watershed.

Gather some information about the watershed in the study area, its uses and its status i.e. whether it is well managed or degraded.

5. Plantation and Farming

Look for the type of plantations (e.g. tea plantation) or farming (e.g. maize, wheat) done artificially on the hill slopes :

- ❖ What type of farming is done ? Is it shifting cultivation, traditional or modernized ? What would be there impact ?
- ❖ Do you observe terrace farming, contour or strip cropping? Why is such cropping helpful in hills ?
- ❖ Find out the water and nutrient requirements of these crops. Do you find these crops/plantations well suited to hill environment or do you think they can have some damaging effects later on ? Discuss with local people.

6. Anthropogenic Activities

How much anthropogenic activities do you observe on the mountains/hills ?

These activities usually include mining, quarrying, tourism, construction, hydro-electric projects etc. What major impacts do you observe or predict in future ?

II. Visit to Some Local Polluted Site

Human activities related to urbanization and industrialization has led to large scale pollution of the environment. Agricultural practices have also led to pesticide pollution, waterlogging and salinization.

A. Study of an Industrially Polluted Area

1. General Information

Note down the name of the industry, year of establishment, its capacity, the type of product and type of wastes/emission produced by it.

2. Pollution Aspects

Look at the stacks (chimneys) in the area which might be given certain emissions. What are toxic gases present in them ? As the wind blows, do they move in the direction that is towards a city or in other direction ?

Find out if there is any effluent treatment plant (ETP) within the industry to treat the wastes before discharging them. You can also see the working of an ETP with prior permission of the industry people.

3. Greenbelt

Do you observe a green belt planted around the industry ? It has now become mandatory for all big industries to plant green trees around the industries.

This is because the tree canopy (leaves) has got an excellent capacity to absorb various pollutants and also reduce noise. They also release oxygen to make the atmosphere pure.

4. Health Aspects

Try to get information about any serious health impacts in the people living in the vicinity of the industry e.g.

- The water drawn from tubewells/handpumps may be contaminated with some toxic substances/dyes, etc. which on drinking may cause health problem.
- The toxic gases and suspended particulate matter realised by the industries is inhaled by the people nearby which might cause skin irritation/ allergy/ respiratory problems.

B. Study of a waterlogged/saline land

1. General Information

Visit a waterlogged and salt affected land in some rural agriculture areas. An area having permanently standing water on the soil is known as waterlogged area.

Gather information from the local people about its historical background i.e. how much irrigation was being done in these areas and for how long? Was the area fertile some years ago and has gradually become waterlogged and saline? What was the crop grown earlier? Try to corelate the problems with the irrigation practices followed there.

2. Salinity and the crop growth

- Find out the salinity level (Electrical conductivity, EC) of the soil. For this you can take 10 grams of soil and dissolve it in 20 ml of water in a beaker. Dip an EC probe into it which will indicate the EC of the soil. The non-saline normal soil has EC< 4Ds/m. If EC exceed 4, it is saline. The EC can be as high as 20–40 Ds/M also. But then it would hardly support any vegetation.
- Do such soils support any crops? Note down the names of the salt-tolerant and salt sensitive crops.

3. Recommendation

Find out what remedial measures are taken by the farmers to deal with the problem. What measures can you suggest?

III. Study of Common Plants, Insects and Birds

Biodiversity is the sum of all the different species of animals, plants, fungi, and microbial organisms living on Earth and the variety of habitats in which they live. It has tremendous potential in terms of its consumptive, productive, social, ethical and ecological value. It is worthwhile to know about some common plants, insects and birds of our locality.

A. Plants

Study the common plants of your locality, including trees, shrubs and herbs. You can study them mainly in relation to their value.

- *Medicinal plants* : Local people often have indigenous knowledge about the medicinal value of various plants. Find out which of the plants have medicinal importance in your locality.
- *Timber wood trees* : Note down the importance of the trees of your locality which yield timber wood.
- *Miscellaneous* : Note down the names of the plants which have the other uses like producing gum, resins, tannins, dye, rubber, fibre, etc.

B. Insects

Identify some common insects of your locality :

- Which may be spreading diseases;
- Which are crop-pests or animal pests; and
- Which help in pollination of ornamental/crop flowers.

C. Birds

Identify some common birds of your locality. Find out how some of them are useful to us and some cause damage to our crops/fruits. Observe small birds with long beaks pollinating flowers. Observe the birds in the ploughed fields eating insects/ larvae.

Glossary

Acid rain — The precipitation of dilute solutions of strong mineral acids, formed by the mixing in the atmosphere of various industrial pollutants — primarily sulphur dioxide and nitrogen oxides — with naturally occurring oxygen and water vapour.

Act — In the legislative sense, a bill or measure passed by both Houses of Congress; a law.

Adjournment — The end of a legislative day or session.

Aerosol — A suspension of small liquid or solid particles in gas.

Air pollution — Toxic or radioactive gases or particulate matter introduced into the atmosphere, usually as a result of human activity.

Alternative energy — Energy that is not popularly used and is usually environmentally sound, such as solar or wind energy (as opposed to fossil fuels).

Alternative fibres — Fibres produced from non-wood sources for use in paper making.

Alternative fuels — Transportation fuels other than gasoline or diesel. Includes natural gas, methanol, and electricity.

Alternative transportation — Modes of travel other than private cars, such as walking, bicycling, rollerblading, carpooling and transit.

Amendment — A change or addition to an existing law or rule.

Ancient forest — A forest that is typically older than 200 years with large trees, dense canopies and an abundance of diverse wildlife.

Apportionment — The process through which legislative seats are allocated to different regions.

Appropriation — The setting aside of funds for a designated purpose (e.g., there is an appropriation of $ 7 billion to build 5 new submarines).

Aquaculture — The controlled rearing of fish or shellfish by people or corporations who own the harvestable product, often involving the capture of the eggs or young of a species from wild sources, followed by rearing more intensively than possible in nature.

Aquifer — Underground source of water.

Arms control — Coordinated action based on agreements to limit, regulate, or reduce weapon systems by the parties involved.

Ash — Incombustible residue left over after incineration or other thermal processes.

Asthma — A condition marked by laboured breathing, constriction of the chest, coughing and gasping usually brought on by allergies.

Atmosphere — The 500 km thick layer of air surrounding the earth which supports the existence of all flora and fauna.

Atomic energy — Energy released in nuclear reactions. When a neutron splits an atom's nucleus into smaller pieces it is called fission. When two nuclei are joined together under millions of degrees of heat it is called fusion.

Beach closure — The closing of a beach to swimming, usually because of pollution.

Bill — A proposed law, to be debated and voted on.

Billfish — Pelagic fish with long, spear-like protrusions at their snouts, such as swordfish and marlin.

Biodegradable — Waste material composed primarily of naturally-occurring constituent parts, able to be broken down and absorbed into the ecosystem. Wood, for example, is biodegradable, for example, while plastics are not.

Biodiversity — A large number and wide range of species of animals, plants, fungi, and microorganisms. Ecologically, wide biodiversity is conducive to the development of all species.

Biomass — (1) The amount of living matter in an area, including plants, large animals and insects; (2) plant materials and animal waste used as fuel.

Biosphere — (1) The part of the earth and its atmosphere in which living organisms exist or that is capable of supporting life; (2) the living organisms and their environment composing the biosphere.

Biosphere Reserve — A part of an international network of preserved areas designated by the United Nations Educational, Scientific and Cultural Organization (UNESCO). Biosphere Reserves are vital centres of biodiversity where research and monitoring activities are conducted, with the participation of local communities, to protect and preserve healthy natural systems threatened by development. The global system currently includes 324 reserves in 83 countries.

Biotic — Of or relating to life.

Birth control — Preventing birth or reducing frequency of birth, primarily by preventing conception.

Birth defects — Unhealthy defects found in newborns, often caused by the mother's exposure to environmental hazards or the intake of drugs or alcohol during pregnancy.

Birth rate — The number of babies born annually per 1,000 women of reproductive age in any given set of people.

Bloc — A group of people with the same interest or goal (usually used to describe a voting bloc, a group of representatives intending to vote the same way).

Blood lead levels — The amount of lead in the blood. Human exposure to lead in blood can cause brain damage, especially in children.

Bottled water — Purchased water sold in bottles.

Brownfields — Abandoned, idled, or under-used industrial and commercial facilities where expansion or redevelopment is complicated by real or perceived environmental contamination.

Budget — A formal projection of spending and income for an upcoming period of time, traditionally submitted by the President or Executive for consideration and approval.

Budget reconciliation — Legislation making changes to existing law (such as entitlements under Social Security or Medicare) so that it conforms to numbers in the budget resolution.

Budget resolution — The first step in the annual budget process. This resolution must be agreed to by the House and Senate. It is not signed by the President and does not have the effect of law, but instead sets out the targets and assumptions that will guide Congress as it passes the annual appropriations and other budget bills.

Bycatch — Fish and/or other marine life that are incidentally caught with the targeted species. Most of the time bycatch is discarded at sea.

Bycatch reduction device (brd) — A device used to cut bycatch while fishing. These gear modifications are most commonly used with shrimp trawls. They are also called "finfish excluder devices" (feds) or, when specifically designed to exclude sea turtles, they are called "turtle excluder devices" (teds).

Cairo Plan — Recommendations for stabilizing world population agreed upon at the U.N. International Conference on Population and Development, held in Cairo in September 1994. The plan calls for improved health care and family planning services for women, children and families throughout the world, and also emphasizes the importance of education for girls as a factor in the shift to smaller families.

Calendar — In the legislative sense, a group of bills or proposals to be discussed or considered in a legislative committee or on the floor of the House or Senate.

Cancer — Unregulated growth of changed cells; a group of changed, growing cells (tumor).

Carbon dioxide (CO_2) — A naturally occurring greenhouse gas in the atmosphere, concentrations of which have increased (from 280 parts per million in preindustrial times to over 350 parts per million today) as a result of humans' burning of coal, oil, natural gas and organic matter (e.g., wood and crop wastes).

Carbon tax — A charge on fossil fuels (coal, oil, natural gas) based on their carbon content. When burned, the carbon in these fuels becomes carbon dioxide in the atmosphere, the chief greenhouse gas.

Carcinogens — Substances that cause cancer, such as tar.

Carpooling — Sharing a car to a destination to reduce fuel use, pollution and travel costs.

Caucus — A meeting of a political party, usually to appoint representatives to party positions.

Chamber — As regards the U.S. government, either the House of Representatives or the Senate.

Chlorination byproducts — Cancer-causing chemicals created when chlorine used for water disinfection combines with dirt and organic matter in water.

Chlorine — A highly reactive halogen element, used most often in the form of a pungent gas to disinfect drinking water.

Chlorofluorocarbons (CFCs) — Stable, artificially-created chemical compounds containing carbon, chlorine, fluorine and sometimes hydrogen. Chlorofluorocarbons, used primarily to facilitate cooling in refrigerators and air conditioners, have been found to damage the stratospheric ozone layer which protects the earth and its inhabitants from excessive ultraviolet radiation.

Clayoquot Sound — One of the last remaining unlogged watersheds on the west coast of Canada's Vancouver Island.

Clean fuel — Fuels which have lower emissions than conventional gasoline and diesel. Refers to alternative fuels as well as to reformulated gasoline and diesel.

Cleanup — Treatment, remediation, or destruction of contaminated material.

Clearcutting — A logging technique in which all trees are removed from an area, typically 20 acres or larger, with little regard for long-term forest health.

Climate change — A regional change in temperature and weather patterns. Current science indicates a discernible link between climate change over the last century and human activity, specifically the burning of fossil fuels.

Cloture — The formal end to a debate or filibuster in the Senate requiring a three-fifths vote.

Coastal pelagic — Fish that live in the open ocean at or near the water's surface but remain relatively close to the coast. Mackerel, anchovies, and sardines are examples of coastal pelagic fish.

Commercial extinction — The depletion of a population to the point where fisherman cannot catch enough to be economically worthwhile.

Communities of colour — Hispanic, black or Asian people or groups living together or connected in some way.

Community right-to-know — Public accessibility to information about toxic pollution.

Compact fluorescents — Flourescent light bulbs small enough to fit into standard light sockets, which are much more energy—efficient than standard incandescent bulbs.

Compost — Process whereby organic wastes, including food wastes, paper, and yard wastes, decompose naturally, resulting in a product rich in minerals and ideal for gardening and farming as a soil conditioners, mulch, resurfacing material, or landfill cover.

Congressional Record — A document published by the government printing office recording all debates, votes and discussions taking place in the Congress; available for free inspection at all government document repositories, as well as in some major libraries.

Contamination — Pollution.
Contraceptive — Preventing conception and pregnancy.
Creek — A watercourse smaller than, and often tributary to a river.
Critical mass — The minimum mass of fissionable material that will support a sustaining chain reaction.
Crop dusting — The application of pesticides to plants by a low-flying plane.
Cryptosporidium — A protozoan (single-celled organism) that can infect humans, usually as a result of exposure to contaminated drinking water.
Demand Side Management (DSM) — An attempt by utilities to reduce customers' demand for electricity or energy by encouraging efficiency.
Demersal — Fish that live on or near the ocean bottom. They are often called benthic fish, groundfish, or bottom fish.
Development — (1) A developed tract of land (with houses or structures); (2) The act, process or result of developing.
Diesel — A petroleum-based fuel which is burned in engines ignited by compression rather than spark; commonly used for heavy duty engines including buses and trucks.
Diesel engine — An internal combustion engine that uses diesel as fuel, producing harmful fumes.
Dioxin — A man-made chemical by-product formed during the manufacturing of other chemicals and during incineration. Studies show that dioxin is the most potent animal carcinogen ever tested, as well as the cause of severe weight loss, liver problems, kidney problems, birth defects, and death.
Double hulled tankers — Large transport ships with two hulls with space between them, protecting the cargo (in most cases, oil) from spilling in case of a collision.
Dredge — A fishing method that utilizes a bag dragged behind a vessel that scrapes the ocean bottom, usually to catch shellfish. Dredges are often equipped with metal spikes in order to dig up the catch.
Driftnet — A huge net stretching across many miles that drifts in the water; used primarily for large-scale commercial fishing.
Dump sites — Waste disposal grounds.
Factory farming — Large-scale, industrialized agriculture.
Factory ships — Industrial-style ships used for the large-scale collection and processing of fish.
Family planning — A system of limiting family size and the frequency of childbearing by the appropriate use of contraceptive techniques.
Fauna — The total animal population that inhabits an area.
Federal land — Land owned and administered by the federal government, including national parks and national forests.
Feedlots — A plot of ground used to feed farm animals.
Fertility — The ability to reproduce; in humans, the ability to bear children.
Fertility rates — Average number of live births per woman during her reproductive years, among a given set of people.

Filibuster— A tactic used to delay or stop a vote on a bill by making long floor speeches and debates.

Fiscal year — A financial term referring to any twelve—month period, usually to set a budget. The federal government's fiscal year begins from October 1.

Fisheries — An established area where fish species are cultivated and caught.

Fissile material — Material fissionable by slow neutrons. The fission process and the fissile isotopes are the source of energy in nuclear weapons and nuclear reactors.

Fission — The process whereby the nucleus of a particular heavy element splits into (generally) two nuclei of lighter elements, with the release of substantial amounts of energy.

Flora — The total vegetation assemblage that inhabits an area.

Florida Bay — Bay at southern tip of Florida which is bounded by the Florida Keys.

Forest certification — A process of labeling wood that has been harvested from a well-managed forest.

Forests — Lands on which trees are the principal plant life, usually conducive to wide biodiversity.

Fossil fuel — A fuel, such as coal, oil, and natural gas, produced by the decomposition of ancient (fossilized) plants and animals; compare to alternative energy.

Fresh Kills — New York City's only operating landfill, located in Staten Island. Infamous as the largest landfill in the world.

Gas — Natural gas, used as fuel.

Gasoline — Petroleum fuel, used to power cars, trucks, lawn mowers, etc.

Geothermal — Literally, heat from the earth; energy obtained from the hot areas under the surface of the earth.

Gillnets — Walls of netting that are usually staked to the sea floor. Fish become entangled or caught by their gills. (See also driftnets).

Global warming — Increase in the average temperature of the earth's surface.

Golden Carrot — An incentive programme that is designed to transform the market to produce much greater energy efficiency. The term is a trademark of the Consortium for Energy Efficiency.

Grassroots — Local or person-to-person. A typical grassroots effort might include a door-to-door education and survey campaign.

Grazing — The use of grasses and other plants to feed wild or domestic herbivores such as deer, sheep and cows.

Green design — A design, usually architectural, conforms to environmentally sound principles of building, material and energy use. A green building, for example, might make use of solar panels, skylights, and recycled building materials.

Greenhouse — A building made with translucent (light transparent, usually glass or fibreglass) walls conducive to plant growth.

Greenhouse effect — The process that raises the temperature of air in the lower atmosphere due to heat trapped by greenhouse gases, such as carbon dioxide, methane, nitrous oxide, chlorofluorocarbons, and ozone.

Greenhouse gas — A gas involved in the greenhouse effect.

Greenway — Undeveloped land usually in cities, set aside or used for recreation or conservation.

Groundfish — A general term referring to fish that live on or near the sea floor. Groundfish are also called bottom fish or demersal fish.

Groundwater — Water below the earth's surface; the source of water for wells and springs.

Growth overfishing — The process of catching fish before they are fully grown resulting in a decrease in the average size of the fish population.

Habitat — (1) The natural home of an animal or plant; (2) The sum of the environmental conditions that determine the existence of a community in a specific place.

Harpooning — A surface method of fishing that requires considerable effort in locating and chasing individual fish. Harpoons are hand-held or fired from a harpoon gun and aimed at high-value fish, such as giant tuna and swordfish.

Haze — An atmospheric condition marked by a slight reduction in atmospheric visibility, resulting from the formation of photochemical smog, radiation of heat from the ground surface on hot days, or the development of a thin mist.

Hearings — Testimony (sworn Statements like those given in court) given before a Congressional committee.

High seas — International Ocean water under no single country's legal jurisdiction.

Highly migratory fish — Fish that travel over great areas.

Household hazards — Dangerous substances or conditions in human dwellings.

Hydroelectric — Relating to electric energy produced by moving water.

Hydrofluorocarbons — Used as solvents and cleaners in the semiconductor industry, among others; experts say that they possess global warming potentials that are thousands of times greater than CO_2.

Hydropower — Energy or power produced by moving water.

Hypoxia — The depletion of dissolved oxygen in water, a condition resulting from an overabundance of nutrients of human or natural origin that stimulates the growth of algae, which in turn die and require large amounts of oxygen as the algae decompose. It was the most ICBM (Intercontinental Ballistic Missile) — a land-based or mobile rocket-propelled missile capable of delivering a nuclear warhead to a range greater than 5,500 kilometres.

ICPD — International Conference on Population and Development.

Incinerators — Disposal systems that burn solid waste or other materials and reduce volume of waste. Air pollution and toxic ash are problems associated with incineration.

Industrialized countries — Nations whose economies are based on industrial production and the conversion of raw materials into products and services, mainly with the use of machinery and artificial energy (fossil fuels and nuclear fission); generally located in the northern and western hemispheres (e.g., U.S., Japan, the countries of Europe).

Insecticides — Substances used to kill insects and prevent infestation.

International Conference on Population and Development — A conference sponsored by the United Nations to discuss global dimensions of population growth and change in Cairo, Egypt in September 1994. The conference is generally considered to mark the achievement of a new consensus on effective ways to slow population growth and improve quality of life by addressing root causes of unwanted fertility.

International Planned Parenthood Federation (IPPF) — An international organization made up of national level affiliates representing every region of the world. IPPF receives and distributes funds from international donor nations to its affiliates, who in turn provide services (prenatal care, contraceptive counselling and service provision, and other reproductive health services) within a country. Some national level organizations provide abortion services, others do not. IPPF sets and supports policies encouraging governmental provision of comprehensive reproductive health care.

Lakes — Substantial inland bodies of standing water.

Landfill — Disposal area where garbage is piled up and eventually covered with dirt and topsoil.

Landings — The amount of fish brought back to the docks and marketed. Landings can describe the kept catch of one vessel, of an entire fishery, or of several fisheries combined.

Land use — The way in which land is used, especially in farming and city planning.

Law — An act or bill which has become part of the legal code through passage by Congress and approval by the President (or via Congressional override).

Lead — A naturally-occurring heavy, soft metallic element; human exposure can cause brain and nervous system damage, especially in children.

Lead poisoning — Damaging the body (specifically the brain) by absorbing lead through the skin or by swallowing.

Least-cost planning — A process for satisfying consumers' demands for energy services at the lowest societal cost.

Leukemia — A form of bone marrow cancer marked by an increase in white blood cells.

Life cycle assessment — Methodology developed to assess a product's full environmental costs, from raw material to final disposal.

Light pollution — Environmental pollution consisting of harmful or annoying light.

Litter — Waste material which is discarded on the ground or otherwise disposed of improperly or thoughtlessly.

Logging — Cutting down trees for commodity use.

Longlines —Fishing lines stretching for dozens of miles and baited with hundreds of hooks. Longlines are indiscriminate and unintentionally catch and kill immature fish along with a wide variety of other animals in the Atlantic including tunas, sharks, marlins, sailfish, sea turtles and occasionally pilot whales and dolphins.

Low-emission vehicles — Vehicles which emit little air pollution compared to conventional internal combustion engines.

Low-impact camping — Camping that does not damage or change the land, where campers leave no sign that they were on the land.

Lumber — Wood or wood products used for construction.

Lung diseases — Any disease or damaging conditions in the lung or bronchia such as cancer or emphysema.

Lymphoma — A tumor marked by swelling in the lymph nodes.

Majority leader — The leader of the majority party in either the House or the Senate.

Malthusian — Based on the theories of British economist Thomas Robert Malthus (1766-1834), who argued that population tends to increase faster than food supply, with inevitably disastrous results, unless the increase in population is checked by moral restraints or by war, famine, and disease.

Mammal — An animal that feeds its young with milk secreted from mammary glands and has hair on its skin.

Managed growth — Growth or expansion that is controlled so as not to be harmful.

Manatee — A plant-eating aquatic mammal found in the waters of Florida, the Caribbean, and off the coast of West Africa.

Marbled murrelet — A rare and imperilled bird that nests in ancient forests on the west coast of the U.S.

Marine mammal — A mammal that lives in the ocean, such as a whale.

Mark-up — Action by a Congressional Committee to amend and/or approve a bill; following mark-up the bill is "reported" out of committee and is ready for consideration by the entire House or Senate.

Marsh — Wetland, swamp, or bog.

Mass transit — *See* public transportation.

Medfly — The Mediterranean fruit fly, a flying insect.

Megalopolis — A large city expanding so fast that city government cannot adjust to provide services (such as garbage disposal).

Methyl bromide — The gaseous compound CH_3Br used primarily as an insect fumigant; found to be harmful to the stratospheric ozone layer which protects life on earth from excessive ultraviolet radiation.

Mining — The removal of minerals (like coal, gold, or silver) from the ground.

Minority leader — The leader of the minority party in either the House or the Senate.

Minuteman — An American-made ICBM; 500 Minuteman III ICBMs are deployed currently in the United States.

Moratorium — Legislative action which prevents a federal agency from taking a specific action or implementing a specific law.

Mulch — Leaves, straw or compost used to cover growing plants to protect them from the wind or cold.

National Recreation Areas — Areas of federal land that have been set aside by Congress for recreational use by members of the public.

Nitrogen oxides — Harmful gases (which contribute to acid rain and global warming) emitted as a byproduct of fossil fuel combustion.

Noise pollution — Environmental pollution made up of harmful or annoying noise.

Nuclear energy — Energy or power produced by nuclear reactions (fusion or fission).

Nuclear power — Nuclear energy.

Nuclear reactor — An apparatus in which nuclear fission may be initiated, maintained, and controlled to produce energy, conduct research, or produce fissile material for nuclear explosives.

Nuclear tests — Government tests carried out to supply information required for the design and improvement of nuclear weapons, and to study the phenomena and effects associated with nuclear explosions.

Oceanography — The study of the ocean and ocean life.

Oil — A black, sticky substance used to produce fuel (petroleum) and materials (plastics).

Oil spills — The harmful release of oil into the environment, usually in the water, sometimes killing flora and fauna of the area. Oil spills are very difficult to clean up.

Old growth forests — Ancient forests.

Omnibus spending bill — A bill combining the appropriations for several federal agencies.

Over development — Expansion or development of land to the point of damage.

Over fishing — Fishing beyond the capacity of a population to replace itself through natural reproduction.

Over grazing — Grazing livestock to the point of damage to the land.

Ozone — A naturally occurring, highly reactive gas comprising triatomic oxygen formed by recombination of oxygen in the presence of ultraviolet radiation. This naturally occurring gas builds up in the lower atmosphere as smog pollution, while in the upper atmosphere it forms a protective layer which shields the earth and its inhabitants from excessive exposure to damaging ultraviolet radiation.

Ozone depletion — The reduction of the protective layer of ozone in the upper atmosphere by chemical pollution.

Ozone hole — A hole or gap in the protective layer of ozone in the upper atmosphere.

Paper — Thin sheet of material made of cellulose pulp, derived mainly from wood, but also from rags and certain grasses, and processed into flexible leaves or rolls. Used primarily for writing, printing, drawing, wrapping, and covering walls.

Paper mills — Mills (factories) that produce paper from wood pulp.

Paper products — Materials such as paper and cardboard, produced from trees.

Particulate — Of or relating to minute discrete particles; a particulate substance.

Particulate pollution — Pollution made up of small liquid or solid particles suspended in the atmosphere or water supply.

Passive solar — Using or capturing solar energy (usually to heat water) without any external power.

Pelagic species — Fish that live at or near the water's surface. Examples of large pelagic species include swordfish, tuna, and many species of sharks. Small pelagics include anchovies and sardines.

Pesticides — Chemical agents used to destroy pests.

Plastics — Durable and flexible synthetic-based products, some of which are difficult to recycle and pose problems with toxic properties, especially PVC plastic.

Plutonium — A heavy, radioactive, man-made, metallic element (atomic number 94) used in the production of nuclear energy and the explosion of nuclear weapons; its most important isotope is fissile plutonium-239, produced by neutron irradiation of uranium-238.

PM10 — Particulate matter less than 10 microns in diameter.

Poison runoff — *See* polluted runoff.

Poison — A chemical that adversely affects health by causing injury, illness, or death.

Polluted runoff — Precipitation that captures pollution from agricultural lands, urban streets, parking lots and suburban lawns, and transports it to rivers, lakes or oceans.

Pollution prevention — Techniques that eliminate waste prior to treatment, such as by changing ingredients in a chemical reaction.

Population — (1) The whole number of inhabitants in a country, region or area; (2) A set of individuals having a quality or characteristic in common.

Post consumer waste — Waste collected after the consumer has used and disposed of it (e.g., the wrapper from an eaten candy bar).

Power plants — Facilities (plants) that produce energy.

Public eState — Public land

Public health — The health or physical well-being of a whole community.

Public land — Land owned in common by all, represented by the government (town, county, State, or federal).

Public transportation — Various forms of shared-ride services, including buses, vans, trolleys, and subways, which are intended for conveying the public.

Pulp — Raw material made from trees used in producing paper products.

Quorum — Minimum number of people who must be present before a specified event can commence (for Congress to vote, at least half the members must be present).

Radioactive — Of or characterized by radioactivity.

Radioactive waste — The byproduct of nuclear reactions that gives off (usually harmful) radiation.

Radioactivity — The spontaneous emission of matter or energy from the nucleus of an unstable atom (the emitted matter or energy is usually in the form of alpha or beta particles, gamma rays, or neutrons).

Radon — A cancer-causing radioactive gas found in many communities' groundwater.

Rainforest — A large, dense forest in a hot, humid region (tropical or subtropical). Rainforests have an abundance of diverse plant and animal life, much of which is still uncatalogued by the scientific community.

Ranking member — The lead member of a Congressional committee from the minority party, usually chosen on the basis of seniority.

Recess — Ending a legislative session with a set time to reconvene.

Recycling — System of collecting, sorting, and reprocessing old material into usable raw materials.

Reduce — Act of purchasing or consuming less to begin with, so as not to have to reuse or recycle later.

Refrigerants — Cooling substances, many of which contain CFCs and are harmful to the earth's ozone layer.

Renewable energy — Energy resources such as windpower or solar energy that can keep producing indefinitely without being depleted.

Reservoir — An artificial lake created and used for the storage of water.

Resolution — A formal statement from Congress.

Reuse — Cleaning and/or refurbishing an old product to be used again.

Rider — Usually unrelated provisions tacked onto an existing Congressional bill. Since bills must pass or fail in their entirety, riders containing otherwise unpopular language are often added to popular bills.

Riparian — Located alongside a watercourse, typically a river.

Risk assessment — Methods used to quantify risks to human health and the environment.

Run-off — Precipitation that the ground does not absorb and that ultimately reaches rivers, lakes or oceans.

Sagebrush Rebellion — A movement started by ranchers and miners during the late 1970s in response to efforts of the Bureau of Land Management (BLM) to improve management of federal lands. While its announced goal was to give the lands "back" to the western States, its real goal — and the one it achieved — was to force the BLM to abandon its new approach to public land management.

Salvage logging — The logging of dead or diseased trees in order to improve overall forest health; used by timber companies as a rationalization to log otherwise protected areas.

Second-growth forests — Forests that have grown back after being logged.

SERP (Super Efficient Refrigerator Programme) — An organization of 24 U.S. utilities that developed a $ 30 million competition to produce a refrigerator at least 25 per cent lower in energy use and 85 per cent lower in ozone depletion than projected in 1994 models. The winning product, produced by Whirlpool, cut energy use by 40 per cent in 1995.

Sick building syndrome — A human health condition where infections linger, caused by exposure to contaminants within a building as a result of poor ventilation.

Silos — Fixed vertical underground structures made of steel and concrete that houses an ICBM and its launch support equipment.

SIP (State Implementation Plan) — Mandate for achieving health-based air quality standards.

SLBM (Submarine Launched Ballistic Missile) — A ballistic missile carried by and launched from a submarine.

Smog — A dense, discoloured radiation fog containing large quanities of soot, ash, and gaseous pollutants such as sulphur dioxide and carbon dioxide, responsible for human respiratory ailments. Most industrialized nations have implemented legislation to promote the use of smokeless fuel and reduce emission of toxic gases into the atmosphere.

Solar energy — Energy derived from sunlight.

Solid waste — Non-liquid, non-gaseous category of waste from non-toxic household and commercial sources.

Soot — A fine, sticky powder, comprised mostly of carbon, formed by the burning of fossil fuels.

Speaker — The leader of the House of Representatives, who controls debate and the order of discussion; chosen by vote of the majority party.

Spotted owl — Reclusive bird, found in the American West, requiring old-growth forest habitat to survive.

Sprawl — The area taken up by a large or expanding development or city.

State land — Land owned and administered by the State in which it is located.

State parks — Parks and recreation areas owned and administered by the State in which they are located.

Stockpile — Nuclear weapons and components under custody of the U.S. Department of Defense.

Straddling stocks — Fish populations that straddle a boundary between domestic and international waters.

Stratosphere — The upper portion of the atmosphere (approximately 11 km to 50 km above the surface of the earth).

Strip mining — Mining technique in which the land and vegetation covering the mineral being sought are stripped away by huge machines, usually damaging the land severely and limiting subsequent uses.

Sulphur dioxide (SO_2) — A heavy, smelly gas which can be condensed into a clear liquid; used to make sulphuric acid, bleaching agents, preservatives and refrigerants; a major source of air pollution in industrial areas.

Surface water — Water located above ground (e.g., rivers, lakes).

Sustainable communities — Communities capable of maintaining their present levels of growth without damaging effects.

Table — In the legislative sense, an action taken to halt debate on a bill.

Tap water — Drinking water monitored (and often filtered) for protection against contamination and available for public consumption from sources within the home.

Tax shift — Replacing one kind of taxes with another, without changing the total amount of money collected. For example, replacing a portion of income taxes with carbon tax or other pollution taxes.

Telecommuting — Working with others via telecommunications technologies (e.g., telephones, modems, faxes) without physically travelling to an office.

Thermonuclear — The application of high heat, obtained via a fission explosion, to bring about fusion of light nuclei.

Threatened species — Species of flora or fauna likely to become endangered within the foreseeable future.

Three Gorges — A project along the Yangtze river in China to build the largest hydroelectric dam in the world.

Timber — Logged wood sold as a commodity.

TNT Equivalent — A measure of the energy released in the detonation of a nuclear weapon, expressed in terms of the quantity of TNT which would release the same amount of energy.

Tongass — A national forest in southeast Alaska comprising one of the United States' last remaining temperate rainforests.

Toxic — Poisonous.

Toxic emissions — Poisonous chemicals discharged to air, water, or land.

Toxic sites — Land contaminated with toxic pollution, usually unsuitable for human habitation.

Toxic waste — Garbage or waste that can injure, poison, or harm living things, and is sometimes life-threatening.

Toxification — Poisoning.

Traffic calming — Designing streets to reduce automobile speed and to enhance walking and bicycling.

Transit — *See* public transportation.

Transportation — Any means of conveying goods and people.

Transportation planning — Systems to improve the efficiency of the transportation system in order to enhance human access to goods and services.

Trash — Waste material that cannot be recycled and reused (synonymous with garbage).

Trawls — Nets with a wide mouth tapering to a small, pointed end, usually called the "cod end." Trawls are towed behind a vessel at any depth in the water column.

Trip reduction — Reducing the total numbers of vehicle trips, by sharing rides or consolidating trips with diverse goals into fewer trips.

Trolling — A method of fishing using several lines, each hooked and baited, which are slowly dragged behind the vessel.

Turtle excluder device (TED) — A gear modification used on shrimp trawls that enables incidentally caught sea turtles to escape from the nets.
Urban planning — The science of managing and directing city growth.
Uranium — A heavy, radioactive metal (atomic number 92) used in the explosion of nuclear weapons (especially one isotope, U-235).
Urban parks — Parks in cities and areas of high population concentration.
Utilities — Companies (usually power distributors) permitted by a government agency to provide important public services (such as energy or water) to a region; as utilities are provided with a local monopoly, their prices are regulated by the permitting government agency.
Veto — A Presidential action rejecting a bill as passed by the U.S. Congress. The President can also effect a "pocket veto" by holding an unsigned bill past the signing period.
Virgin forest — A forest never logged.
Voice vote — A vote where members vote by saying either "yes" or "no" together; individual member's votes are not placed on record.
Warhead — The part of a missile which contains the nuclear explosive.
Waste — Garbage, trash.
Waste site — Dumping ground.
Waste stream — Overall waste disposal cycle for a given population.
Waterborne contaminants — Unhealthy chemicals, microorganisms (like bacteria) or radiation, found in tap water.
Water filters — Substances (such as charcoal) or fine membrane structures used to remove impurities from water.
Water quality — The level of purity of water; the safety or purity of drinking water.
Water quality testing — Monitoring water for various contaminants to make sure it is safe for fish protection, drinking, and swimming.
Watershed — A region or area over which water flows into a particular lake, reservoir, stream, or river.
Well — A dug or drilled hole used to get water from the earth.
Wetland — Land (marshes or swamps) saturated with water constantly or recurrently; conducive to wide biodiversity.
Wilderness — Land remaining in basically wild (i.e., undisturbed) condition, with few if any traces of human activities.
Wilderness area — A wild area that Congress has preserved by including it in the National Wilderness Preservation System.
Wildlife — Animals living in the wilderness without human intervention.
Wildlife refuges — Land set aside to protect certain species of fish or wildlife (administered at the federal level in the U.S. by the Fish and Wildlife Service).
Windpower — Power or energy derived from the wind (via windmills, sails, etc.).
Wise use movement — A loosely-affiliated network of people and organizations throughout the U.S. in favour of widespread privatization and opposed to environmental regulation, often funded by corporate dollars.

Woods Hole — A town on Cape Cod where several important ocean research institutes are located.

Zero emission vehicles — Vehicles (usually powered by electricity) with no direct emissions from tailpipes or fuel evaporation.

Zoning — The arrangement or partitioning of land areas for various types of usage in cities, boroughs or townships.

Index

Abrasion, 94
Acid rain, 193-94, 251-252
  causes of, 252-53
  effect and problems of, 252-53
  possible solutions, 253-54
Acute Respiratory infections, control of, 280
Afforestation, 27
Age pyramids, types of, 276
Agriculture, 55-56
  expansion of, 145
  freshwater for, 36
  global extent of, 57-58
  intensification of, 58-59
  production trends in, 61-62
Agricultural conversion, 145
Agricultural labour, 56
Agricultural produce, solar dryer for, 75-76
Agricultural productivity, 89-90
  losses, 88-89
Agricultural water, 31-33
Agro-ecosystems, 59-60
Air pollution, 191-93
  effects of, 196
  sources of, 193-94
  suspended particulate matter, 195
  units and methods, measurement of, 194-95
Air Pollution and Control of Pollution, 261-62
Airborne movements, 39
Amazonia, 22
Anaerobic digestion, 15
Animal husbandry, 36
Antarctica, 143
Anthropogenic activities, 314-15
Aphotic zone, 6
Aquatic animals, 183-84
Aquatic ecosystem, 135
  functions of, 141-42
Aquatic life, observation of, 311-12
Arctic Ocean, 5, 143
Armstrong, Neil, 27
ASEAN Agreement on Transboundary Haze pollution, 263-64
Atlantic ocean, 5
  layers of, 7-8
  thickness of, 8-9
Atomic power stations, 70
Attrition, 95
Automatic Airquality Monitoring Stations, 198
Autotrophic organisms, 135
Awareness, 8-9

Bhakra Nagal Project, 78
Bhopal disaster, 193
Biodiversity, 137-38
  benefits of, 152
  conservation of, 183-84
  current trends in, 164-65
  evolution of, 153-54
  hotspots of, 166-68

indirect drivers of, 162-63
levels of, 150-51
medicinal importance of, 153-54
spatial patterns of, 157-58
temporal patterns of, 159-60
value of, 182-83
Bioful, 82-84
Biogas plants, types of, 81-82
Biogeochemical cycles, 119-20
Biogeographical realms, 158
Biological diversity, 264
Biological processes, 15
Biomass, produces of, 109-10
pyramid of, 116-17
Biomass-To-Liquids (BTL), 82
Biometer energy, 82
Biosphere reserves, 5-7, 184-85
Birds, 181-82
Blue energy, 71
Bonn convention, 264
Brahmaputra valley, 33, 41
semi-evergreen forests, 170
Broadleaf forest, 168
Brundtland Commission, 241

Cambrian explosion, 153
Carbon cycle, 22, 120-21
Carbon, Rachel, 4
Cauvery water dispute, 40
CFC emissions, 4
Central Pollution Control Board (CPCB), 208, 211, 213, 218
Challenges, 62
Chambal Project, 78
Chandra Gupta Maurya, 27
Chotanagpur dry deciduous forests, 174
Child welfare, components of, 288-89
China, one-child policy of, 288
reforestation campaign, 21
Chipko movement, 269
Common plants, insects and birds, 316
Computerization, 305
Control air pollution, measures to, 199
Control noise pollution, measures to, 203-04
Clapham, Roy, 107
Climate change, 2-4, 138-39, 160-61
Coal, consumption pattern of, 68
varieties of, 68-69
Coastal biodiversity, 139-40
Coastal ecosystem, 136-37
modification in, 139-40
pressures on, 138
Coastal Zone, 262
Cochin Port Trust, 142
Commercial logging, 20
Comprehensive Nuclear, 260-62
Conifer forests, 24
Constraints, 33
Consumerism, 258-60
Consumption, disparities in, 102
Continental land area, 6-7
Contour planning, 96
Control global warming, 251
Cooking/Heating stoves, 74-75
Core reefs, 139
Corona discharge, 255
Corrosion, 94
Current environmental issues, 240-41
Cyclones, 231-32
accounts of, 234-35
destruction caused by, 233-34
prevention/preparedness from, 235-36
Cyclones Distress Mitigation Committee (CDMC), 235

Dams, benefits of, 42-42
 problems of, 42
Damodar Valley Project, 78
Deciduous forests, 17
Deforestation, 20-22, 242-44
 causes of, 20-22
 consequences of, 22-24
 wood consumption, 22
Degraded forests, 17, 25
Demographic Transition Model (DTM), 228
Dense forests, 16
Deserts, 133-34
 birds, 132-33
 camels, 134
 insects and arachnids, 152
 mammals, 133
 reptiles, 133
Deserts ecosystem, 131-32
Desertification, 22-23, 97-98, 242
 causes of, 98
 control of, 99
 effecting extent of, 98-99
Detritus food chain, 114
Dhani Panch Mauza Jungle Surakhya Committee, 28
Diarrhoeal Disease Control programmes, 290
Disasters, 225-26
 planning and management, 236-27
Domestic animals, 55
Drinking water, 29-30
Drought control, 39
Drought Prone areas, 38-39
Dry cooling tower, 216
Dry farming projects, 39

Earth, conviction system, 6
 geological history of, 10-11
 structure of, 9-10
Earthquakes, 10, 226-28
 significant of, 229
Eastern highland moist deciduous forests, 170
Eastern Himalayas, 168
Ecolabelling, 258-60
Ecological adoption, 122-23
Ecological pyramid, 115-16
Ecological succession, 122
 processes of, 122-23
Ecomark, 259
Economic activities, 85
Ecosystem, abiotic components, 109
 benefits of, 123-24
 balance in, 121-22
 concepts of, 107-08
 functional attribute, 111-12
 grazing food chain in, 112-13
 primary goods and service of, 125-26
 primary human-induced pressures on, 146
 structure of, 108-09
 types of, 124-25
Education programmes, 9
Employment, 137
Energy, budget, 118
 conservation, 100-01, 118
 consumption of, 64-65
 flow of, 117-18
 generating mineral, 50-51
 non-renewable resources, 67-68
 pyramid, 117
 renewable resources, 67-68
 resources of, 64-65
  types of, 67

use of alternative source of, 84-85
Environmental awareness, 8
Environmental conservation, 8
Environmental education, 9-10, 268-70
categories of, 2-4
objectives of, 3-4
importance of, 4-5
Environmental functions, 141-42
Environmental Information System (ENVIS), 247
Environmental Law, 259-63
Eniviromental Modification Techniques (Convention), 265
Environmental pollution, 3, 190-230
Environmental problem, 136
Environmental Protection Act (EPA), 261
Environmental Science, issues of, 2-3
Environmental sustainability, 242
Environmental treaties, 263-64
Epicenter, 226
Epidemic diseases, 207
Erosion control, methods of, 96-97
Estuary, detritus food chain in, 114
Evergreen forests, 16-17

Family welfare programmes, evolution of, 284-85
Fertility, mortality and population growth, planning for, 290-91
Five Year Plans, 243
Flood, affected area, 38-39
causes of, 38
control of, 38
Flooded grasslands, 178-79
Food resources, 52-63
sources of, 54-55
Food chain, 111-13
significance of, 114-15
types of, 112-113
Food plants, 54-55
Food processing, 31-32
Food security, 52-54, 63-65
Food web, significance of, 114-15
Food and Agriculture Organization (FAO), 52, 63
Foodgrain production, 62-64
Forests, species of, 24-25
Forests conservation, 27-28
Forest cover, 20-22
assessment of, 24
Forest degradation, 24-25
Forest deforestation, 24
Forest ecosystems, 116, 126-28
areas of, 19-20
Forest environment, 312-13
Forest Lains, 260
Forest products, 18-19
Forest resources, 16-27
global situation of, 19-20
importance of, 17-18
Fossil fuels, 15-16, 67-68
Fresh water ecosystems, 36, 140
resources of, 33-34
Future food problems, 282-83

Ganga basin, 33, 41, 210
groundwater resource, 44-45
pollution, sources of, 210
Ganga Action Plan (GAP), 211-12
Garampani, 29
Geothermal energy, ways of, 79-80
Global Assessment of Soil Degradation (GLASOD), 87-90
Global Biodiversity, 157-58, 162-67
loss of, 159-60
Global warming, 84, 121-22, 248

causes of, 249-50
effects of, 250-51
Global wood consumption, 282
Global Wood Energy Council, 76
Godavari, 41
Gravity erosion, 93
Grassland ecosystem, 116, 130-31
characteristics of, 130-31
environmental aspects of, 312-13
Green house effect, 16
Green house gases, emissions, 249-50
Green marketing, 259
Groundwater, uses of, 36-37
Groundwater resource potential, 36-37, 44-45
Gross-Domestic Product (GDP), 18, 25, 55-56, 89-90
Gujarat, coastal marine environment, 213-14
Gully erosion, 94

Hazardous Substances Act, 226
Hazardous wastes, 226
Heterotrophic Organism, 135
Hirakud Project, 88
HIV/AIDS, 294-96
current estimates and future projection, 296-97
Hospital waste, 220-21
Household food demand, projections of, 62-63
Human nutrition, 56-57
Human health, 292-92
Human Rights, 297
right to equality, 301-02
universal declaration of, 297-98
Hydel Power Projects, 78
Hydrogen biofuel, 83-84
Hydro power, 77-78

Ice erosion, 95
Immunization, 289
Increasing human consumption, 281-82
India, air pollution in, 196-97
atomic power stations, 70
biodiversity in hotspots of, 166-68
biogeographic regions, 167
eco-regions in, 168-69
energy consumption of, 65-66
family welfare programmes, 284-85
food demand in, 61-62
forest areas of, 13-24
land degradation in, 88-90
national parks in, 185-86
petroleum product in, 69-70
pollution problems areas, 218-19
solid waste in, 221-22
sustainable development in, 241-43
water conflicts in, 39-40
water use in, 37-38
water pollution in, 208-10
water resources in, 33-35
wildlife in, 180-81
Zoo in, 186
Indian Council of Forestry Research and Education (ICFRE), 26
Indian Ocean, cyclones in, 232-33
Indian Plywood Industries Research and Training Institute, Bangalore, 26
Indian Remote Sensing Satellite (IRS), 306
Indigenous forests, 20
Indira Gandhi Institute of Development Research, 286
Indo-Gangatic Plans, 91
Indus Water Treaty, 39-40

Industrial development, minerals for, 50-51
Industrial polluted area, 375-76
Industrial and Hazardous waste, 224-25
Industrial revolution, 68
Industrialized countries, 88
Information Technolohy and Environment, 305-307
Inland water resources, 35
Insects, 127
Integrated Child Development Services (ICDS) programmes, 285
Inter-governmental Panel on Climate Change (IPCC), 160
International policy agreement, 32

Jammu & Kashmir, 36
Japan, solar energy investment in, 84
Jharkhand, 68, 70
Jhum cultivation, 25
Joint Forest Management (JFM), 248

Kathiarbar-Gir dry deciduous forets, 174-75
Kerala, back water, 142
Kerala Forest Research Institute, 26
Kyoto Protocol, 251, 266

Lake ecosystems, 140
Land degradation, global situation of, 87-88
  causes of, 86-87
  reasons of, 86-87
Landholding, categories of, 43
Land resources, 85-86
  functions of, 85-86
Landslides, 99-100, 229-32, 319-15
  causes of, 229-30
  types of, 230
Laws to protect the wildlife, 260
Life expectancy, 277
Linear Expansion System (LES), 61
Liquid biofuel, 82-83
Lithosphere, types of, 6-7
Living plants, 89-90
Living Plants Index, 89-90, 165
Local Agenda, 21, 243
Long Range Transboundary Air Pollution, 264-65
Lower Gangetic Plains, most deciduous forests, 171

Macro and Micro consumers, 110-11
Mahabharata, 186
Maharashtra, coastal marine environment, 213-14
Mahatma Gandhi, 14
Malabar coast's moist forests, 171-72
Malthusian theory, 60-61
Mammals, 128, 182-83
Mangrover, 139-40
  forests, 17, 142
  plants, 179-80
Marine ecosystem, 135-36, 161-62
Marine fisheries, 137
Marine pollution, 212-13
  causes of, 213
  control of, 214-15
Mass Media, 268
Mass wasting processes, 93
Meghalaya subtropical forests, 169-70
Mesosphere, 8
Minerals, kinds of, 45-46
  classifications of, 45-46
  conservation of, 51-52
  resources of, 45-46, 50-52
  uses and exploitation of, 45-46

Mining activities, environmental damages caused by, 49-80
Modern agriculture, effects of, 52-80
Modern artificial environment, 201-02
Moist decidous forests, 171
Montane grasslands and shrublands, 178-79
Montreal Protocol, 4, 266
Mountain/Hilly area, 313-14
M.S. Swaminathan Research Foundation (MSSRF), 63
Multidisciplinary nature, 1-2
Municipal solid waste, 220-21

Narmada, 24, 41
Narmada Bachao Andolan, 269
Narmada valley dry deciduous forests, 175
National Ambient (Surrounding) Air Quality Standards, 195
National Anemic Prophylaxis Programmes, 285
National Council for Environmental Policy and Planning, 243
National Environment Council (NEC), 245
National Environmental Information System, 246
National Five Year Planning, 243-44
National Green Corps (NGC) programme, 247
National Human Rights Commission, 302-05
 challenges of, 305-06
 foundations of, 303
National Lake Conservation Plan, 209
National Natural Resources Management System (NNRMS), 9
National Parks, 185-86
National Population Policy and Family Welfare, 287-88
National River Conservation Plan,209-10
National Sustaniable Development Stretegy, aspects of, 245-50
 development and institutional aspects, 245-46
 monitoring aspects, 246-47
 participation aspect, 246
 implementation aspect, 247-48
 specific initiatives aspect, 247-48
National Waste Management Council (NWMC), 222
Natural calamities, 137
Natural ecosystems, conversion of, 144-45
Natural resources, 2, 104-06
 classification of, 14-18
 conservation of, 100-101
Natural vegetation, 314
Nitrogen cycles, 119-20
Nitrogen dioxide, 195
Noise pollution, 199-02
 causes of, 199-200
 effect on human health, 201-02
 government policies, 202-03
 sources of, 200-01
Noise Pollution (Regulation and Control) Rules, 262
No-till farming, 96
Non-conventional energy potential, 84
Non-Governmental Organizations (NGOs), 27, 269-70
Non-renewable resources, 18-16
North-western Ghats, moist deciduous forests, 172
Nuclear energy, 70-72

Nuclear Non-Proliferation Treaty (NPT), 267
Nuclear pollution, 216-18
  control of, 217-18
Nuclear power plants, 70
Nutrients cycles, 119

Oceans, 136
Ocean Thermal Energy Conservation (OPTEC), 77, 79
Oceanic litthosphere, 7
On-going natural processes, 15-17
Operation biosphere resources,185
Organism, classes of, 136
Organisation of Petroleum Explorting Countries (OPEC), 69
Orissa Semi-evergreen forests, 171
Over harvesting, 138
Overgrazing, 98
Overpopulation, problems of, 280-81
Ozone layer, 245, 255-56
  application of, 256
  depletion, 255, 257-58
  industrial production of, 255-56

Pacific ocean, 5
Parasitic food chain, 116
Petroleum production, 69-70
Photic Zone, 6
Phytoplankton, 11-12, 117-18
Pilot Analysis of Global Ecosystem (PAGE), 124
Planning Commission, 243, 247
Plant Genetic Resources, international treaty on, 265-66
Plastic and waste management issues, 223
Polar regions, 141-42
Pollution, 1, 34-35, 102-04, 138-40, 190-92
  load, assessment of, 213-14
  problem areas, 218-19
  role of man in prevention of, 219-20
  types of, 191-92
Pollution Control Board, 197-98
Pollution material, categories of, 190-91
Pollution Under Control (PUC) certificate system, 198
Pond ecosystem, 140-41
Population characteristics, 275-76
Population growth, 273-75
Poverty, 303
Poverty alleviation, 53
Power generation, 31-32
Prevention of Marine Pollution, 265
Primates, 129
Propagate Environmental awareness, methods of, 268-69
Promote sustainable agriculture, 101
Public awareness, 8-9
Public environmental awareness, 267-68
Pure polio immunization, 259-90
Pyramids, types of, 116-17

Radioactivity, sources of, 217
Rainfall, 37-38
Rain forests, 127, 168-70
Rainwater harvesting, 42
  objectives of, 43
Ramayana, 186
Rann of kutch, 178-79
Rao, K.L., 33
Reforestation, 21-23, 27, 97-98
Regenerating forests, 28-29
Remote sensing data, 9, 306
Renewable energy resources, 14-15, 71-72

Reproductive and Child Health (RCH) programme, 286-87
Reptiles, 128, 181
Reserve forests, 27
Rivers, categories of, 33-34
  interlinking of, 40-41
  problems of, 34-35
River ecosystems, 310
Riprap, 97
Rural Water Programme (RWP), 39

Sacred grooves, 27
Salinization, 60
Salt water oceans,5-6
Sardar Sarovar Dam, 26
Savannas Rann of Kutch, 178-79
Schumachar, E.F., 14
Second Five Year Plan, 39
Shallow landslide, 230
Sheat erosion, 94
Shifting cultivation, 24
Shoreline erosion, 94-95
Sixth Five Year Plan, 23
Slumping, 93
Soil, forms of, 89-90
  formation of, 89-91
  horizons of, 90-91
  management of, 99-100
  problems of, 91-92
  types of, 91-92
Soil contamination, micro analysis of, 212
Soil degradation, 59-60, 87, 89-90
Soil erosion, 22, 91, 242
  causes of, 92
  processes of, 93-94
Soil pollution, 211-13
  causes of, 211-12
  control of, 212-13
Solar dryer, 75-76
Solar energy, 15, 71-72
  technology used for, 72-73
Solar Passive Space Heating System, 73-74
Solar Photovoltaic (SPV) Cell, 72-73
Solid Biomass, 83
Solid waste, 220
  types of, 220-21
  health impacts of, 221-22
  prevention measures of, 225-26
South Western Ghats moist deciduous ghats, 172
Splash erosion, 93
Stakeholders, 269
Stockholm, 242, 266
Stratozphere, 8
Strip farming, 96
Sturgstrom, 230
Sulphur dioxide, 194-95
Sunderbans freshwater swamp forests, 170-71
Surface water, 33-34
Surge prone coasts, 234
Sustainable development issues, 245
  concept of, 241-45
  principles, 244-45
Sustainable Development Networking Programme, 246
Sustainable tourism, 36
Sutluj-Yamuna Link (SYL) canal dispute, 40-41

Taiga biome, 143
Tansley, Arthur, 107
Tata Energy and Resource Institute (TERI), 245

Tectonic plates, 6
Temperate Coniferous forests, 177
Temperate Broadleaf and Mixed Forests, 176-77
Temperature forest ecosystem, 129-30
Tenth Five Year Plan, 244, 246, 247
 targets of, 244-45
Terrestrial ecosystem, 161
Thermal Pollution, causes of, 214-15
 Control methods of, 216-17
 effects of, 214-15
Thermal Transfer agent, 30-31
Thermosphere, 8
Thompson, Warren, 288
Tidal energy, 79
Total Fertility Rate (TFR), 275-76
Tourism, 137-38
Tree breeding, 27
Tropical areas, reforestation in, 21-22
Tropical Cyclone Project (TCP), 235
Tropical Rain forest ecosystem, 126-27
Tropical and Subtropical Dry Broadleaf Forest, 168-69, 173-74
Tropical and subtropical grasslands, 177-78
Tropical wet forests, 169
Tsunami, 228-29
Tundra ecosystem, 134-55

Udaipur, climax of malnutrition, 164-65
U.N. Environmental programmes, 22
U.N. Food and Agriculture Organization, 21
UNESCO, 3
Underground water, over use of, 37
Unequal geography, 101-02
United Nations Division, Sustainable development of, 241
Upper Gangetic plains, moist deciduous forests, 171
Urban agglomeration, 277
Urban forestry, 27
Urban India, food security in, 63-64
Urban and pollution, 192
Urban air quality, 196
Urbanization, 277
Uttrakhand, 29

Valley or Stream erosion, 94
Van Mahotsav, 27
Vagetation, kinds of, 92-93
Vinson Massif, 143
Vizhinjam Harbour, 79

Waste water treatment, 206-207
Water, consumption of, 29-30
 distribution of, 32-33
 forms of, 19-30
 human use of, 30
 importance of, 29-30
 solvating power of, 30
 use for food processing, 31-32
 use for industrial applications, 31
 use for recreation purposes of, 30-31
Water conservation, 100
Water cycle, 22
Water erosion, 92-94
Water harvesting, objectives of, 43-44
 system of, 43
Water pollution, 37, 49-50
 causes of, 204-06
 effects of, 207-08
 problems of, 99-100
 sources of, 204-06
Water Pollution Prevention Laws, 260-61

Water Power, forms of, 78-77
Water quality observation, 310-11
Water resources, 27-52
    conservation of, 42-43
Waterlogging, 59-60, 315-16
Watersheds, 314-15
    development programmes, 43-44
Wave energy, 78-79
Weathering, 90
Wet Cooling Tower, 210
Wetlands, 141-42
    areas, 35-36
    environmental sources, 36
Wild animals, migratory specious of, 264-68
Wildlife, 80-81'
    sanctuaries, 187
Wind energy, 76-77
Wind erosion, 95-96
Women and children, sexual exploitation of, 305
World agro-ecosystem, 56
World Bank, 52
World Energy Consumption, 64-67
World Food Demand, 57
Wold Food Problems, causes of, 52-54
Wold Food Programme (WFP), 63
World Resources Institute (WRI), 130
World Summit for Sustaisable Development (WSSD), 246
World Water Assessment Programme, 29
Worldwide earthquakes, 227-28

Xeric shrublands, 179-80
Xerophytes, 123

Yellowstone National Park, USA, 29
Yield growth, changes in, 59-60
Yokihama Stretegy for Natural Disaster Reduction, 237

Zambia, 21
Zero Population Growth (ZPG), 277
Zoo, 186
Zooplankton, 117-18